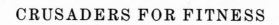

CRUSADERS FOR FITNESS

CRUSADERS FOR FITNESS

☆☆☆☆☆☆☆☆☆☆☆☆☆☆☆☆☆☆☆☆☆☆☆☆☆☆☆☆☆☆☆☆☆

THE ★ HISTORY ★ OF

AMERICAN

HEALTH REFORMERS

☆☆☆☆☆☆☆☆☆☆☆☆☆☆☆☆☆☆☆☆☆☆☆☆☆☆☆☆☆☆☆☆☆

JAMES C. WHORTON

PRINCETON UNIVERSITY PRESS

For Sue

Contents

List of Illustrations

Acknowledgments

I feel a special obligation to Professor James Harvey Young of Emory University for his service as a critic and a model. I am indebted to the National Library of Medicine for the grant (LM 02360) that supported most of the research for this study, and to the University of Washington for granting me a quarter's leave to complete the manuscript. The staff of the University's Health Sciences Library, especially Dale Middleton and Ellen Howard, also earned my gratitude for their resourcefulness (and patience) in helping me locate and procure needed materials. Finally, my wife Sue, while she neither criticized, nor typed, nor proofread a page of the manuscript (I insisted on sparing her the ordeal this time), is entitled to a large share of whatever credit this work deserves. Its completion was obviously facilitated by her uncomplaining acceptance of an author's selfish schedule and daily tolerance of his day-end frustrations. But of more subtle and inestimable value was her joyful and loving spirit that made the project's every day, work and play, one of excitement, happiness, and satisfaction.

CRUSADERS FOR FITNESS

☆☆☆☆☆☆☆☆☆☆☆☆☆☆☆☆☆☆☆☆☆☆☆☆☆☆☆☆☆☆☆☆☆☆

INTRODUCTION
THE KINGDOM OF HEALTH

☆☆☆☆☆☆☆☆☆☆☆☆☆☆☆☆☆☆☆☆☆☆☆☆☆☆☆☆☆☆☆☆☆☆

ONE OF THE CLASSIC CHARACTERS BRED BY AMERICAN CUL-
ture of the past century and a half is the health fanatic, the
man who (in Twain's phraseology) eats what he doesn't
want, drinks what he doesn't like, and does what he'd
druther not, all the while smugly announcing himself to be
energetic, joyful, and certain of long life, and exhorting his
errant neighbor to reform.[1] The comic stature he has
achieved is well deserved, but he has also a serious side that
has been badly neglected. Until recently at least, historians
have recognized health faddism primarily for its rich store
of anecdotes for illustrating human credulity and the possibilities for distorting scientific thought. As a subject for serious intellectual history it has gone begging, except for scattered articles in scholarly journals and two recent
book-length studies: Ronald Numbers, *Prophetess of Health:
a Study of Ellen G. White,* and Stephen Nissenbaum, *Sex,
Diet and Debility in Jacksonian America: Sylvester Graham
and Health Reform.* Those volumes are valuable but still
leave much room for elaboration on health faddism as an
evolving, persistent phenomenon in American society.

In attempting to enlarge that theme, one must first object
to the term "health faddism," which connotes little more
than foolishness and ephemerality. As naive and short-lived
as health reform crusades have often been, their leaders have
too frequently attracted sizeable followings, including well-
educated and otherwise critical minds, to be dismissed so
flippantly as "the nuts among the berries."[2] When any

[1] Samuel Clemens, *Following the Equator,* two vols. New York, 1906, 2:
151.
[2] Ronald Deutsch, *The Nuts Among the Berries,* New York, 1961.

health reformer's popularity is lazily explained by nothing
more than human gullibility, he is reduced to the status of a
mere aberration, a figure whose illusions are idiopathic
rather than symptomatic of his intellectual and social environment. Instead, health reform movements must be understood as hygienic ideologies, idea systems that identify
correct personal hygiene as the necessary foundation for
most, even all, human progress, and that invite acceptance
by incorporating both certain universal feelings about man
and nature, as well as the popular aspirations and anxieties
peculiar to distinct eras. The word ideology also suggests the
radicalism and visionary theorizing that has characterized
these systems of hygiene.

Such levels of devotion, asceticism, and zeal have so often
attended the practice of the ideologies, however, that they
must ultimately be described as hygienic religion. Religious
analogy has in fact commonly been used by health crusaders
(and their detractors) to describe their missions. An antimedical propagandist of the 1920s, Anne Riley Hale, defined the essential creed of health reform as the belief "that
the Kingdom of Health, like the Kingdom of Heaven, is
within you" and is to be gained by hygienic righteousness. A
somewhat more distinguished thinker, William James,
touched upon the same idea in his 1901–1902 lectures on *The
Varieties of Religious Experience*. Two of those lectures
were dedicated to what he called "the religion of healthy-
mindedness," the happy faith that presumes that evil either
does not exist or can be easily ignored, and that was being so
conspicuously advanced by the various expressions of positive thinking elaborated in the late nineteenth century. The
spokesmen for "New Thought," with their several programs
for helping individuals recognize the universal soul within
themselves and achieve oneness with the Divine Mind, were
the special subjects of the lectures. But James was also sur-
rounded by much new thought about the possibility of eliminating all physical evil from the human body, and these
physiologies of perfection could lay equal claim to the label

of healthy-mindedness. In fact, of all the writers available to quote as illustrations of the New Thought, James selected Horace Fletcher, a man who had begun his literary career as a mind curer, but who was emerging at the turn of the century as a leading reformer of physical health.[3]

Indeed, the religions of physical purification have all derived from the same article of faith James discovered at the root of healthy-minded psychology, the assumption that "Nature, if you will only trust her sufficiently, is absolutely good." This unquestioning trust in the wisdom and beneficence of nature stimulates certain beliefs that have typified American hygienic ideologies of all periods. First, health reformers, like the Houyhnhnms encountered by Gulliver, have found it impossible to conceive that, "Nature, who worketh all things to Perfection, should suffer any pains to breed in our Bodies." If nature is absolutely good, illness and incapacity cannot be part of the natural order, but must be evils dragged in by individuals' violations of natural physiological laws. Health reform programs have thus usually been professions of physical Arminianism: bodily happiness is intended by nature (God), but each person must assume responsibility for his physical salvation and earn it by physiological rectitude. By adherence to nature's laws of dress, exercise, and/or diet—especially diet—one may achieve for oneself almost any desired level of vitality, including levels challenging common experience and scientific opinion. Anyone can greatly enhance his ability to enjoy his physical powers, acquire resistance to all disease except graceful aging, and markedly extend his life span.[4]

Glorious as such physical advancements are, they usually comprise but the first step of a perfecting of the whole person. Recognition of the brain as an organ whose molecular composition is affected by diet and observation of the mind-

[3] Anne Riley Hale, *These Cults*, New York, 1926, p. 23; William James, *The Varieties of Religious Experience*, London, 1929, p. 98.

[4] *ibid.*, p. 80; Jonathan Swift, *Gulliver's Travels*, New York, 1977, p. 254.

clearing, tension-relieving effects of strenuous exercise have made it easy to suppose good hygiene must elevate mental ability. Further, since mental growth implies strengthened will power, and immorality is often the result of weak-willed submission to appetites and passions, hygiene might be expected to exalt the individual's moral character as well. This hope has been buttressed, of course, by faith in natural beneficence. Most hygienic ideologists have espoused Christianity, and have seen nature as good because it is designed by God, who is also the author of the laws of morality. It is but a short jump from the self-evident proposition that the two sets of laws (physical and moral) of an omniscient creator cannot conflict, to the assumption they must mutually promote one another. According to nineteenth-century phrenologist and health enthusiast Orson Squire Fowler, "by a law of things, whatever depraves or vitiates the body, thereby depraves the NERVOUS system, and through it the BRAIN, and thereby the MIND. To disease any part of the body, especially the nerves, is to disease the brain, and thereby to produce a SINFUL state of mind. Mental purity is compatible only with physical health." The derivation of this "law of things" has rarely been presented with any more clarity, yet it has been regularly used to promise improved morals from improved hygiene, and, by inference, to conclude that any indulgence which is immoral (e.g., whiskey, meat) must be also, "by a law of things," unphysiological. This insistence on blending physiology and ethics is what prompted Mencken to sneer that "hygiene is the corruption of medicine by morality. It is impossible to find a hygienist who does not debase his theory of the healthful with a theory of the virtuous. The whole hygienic art, indeed, resolves itself into an ethical exhortation."[5]

But optimistic hygiene has also had secular applications,

[5] Fowler quoted in Joel Shew, *Tobacco: Its History, Nature, and Effects on the Body and Mind,* New York, 1854, p. 111; H. L. Mencken, *Prejudices. Third Series,* New York, 1922, p. 269.

in which case it has resolved itself into a social exhortation, an assertion that an ideal society will arise from the physical renovation of all individual citizens. The path to social perfection may lead backward, be a return to Eden; but more commonly it has stretched toward the future, to a civilization redesigned to accommodate nature. Most hygiene reformers have acknowledged physiological, and moral, amenities in industrialized society, and have sought to preserve these while casting aside the insults of luxurious diet, sedentary habits, and nerve-jangling pace. The kingdom of health has been a city, not a garden.

Confidence that humanity will seek the kingdom has stemmed from the faith that man, as a product of nature, is essentially good. People have fallen into error by a misguided surrender to appetite, but they can yet be restored to strength and wholesomeness, and, once there, will become so appreciative of the joys of health as to never again backslide. Furthermore, with a carrot so appetizing as health, a stick should not be necessary. Health evangelists have typically eschewed coercion and prohibition in favor of education and persuasion, confident that once the light is seen, individuals will voluntarily follow it. And as individuals improve, institutions will become better as a matter of course. Hygienic ideologists have consistently blamed people rather than the organization of the social system for the ills of society, and consequently their utopias have been familiar structures, purified versions of the status quo.

The quest for purity of society and the individual and the equation of physiological propriety with spiritual virtue have forced health reformers to present good hygiene as a moral obligation. The obligation may be to God, to the race, the nation, nature, or simply to self. But whatever the direction of the obligation, failure to fulfill it constitutes immorality: bad hygiene is evil, disease is a sin. Preachers of hygiene have thus commonly regarded themselves as physiological missionaries, bearers of a light man's burden to spread the gospel of health to the gluttonous and indolent heathen of the world. Too often, solemn devotion to that mission has made the bearer such a physical prude as to destroy any hope of rapport with most of his potential converts. It has been a rare health missionary indeed who might have seen the humor, let alone the truth, in W. C. Fields' reputed denunciation of life "on the wagon": "Why, they expect a man to live on nothing but food and water." Rather, most hygienic ideologists have been of a mind with Irving Fisher, the Progressive period's brilliant economist and tireless hygienist, who felt profound disgust at being served beer and cigars at a University of California faculty smoker, and happily congratulated himself for having "a taller moral stature than they" (the California faculty).[6]

The mental stature of health reformers has been another matter entirely. They have not, as a rule, been the dolts of popular stereotype. But they have lacked the critical faculties needed to temper their congenital optimism. They have been precisely the type described by James, people "passionately flinging themselves upon their sense of the goodness of life." They have generally been well-read and progressive individuals, conscientious about staying abreast of developing science, but unable to recognize any implications of that science running contrary to their fundamental faith in human perfectibility. As Oliver Wendell Holmes said of the phrenologists, they have juggled with nature; each one's system has been "so adjusted as to soak up all evidence that helps it, and shed all that harms it."[7]

This cavalier handling of theory has been abetted by at least two other forces. The first is the arrogance of the true believer, pure and simple. Consider the comment of an 1850s vegetarian dismissing his adversaries: "It often happens that what is plain and clear to the mental perception of a vegetarian, is obscure, if not wholly incomprehensible to the

[6] Fisher quoted in Irving Fisher [Jr.], *My Father, Irving Fisher,* New York, 1956, pp. 176–177.

[7] James (n. 3), p. 79; Oliver Wendell Holmes, *Medical Essays,* Boston, 1891, p. 245.

mind of the flesh-eater."[8] Secondly, there is the fact that hygienic systems have been empirical discoveries, and rationalizing them has been attempted only after the discoverer had become convinced of their validity through his own experience. To admit that the flesh eater had theoretical evidence on his side would have forced the vegetarian to deny that he had improved in health on his restricted diet.

And most health reformers have had to reform themselves first. They have a standard biography, from which few have deviated. Due to a weak constitution and/or bad habits, the individual's early years are a steady descent through levels of vitality, until semi-invalidism is approached. A shock of realization of poor health at last fires a renunciation of self-indulgence and a search for hygienic truth. Reading and self-experimentation reveal one or a few dietary (or other physical) practices to be the required tool(s) with which to rebuild health. The well-being following his reform convinces the hygienist his program is the secret to all self and social improvement, and gives him the energy to compose the articles and books of health wisdom with which he philanthropically bombards the public until his death. It is a rare individual who can allow mere scientific facts to unseat his faith in a regimen that he believes to have been his personal salvation.

That certainty of having been saved makes public indifference to his message all the more infuriating to the health crusader. Like the reformed drunkard, he is apt to exaggerate the continuing vices of those who have not yet turned to the straight and narrow. The majority of humankind have never been distinguished for strength or energy or vigorous longevity, but does that justify such statements as the remark of a weightlifter of the 1880s, that "General debility is heard of nowadays almost as often as General Grant?"[9]

---

[8] *Water Cure J., 16*, 11 (1853).

[9] William Blaikie, *How to Get Strong and How to Stay So*, New York, 1884, p. 57.

On the other hand, debility is in the eye of the beholder, and in health reformers' eyes, debility has been seen not as the presence of disease, but as the absence of full vitality. For one hundred fifty years they have campaigned for the concept of health as the positive end of a spectrum of well-being and not merely the absence of clinical symptoms. That the current promotion of "high level wellness" seems so novel to the proponents of holistic health is testimony to the failure of previous generations of health reformers to persuade the public that true health is a wonderful condition far above the level ordinarily intended by the term.

And the first step, persuasion, is actually easier than the second. "Though I should *Convince* the World," an eighteenth-century hygienist despaired, "I must not expect to *Convert* it: Lessons of *Abstinence* and *Self-denial* loose their *Weight,* when offered to strong *Passions,* and *high Spirits.*" Corrupted human nature, with its appetites and love of luxuries, has ever been the rock on which health reform plans have foundered. When pleasures are immediate and penalties remote, it is difficult to gain the sensualist's ear. "Mary had a little lamb," a twentieth-century reformer sang in resignation,

> With gravy and mint sauce,
> Potatoes, cabbage, and green peas.
> (She ate the lot, of course.)
> She followed up with cherry tart
> —'Twas not against *her* rule;
> A second helping, cheese, and bread,
> Just packed her nicely full. . . .
> Oh! Mary had a little lamb
> And eke a great deal more.
> Yet Mary wonders *why* she's ill
> —And votes this book a bore![10]

[10] George Cheyne, *The Natural Method of Cureing the Diseases of the Body,* London, 1742, p. A4; C. H. Collings, *How Food Poisons Us,* London, 1917, p. 56.

As unexciting as the health reform message has been, it has nevertheless made its public impact. While few have adopted any hygienic gospel completely and for life, elements of many systems have at least modified the behavior of the masses. Despite their extremism, they have contained much common sense and beneficial advice, from daily bathing to consumption of more vegetables to more thorough chewing of all food. And where health reform programs are concerned, half a loaf is generally better than the whole. If people are encouraged to adopt only the substantial elements of a reform, without swallowing the trifles, they will still improve. They may fall short of the promised perfection, but there will be consolation in the joys of the good food and drink they have retained. A Welsh miner responding to one of Bernarr Macfadden's muscle-flexing demonstrations put the value of radical hygiene in proper perspective: "I'll have me Guinness and 'alf-and-'alf, but the old boy's right about buildin' up the body."[11]

Exhaustive coverage of the history of America's hygienic religions would probably be impossible, and certainly be tedious. While it would be a glib exaggeration to say that if you have seen one health reformer you have seen them all, there is nevertheless a great deal of overlap between the philosophies of health extremists, and encyclopedic coverage of individuals and ideas would make "this book a bore." A more effective tactic is to identify the major themes of health extremism as they evolved between 1830 and 1920, and elucidate them by focussing on individuals who were vital and unique participants in that evolution. The chronological boundaries are suggested by the pattern of evolution. Radical schemes of hygiene have been a constant feature of American life since the early 1800s, but they have naturally flourished in periods of general reformist ferment and social optimism when an expanding public spirit enlarged the con-

[11] Mary Macfadden and Émile Gauvreau, *Dumbbells and Carrotstrips,* New York, 1953, p. 15.

stituency for perfectionist campaigns. Thus the Jacksonian
1830s and 1840s and the Progressive 1900s and 1910s were
years of extraordinary reform activity, and the Gilded Age a
relatively quiescent transition period. The second transition, from the Progressive era to the current "holistic health
explosion" (so dubbed by Norman Cousins) is sufficiently
complex to require a separate study. Such a study would
show how hygiene turned inward during those years, and
became increasingly occupied with the individual (inevitably following the larger cultural trend). But in shifting to
that modern orientation, hygienic extremism did not disin-
herit all the beliefs and prejudices of its earlier years. The
ends of radical hygiene have changed to some extent, but the
means have remained much the same. Anyone who would
understand present-day health reformers, would "know
where they're coming from," as the current idiom has it,
must be familiar with the development of hygienic religion
in the nineteenth and early twentieth centuries.

☆☆☆☆☆☆☆☆☆☆☆☆☆☆☆☆☆☆☆☆☆☆☆☆☆☆☆☆☆☆☆

CHAPTER ONE
A FIG FOR THE DOCTORS

☆☆☆☆☆☆☆☆☆☆☆☆☆☆☆☆☆☆☆☆☆☆☆☆☆☆☆☆☆☆☆

ONE OF THE CLEAREST SIGNALS OF THE ARRIVAL OF THE Jacksonian era for medicine was the launching, in the year of the president's inauguration, of the *Journal of Health*. Edited by an association of Philadelphia physicians who preferred to remain anonymous, the periodical was addressed to the public and sought to instruct it on "the means of preserving health and preventing disease." The editors modestly described their style as "familiar and friendly," but they should also be recognized as selflessly democratic, offering as they did advice which could allow common folk to achieve independence from the medical elite. An anecdote near the close of the first volume was especially telling. A celebrated physician who desired to share with posterity all the wisdom gleaned from his many years of practice left behind a book which, when opened, was found to contain but a single sentence: *"Keep the feet dry—the skin clean—the head cool—the digestion regular—and a fig for the Doctors."*[1]

To be sure, the moral of the tale was hardly new. That disease was a consequence of careless living and health a benefit to be earned by the individual rather than conferred by the physician, had been elements of medical philosophy since antiquity. Dryden's lines—

> The first physicians by debauch were made;
> Excess began and sloth sustains the trade[2]

---

[1] *J. Health, 1*, 326 (1829–1830).

[2] John Dryden, "Epistle to John Dryden of Chesterton," in *The Poetical Works of John Dryden*, ed. George Gilfillion (Edinburgh, 1855).

—were, for all their wit, commonplace. And their truth, furthermore, was wisdom at which people had always winked. Ideally, doctors might not be needed, but there were few who could look upon the ideal as a prize if excess and sloth had to be abandoned. By the 1830s, however, that nonchalance was being shaken. Not only did morbidity and mortality seem to be on the rise, but the course of medicine over the previous half century had been so turbulent as to erode the public's confidence in the ability of doctors to rescue them from the effects of their self-abuse. At the same time, other medical and broader cultural trends were making the ideal of health look more attractive and more attainable. The Jacksonian intellectual environment, in fact, was one that positively encouraged hygienic optimism. And it produced it, with a vengeance, in the popular health reform, or Grahamite (after Sylvester Graham) movement.

As modern as that optimism was, it borrowed heavily from ancient ideas about health. A significant debt to tradition was to be expected, of course, since most rules of healthful living are quickly made obvious by experience and were undoubtedly recognized at an early period of human history. They were formally codified as part of medical thought by Galen, the Greek physician of the second century A.D. Galenic answers to virtually all medical questions dominated theory and practice into the 1600s, but while most features of Galenism were cast aside during that century, the code of hygiene retained its hold. It was, after all, solidly founded on experience, ordered around the individual's careful regulation of those factors of existence over which he had control: air, food and drink, sleep and watch, motion and rest, evacuation and repletion, and passions of the mind. Attention to these "six non-naturals," as they had come to be confusingly called,[3] had been urged by medical writers throughout the

---

[3] For good discussions of non-natural doctrine, and its confusing terminology, see L. J. Rather, "The 'six things non-natural': a note on the origins of fate of a doctrine and a phrase," *Clio Medica*, *3*, 337–347 (1968); and William Coleman, "Health and hygiene in the Encyclopedie:

late Middle Ages and Renaissance, but the matter seemed to assume new importance during the mid-1700s. Enlightenment faith in science, education, and social progress sparked a concern to instruct citizens in the natural laws of health. This educational effort further agreed with the social ethos of the rising bourgeosie: it was an activist move to enhance individual strength and acquire some measure of control over nature.[4] Finally, liberalized theology suggested a physical Arminianism, a belief that bodily salvation might be open to all who struggled to win it, and that disease and early death were not an ineradicable part of the earthly passage. The knowledge required for that salvation was poured forth in a torrent of volumes of health instruction, most written by physicians and all offering essentially the same advice.[5]

The golden rule pressed upon readers was moderation in all things, the avoidance of both too much and too little. "Unerring *Nature* learn to follow close," a poetic physician counselled:

> For *quantum sufficit* is her just Dose;
> *Sufficient,* clogs no wheels and tires no Horse,
> Yet briskly drives the *Blood* around the Course.[6]

His subsequent warning that *"surfeiting* corrups the purple Gore"* betrays the typically greater emphasis placed on excess over deficiency. Overindulgence was the sin stressed, and its wages could be blood chilling merely in the reading. The intemperate, Cornelius Blatchly declared "shall be af-

---

a medical doctrine for the bourgeosie," *J. Hist. Med. Allied Sci.,* 29, 399–421 (1974).

[4] Coleman (n. 3) discusses this phenomenon in France.

[5] John Blake, "Health reform," in *The Rise of Adventism: Religion and Society in Mid-Nineteenth-Century America,* ed. Edwin Gaustad, New York, 1974, pp. 30–32, offers a good condensed treatment of this hygienic literature.

[6] Darby Dawne [Edward Baynard], *Health, A Poem,* Boston, 1724, 4th ed., p. v.

flicted with the gout, racked with the stone, cramped with the colic, drowned with the dropsy, suffocated by asthma and hydrothorax, nauseated with gluttony, vomited with drunkenness, burnt, like Aetna, with lusts or fever, shaken like Sinai with hypochondriac and hysteric terrors and perturbations, or stretched as on a rack with tetanus."[7]

Despite occasional hyperbole, what was preached by these works was a common-sense regimen that nearly all readers could find agreeable in theory, if not always in practice. It was largely a quantitative philosophy, anxious about amount in diet and exercise, but giving only secondary consideration to the quality of food, drink, and exertion. Whole classes of food and activity were not proscribed, temperance was not perverted to abstinence. If an author advised against the drinking of ardent spirits, he would still describe beer and wine as "perfectly wholesome."[8] Similarly, all types of food were acceptable, even intended for human consumption. According to another authority,

> ... heaven has formed us to the general taste
> Of all its gifts; so custom has improv'd
> This bent of nature; that few simple foods,
> Of all that earth, or air, or ocean yield,
> By by excess offend.[9]

Such passages also show a basic assumption common to all this hygienic literature—the idea that health results from individuals living in accord with their natures, natures which have been formed by heaven. Implicit in this is the argument that since the laws of human nature are of divine origin, one has a Christian obligation to observe them, and might regard health as his reward for godliness. Some stated

[7] Cornelius Blatchly, *An Essay on Fasting, and on Abstinence*, New York, 1818, p. 16.

[8] Shadrach Ricketson, *Means of Preserving Health and Preventing Diseases*, New York, 1806, p. 45.

[9] John Armstrong, *The Art of Preserving Health*, Kennebunk, Maine, 1804, p. 33.

that conclusion openly, even proposing physical improvement necessarily contributes to moral perfection, but for the most part that sentiment lay dormant until the 1830s.[10]

Fuller expression was given to a number of other themes that were to be absorbed into health reform ideology. The foundation of Enlightenment reasoning about man's physical nature was a Newtonian view of body structure and function.[11] The body was conceived to be an atomic machine, and human development, decline, and death were explained accordingly. "When life is new," John Armstrong wrote, "the ductile fibres feel / The heart's increasing force"; they stretch and expand, until the individual reaches maturity. Then,

> Life glows ... amid the grinding force
> Of viscous fluids and elastic tubes;
> Its various functions vigorously are plied
> By strong machinery; and in solid strength
> The man confirm'd long triumphs o'er disease.

But nature moves onward,

> the full ocean ebbs. . . .
> Through tedious channels the congealing flood
> Crawls lazily and hardly wanders on;
> It loiters still; and now it stirs no more.[12]

Bad hygiene, intemperance, could thus be analyzed in terms of its bioatomic effects, its wearing of machinery, thickening of fluids, or hardening of elastic tubes.

The Newtonian hygienists also shared a conviction that

[10] George Cheyne, *An Essay on Health and Long Life,* New York, 1813, p. 16; Bernhard Faust, *Catechism of Health,* Philadelphia, 1795, p. 3.

[11] Good impressions of Newtonian physiology can be obtained from Everett Mendelsohn, *Heat and Life. The Development of the Theory of Animal Heat,* Cambridge, Mass., 1964, pp. 67–107; and Robert Schofield, *Mechanism and Materialism. British Natural Philosophy in an Age of Reason,* Princeton, N.J., 1970, pp. 191–232.

[12] Armstrong (n. 9), pp. 49–50.

the human frame was degenerate, had declined from a former glory. The idea was an old one; already in the pre-Christian era, Philo-Judaeus had praised Adam for being "born in the best condition of both soul and body, and to have differed to a great degree from those who succeeded him by his high superiority in both." The premise was repeated, and enlarged, by medieval writers, Hildegard of Bingen even dating the appearance of weakness and disease in the world with the Fall.[13] Literal reading of Biblical accounts of the lives of the patriarchs reinforced the notion, but it was carried to its peak by the disenchantment with civilization, with the luxury and refinement estranging man from nature that accompanied the progress of the eighteenth century. Dryden opened the period complaining of "a pamper'd race of men" whose lives had "dwindled" compared to their toil-seeking, "long-lived fathers."[14] That feeling only gathered strength with the passing decades, as it fed off the general cultural primitivism that was building toward its climax in the second half of the century.[15] And just as social philosophers lamented the loss of the natural moral simplicity of some long-gone golden age, so hygienic writers deplored the state into which physical man had fallen. Our healthy ancestors, according to Cheyne, slid into such lewdness and luxury that they could eventually give "only a diseased, crazy and untuneable carcass to their sons." Consequently, "vicious souls and putrefied bodies, have in this our age, arrived to their highest and most exalted degrees."[16]

Embedded in Cheyne's grumbling is the assumption that debility is hereditary, a concept which, along with the companion belief that "healthy stamina" is also transmitted to

[13] George Boas, *Essays on Primitivism and Related Ideas in the Middle Ages,* New York, 1966, pp. 3, 75.

[14] Dryden (n. 2), pp. 29–30.

[15] For a thorough analysis of this cultural primitivism, see Lois Whitney, *Primitivism and the Idea of Progress in English Popular Literature of the Eighteenth Century,* Baltimore, 1934.

[16] Cheyne (n. 10), p. 192. Also, Armstrong (n. 9), p. 43.

offspring, was common in the hygienic tradition.[17] This idea of inheritance of acquired characteristics was to gain prominence through the nineteenth before declining in the early twentieth century, and was to be regarded by health reformers as a critical principle.

Enlightenment hygienists' regret at human deterioration could nevertheless—as Lovejoy has observed of eighteenth-century primitivism generally—be united with the era's belief in progress.[18] By readopting a natural mode of living, man might be restored to his original state of goodness. Indeed, the certainty that the human race was presently so miserable almost forced hygienic authors to promise extraordinary benefits to those able to return to nature. The promises, furthermore, could be backed up by the personal example of a man who had actually succeeded. The sixteenth-century Italian nobleman Luigi Cornaro was probably the best known of all the pre-1800 health writers. His *Discourses on a Sober and Temperate Life* was an autobiographical account of a man whose sensual indulgences had virtually ruined his health before the age of forty. Warned by physicians that he would have to trim his sails or die, Cornaro immediately converted to a program of extreme moderation, allowing himself only twelve ounces of food and fourteen ounces of wine daily. Abstemiousness not only relieved his ailments, it lifted him to higher levels of physical, and mental, happiness than he had ever known before. At the age of eighty-three, still enjoying remarkable vitality, he began the *Discourses* which he finally completed in his ninety-fifth year—and he lived several years longer. Most of the advice of the work is standard "non-natural" fare, but it also includes certain emphases that were to have long-ranging influence on hygienic thought. First, Cornaro believed right living created immunity to disease; "the holy medicine of the temperate life" has, he asserted, "removed from me

---

[17] Ricketson (n. 8), p. vi.

[18] Arthur Lovejoy, "Foreword," in Whitney (n. 15), p. xiii.

forever all the causes of illness." That same holy medicine produced an uncommon degree of physical strength and energy, as well, and even promoted mental clarity, emotional cheerfulness, and spiritual tranquillity. Eventually the *Discourses* are made tiresome by Cornaro's narcissistic hymns to his own vigor, but he sang along untroubled, confident that his creator had intended such happiness. Presaging a crucial element of health reform ideology, he denied the fatalism that accepted illness as part of the divine plan: "I cannot believe God deems it good that man, whom he so much loves, should be sickly, melancholy and discontented."[19] Rather, health and contentment were God's desire, as was an extended life-span. The last point represents perhaps Cornaro's greatest contribution to hygienic thought. Gruman, the historian of prolongevity ideas, in fact argues that Cornaro "opened the way" for belief in the ability of all (not just those of hardy constitution) to realize an exceptionally long and happy life.[20] A final blessing was that when the healthy life ended, after one hundred or more years, it would be a peaceful and painless event, a "natural death" similar to that of the "lamp which gradually fails."[21] All these expectations of temperance went into a "Cornaro tradition" that colored hygienic literature down to the 1830s. Eighteenth-century health guides regularly assured readers that, were temperance observed, the soul within the body

> Might full a hundred years with comfort *dwell*,
> And drop, when ripe, as Nuts do slip the Shell.[22]

And that was the conservative estimate. The Enlightenment disposition to credit science with omnipotence led some to

---

[19] Cornaro's book has been issued under several titles in addition to the original *Discourses*. I used *The Art of Living Long*, Milwaukee, 1905, pp. 73, 112.

[20] Gerald Gruman, "A history of ideas about the prolongation of life," *Trans. Am. Phil. Soc.*, *56*, 70 (1966).

[21] Cornaro (n. 19), p. 65.

[22] Dawne (n. 6), p. v.

foresee a world in which the ripening process would require far more than a century. Condorcet was an extremist for supposing that the advance of reason would allow such a "perfection of the human species . . . [that] the average span between birth and decay will have no assignable value." But even so sober a thinker as Benjamin Franklin considered it reasonable that through scientific progress "all Diseases may by sure means be prevented . . . and our Lives lengthened at pleasure even beyond the antidiluvian Standard."[23] However much the anticipated increases varied from one hygienist to another, a dramatic lengthening of life was a common goal long before the Grahamite era.

So was a diminishment of the therapeutic activity of physicians. That medical intervention against illness was often unnecessary had been appreciated since the time of Hippocrates, who had recognized an innate power in the body to combat the disequilibrium of disease and restore itself to health. A corollary was that this power—the *vis medicatrix naturae*—was equally effective at keeping a person in health, as long as it was not weakened by intemperance. Cornaro had assured each reader that with temperance, "he would become his own physician, and, indeed, the only perfect one he could have." His sentiments were to be repeated through the 1700s. William Buchan, for example, the author of an immensely popular handbook of domestic medicine, opined that the person who lived by the rule of moderation "will seldom need the physician; and he who does not, will seldom enjoy health, let him employ as many physicians as he pleases."[24]

It was but a step from regarding medicine as frequently useless to recognizing it as sometimes dangerous. The commonly employed treatments of the time were, of course, often injurious, even lethal, and hygiene advocates occasionally took fellow doctors to task for their heroic therapeutics. The

[23] Gruman (n. 20), pp. 74, 87.
[24] Cornaro (n. 19), p. 57; William Buchan, *Domestic Medicine,* Boston, 1813, p. 2.

first American author of a comprehensive health guide, the Quaker physician Shadrach Ricketson, concluded his 1806 work with a section of "Observations on the abuse of medicine." In it he called for physicians and patients alike to avoid strong medication in milder complaints, and discussed specific forms of treatment that, like "edge tools," were of value in skilled hands, but could easily wreak havoc when carelessly used. His list included mercury compounds, opium, strong emetics and cathartics, and bloodletting.[25] But therapy was still less heroic in Ricketson's day than it would be in the 1830s, and as the volume of blood let and the doses of calomel given steadily rose, there was ever more reason to be leery of medicine.

During the interim there accumulated hard data to back up that wariness born of common sense. Under the aegis of the "Paris" or "Clinical School," there occurred a reaction against the excessive rationalism of eighteenth-century medicine and its attendant heroic therapeutics. An outgrowth of Enlightenment sensualist philosophy, the Paris orientation was toward scientific empiricism. Hypothesis was disdained, and physicians enjoined to study disease by close observation of the symptoms of live patients and the pathological anatomy of those that died. The prohibition of theorizing implied a therapeutic skepticism, as most conventional therapy was justified primarily by its agreement with theory. But the skepticism was being made explicit by the 1830s, as statistical evaluation of therapy—Pierre Louis' "numerical method"—was demonstrating that traditional treatments were indeed useless in most cases, and injurious in many.[26] American medical students who flocked to Paris during that era often returned home convinced of the futility of intervening in "self-limited diseases," and fired with admiration for the *vis medicatrix naturae*. Colleagues who had not had

[25] Ricketson (n. 8), pp. 266–289.

[26] Erwin Ackerknecht, *Medicine at the Paris Hospital, 1794–1848*, Baltimore, 1967.

the advantage of Parisian indoctrination attacked expectant treatment as do-nothingism, and there was near constant wrangling around mid-century over the relative merits of nature and art (standard therapy). What Oliver Wendell Holmes described as "the nature trusting heresy" did not truly blossom until the 1850s, but it was opening already by the 1830s and added to the health reform movement's confidence in the power of hygiene. It made sense that America's most active promulgator of the Paris philosophy, Elisha Bartlett, was also in sympathy with the essence of health reform doctrine. His 1838 lecture on "the moral duty of obedience to the physiological or organic laws," in fact, was an address to health reform devotees, and presented their dearest tenets with a clarity and conciseness that few of them ever achieved.[27]

The superiority of empiricism to rationalism, the favorite theme of Bartlett's major works, was also being sounded from beyond the walls of the medical profession and shaping the health reform *milieu*. The eighteenth century had already been marked by lay objections to the theoretical complexity of medicine and the neglect of the empirical evaluation of therapy. But works such as John Wesley's *Primitive Physick*, though popular, had been isolated, unorganized protests.[28] During the early 1800s, though, several alternative systems of healing appeared, each with numerous practitioners and all claiming to be safer and surer than regular medicine. The first of these "irregulars" in America, Samuel Thomson, ran patients through a demanding course of spicy and emetic botanicals, steambaths, and enemas laced with cayenne pepper. The popularity of Thomsonianism, obviously, owed little to therapeutic mildness. It succeeded,

[27] Elisha Bartlett, *Obedience to the Laws of Health, a Moral Duty*, Boston, 1838.
[28] C. Wayne Callaway, "John Wesley's *Primitive Physick:* an Essay in Appreciation," *Mayo Clinic Proc., 49*, 318–324 (1974); Samuel Rogal, "Pills for the Poor: John Wesley's *Primitive Physick,*" *Yale J. Biol. Med., 51*, 81–90 (1978).

rather, through a carefully orchestrated exploitation of popular sentiments. egalitarianism, nationalism, romanticism, and others. Far from the least important was Thomson's insistence that all his remedies had been discovered by empirical determinations of what actually aids nature.[29]

That same tack was followed by the other successful unorthodox groups. Samuel Hahnemann, formulator of homeopathy, stressed that his drugs, each supposed to duplicate the symptoms of the specific diseases it cured, had all been selected by experimental testing of their effects. Likewise his practice of potentizing drugs by diluting them to infinitesimal concentrations, so nonsensical to theoreticians, was the result of repeated clinical experience. Hahnemann laughed at doctors for "inventing systems by stringing together empty ideas and hypotheses," and though he eventually spun some fine theoretical webs of his own, he kept the *vis medicatrix* at the center. His dilutions, he rationalized, operated by a "dynamic," spiritual effect on the body's vital force, "leaving in its primitive state of integrity and health the essence or substance which animates and preserves the body."[30]

Empiricism and trust in the body's innate power to regulate itself were still more marked in the system of hydropathy. Its program of assorted baths and liberal drinking of water was entirely the outgrowth of Vincent Priessnitz's self-experimentation. The flushing of morbid impurities from the body was also presumed to be aided by exercise and fresh air, but both these agencies, as well as the water, were directed by the patient's own inner force. Hydropathy was separated from hygiene by only the thinnest of lines. Not only did the followers of Priessnitz promote exercise and fresh air, but their only "medicine," water, was, after all, an essential for the healthy as well as the ill; it was a physiological element rather than a drug. Indeed, the most difficult ob-

[29] Samuel Thomson, *New Guide to Health; or Botanic Family Physician,* Boston, 1835, pp. 8–9.

[30] Samuel Hahnemann, *Organon of Homeopathic Medicine,* Allentown, Pa., 1836, pp. 79, 90.

stacle to hydropathy's advance was a public unwillingness "to be cured by so simple an article. They had rather be sick and take a potion of delicious calomel."[31] The deliciousness of calomel, and for that matter the necessity of most medicine, was being questioned from all quarters during the early 1830s, and health reform was simply the extreme toward which therapeutic skepticism and nature trusting pointed.

Confidence that hygiene could replace medicine grew also from the expansion of the basic medical sciences, particularly physiology. Although most traditional hygiene was derived from simple experience, it was still rationalized as applied physiology, and clearly the content of a hygienic code and the confidence with which it might be recommended were a reflection of the current state of that science. The 1750 to 1830 period had been one of startling maturation for physiology. Albrecht von Haller's studies on the irritability of muscle and sensibility of nerve tissues, accomplished in the 1750s, opened a new era in physiological research. Subsequent investigations—those, for example, of de Réaumur and Spallanzani on digestion, Lavoisier on respiration, and Bell and Magendie on the sensory and motor nerves—were individually significant, but were even more important for their total impression. The great range of physiological research and its sparkling newness could dazzle hygienists. Like eighteenth-century physicists, they might see their science as virtually complete, requiring only touching up in a few spots. Health reformers were thrilled to witness this climax of scientific progress, and felt blessed by it. It allowed them—called them—to become the first teachers capable of offering thorough and fully effective instruction in the laws of healthful living.[32]

And never had such teaching been so urgently needed.

[31] Nathan Bedortha, *Practical Medication, or the Invalid's Guide*, Albany, N.Y., 1860, p. 65. Also see Harry Weiss and Howard Kemble, *The Great American Water Cure Craze*, Trenton, N.J., 1967.

[32] Fielding Garrison, *An Introduction to the History of Medicine*, Philadelphia, 1914, pp. 246–249, 381.

This young, reckless society was perhaps nowhere more given to excess than in its contemptuous disregard of the non-naturals. Genteel European tourists were disgusted while here, then delighted on returning home to be able to report the brutish habits of the North American provincials. Some deduction must be made from their accounts for snobbery, needless to say, but so much abominable hygiene was corroborated by American observers (and has persisted to the present) that the ridicule has to be accepted as fundamentally valid. The impressions gathered by Anthony Trollope's mother Frances were typical. Coming to the United States in the late 1820s, she stayed for several years of looking down her nose at, then writing about, *The Domestic Manners of the Americans:* "The voracious rapidity with which the viands were seized and devoured," "the incessant use of ardent spirits," and "the incessant, remorseless spitting" of tobacco juice by "George Washington Spitchew" are phrases that echo through mid-nineteenth-century social commentary.[33]

Complaints of dirtiness, sedentariness, and ill temper added to the din, yet one managed to be heard above the rest. Americans' eating—quantity, quality, and speed—struck most critics, foreign and native, as the most general and egregious abuse. The classic portrait of the comfortable Jacksonian at the table depicts him wolfing a mountainous spread of meats and starches, with most of the dishes crudely fried and all dripping with lard or butter. Sad confirmation of the picture is given by the newspaper report of a man who choked to death at dinner and was found to have a wedge of steak one-half by one and one-half by three inches lodged in his throat. Such masticatory impatience was the rule, according to a British witness. "I never saw a Yankee," he marvelled,

> that did not bolt his food whole, like a boa constrictor. How can you expect to digest food that you do not take the

[33] Frances Trollope, *Domestic Manners of the Americans*, ed. Donald Smalley, New York, 1949, pp. lvi, 16, 18, 20.

trouble to masticate? It's no wonder you lose your teeth, for you never use them; nor your digestion, for you overload it; nor your saliva, for you expend it on the carpets instead of on your food. You Yankees load your stomachs as a Devonshire man does his cart, as full as it can hold, and as fast as he can pitch it in with a dungfork and drive off; and then you complain that such a load of compost is too heavy for you. I'll tell you what—take half the time to eat that you do to drawl, chew your food half as much as you do your filthy tobacco, and you'll be well in a month.[34]

Barbaric hygiene was not a Jacksonian innovation; colonial Americans had fallen short of absolute decorum too. But they had at least been forced into much healthful activity by the exigencies of agrarian existence. As a mid-nineteenth-century health writer characterized her own upbringing, "We obeyed the laws of health, not from *principle,* but from *poverty.*"[35] And even those who had the money for dissipation could only hurt themselves so much. Daily labor in the sun and fresh air neutralized a fair amount of self-abuse at the table and tavern. Yet, though the country was still largely rural in 1830, cities had grown markedly during the few decades before and were on the verge of a population explosion. Many Americans, whether employed in factory or countinghouse, were restricted to inactive indoor lives, but had not altered their living habits to compensate. The city had long been vilified as a health destroyer, of course; its foul air and softening luxuries were staple dangers in eighteenth-century health guides. So was the nervous agitation of urban life: "The uncultivated boor," as one hygienist described rural man, "glides along unconscious of the pleasures and unacquainted with the sufferings which necessarily grow out of civic society and intellectual refinement." The type of city that was appearing along the eastern seaboard by 1830, though, was a new sight for Americans, and a

---

[34] *Graham J. Health and Longevity, 2,* 27 (1838); *ibid., 1,* 254 (1837).

[35] Catherine Beecher, *Letters to the People on Health and Happiness,* New York, 1855, p. 113.

profoundly disturbing one to those anxious for the nation's physical and moral vitality. The filth and crowding, drunkenness and debauchery of mangy slum dwellers, as well as the idle intemperance of the Quality, threatened to make debility epidemic. More than a few doctors were worried by the "pale cheeks, and hollow eyes, and early wrinkles, and narrow chests, and lank limbs, and flabby muscles, and tottering steps [that] meet us at every corner."[36]

Still more unsettling was the certainty that such a rundown population must be highly susceptible to more serious acute disease. The eruption of tuberculosis early in the nineteenth century was a particularly terrible substantiation of that concern, but other diseases appeared to be on the increase too. The climax came in 1832, with the first American invasion of Asiatic cholera. With its newness, unpredictable spread, rapid course, horrible symptoms, and extraordinary mortality rate, it was the most terrifying disease of the century. And for that very reason, cholera served as a potent catalyst to the mid-century's nascent public health activity. Dread of a recurrence of such a devastating epidemic drove both physicians and the public to take an interest in the sanitary reform movement developing in England. That movement, which steadily gained momentum through the 1830s and 1840s, was directed by an epidemiology that blamed the outbreak of large-scale disease on air poisoned by miasmatic vapors that had been released from decomposing organic material. Though centuries old, the theory still made sound epidemiological sense at a time when transmission of infection by such subtle vehicles as the water supply, insects, and healthy human carriers was unappreciated, and when urban streets were overflowing with animal and vegetable waste. Statistical correlations of mortality rates and levels of environmental filth strengthened faith in the "sani-

---

[36] James Johnson, *The Influence of Civic Life, Sedentary Habits, and Intellectual Refinement, on Human Health and Human Happiness,* Philadelphia, 1820, p. 110; Bartlett (n. 27), p. 10.

tary idea," and were used to round out arguments for the public financing of efficient systems of drainage and refuse removal. Sanitary reform did not begin to take a firm hold in America until the 1850s, but earlier expressions of interest in this program of environmental hygiene, few as they were, signify the rudimentary preventive mentality already in existence by the health reform era—and which would be fostered by the health reform movement.[37]

But the special health reform approach to prevention was only partly a product of medical trends. It was, in fact, a medical expression of that tide of the Romantic reform spirit rising so rapidly in all areas of American society during the first half of the century. The diverse "New England Reformers" so deftly dissected by Emerson, including those who believed "that we eat and drink damnation," were united by their Rousseauist faith in the automatic elevation of human beings returned to a natural society. Certain that the restoration of such a society required only the demolition of some specific barrier, they allowed their assaults on slavery, capitalism, alcohol, and other evils to become moral crusades. Romantic reform was, in Hulme's vivid phrase, "spilt religion"; it was an excitement about the prospects of human perfection that had overflowed the walls of religious institutions and settled into all the compartments of society.[38]

But the overflowing left the religious institutions themselves filled to the brim, and it was from contemporary Christianity, more than any other source, that health reform ideology drew its inspiration. Even the fundamental hygienic idea that disease might be prevented owed as much to

[37] Wilson Smillie, *Public Health. Its Promise for the Future*, New York, 1955, pp. 120–155; John Duffy, *A History of Public Health in New York City, 1625–1866*, New York, 1968; Charles Rosenberg and Carol Smith-Rosenberg, "Pietism and the Origins of the American Public Health Movement," *J. Hist. Med., 23*, 16–35 (1968).

[38] Ralph Waldo Emerson, *The Works of Ralph Waldo Emerson*, Roslyn, N.Y., n.d., p. 295; Hulme is quoted and discussed by John Thomas, "Romantic Reform in America, 1815–1865," *Am. Q., 17*, 656–681 (1965).

religious considerations as to medical ones. Historically, appreciation of the possibility of prevention of disease on a major scale had been inhibited by the interpretation of epidemics as divine punishment for human sinfulness. Wesley, in the middle of the eighteenth century, began his *Primitive Physick* (a book designed to help people deal with disease) with the reminder that since the Fall, "the Seeds of Weakness and Pain, of Sickness and Death, are now lodged in our inmost Substance.... The Heavens, the Earth, and all Things contained therein, conspire to punish the Rebels against their Creator." And while the collection of remedies that followed might lessen these inconveniences, they could not, he persisted, wholly remove them. Obedient resignation to periodic scourging as part of the natural order dampened any hopes of disease eradication and could even generate active resistance to any preventive efforts which were taken. When smallpox inoculation was first tested in Boston in 1721, for example, it was opposed not just by certain medical objections to its dangers, but by religious misgivings that it might be safe and effective, and thereby thwart the will of God. "It is impossible that any *Humane Means*, or *preventive Physick* should defend us from, or Over-rule a *Judicial National Sickness,*" one casuist argued. If sinners could be made as safe as the most righteous, *"national Judgments* would not have the *Designed Ends* for which they were sent *National Amendment."*[39]

During the later 1700s, though, American religious thought, leavened by the Arminian emphasis on human initiative and freedom to win salvation, began to ferment with new attitudes. This Second Great Awakening involved a steady drift away from the old-line Calvinist world-view preoccupied with human depravity and helplessness before an almighty and vengeful God. As God came to be regarded

---

[39] John Wesley, *Primitive Physick,* Philadelphia, 1764, pp. iii–iv; John Blake, "The Inoculation Controversy in Boston: 1721–1722," *New Eng. Q., 25,* 498 (1952).

more as a loving father than a wrathful sovereign, the concepts of universal salvation (instead of limited election) and the importance of good works gained dominance. This humanized religion was incompatible with an acceptance of disease as deserved and inevitable. It did, however, require man to win salvation from disease for himself, through the exercise of God's gift of reason. If disease were a natural phenomenon, it must be subject to laws that human intelligence could discover and understand. That understanding should suggest measures of prevention allowing man to eliminate disease—with God's blessing. The laws to be understood were those of the environment (the generation of miasmas from filth) and the body (physiology). Study of the latter, in fact, was almost obligatory: the body housed the soul, and, as the most marvelously intricate construction in all nature, provided the most dramatic evidence of divine wisdom. In this light, it was easy to regard physiological knowledge and hygienic living as Christian duties.

This mode of reasoning, the heart of health reform philosophy, is also evident to some extent among precursors. Amherst professor Edward Hitchcock, for instance, had some unpleasant encounters with dyspepsia, recovered through temperance, and decided to share the wisdom gained with his students. The recommendations in his 1830 lectures on *Dyspepsy Forestalled and Resisted* straddled the fence between temperance and abstinence. He was opposed to alcohol in any form and inclined toward a total rejection of meat, but stopped short of demanding vegetarianism. Rather, the suppression of gluttony, a quantitative matter, was his primary object, and in inveighing against that abuse he made it into a sin and tied it to religion in a way prefiguring health reform. "Every Christian is accountable to God for exceeding this standard" of dietary temperance, Hitchcock thundered, "and I tremble for him who persists in following his voracious appetite." In a later lecture, he analyzed for students the connections between dietary restraint and the Christianizing of the world. Respect for the body and its divine laws will encourage piety and expand the population from which ministers can be drawn, he began. The additional ministers, and others eager to do the work of Christianization, will be able to accomplish much more by virtue of the greater strength and longevity granted them by temperance. Finally, the money to be saved from expenditures on whiskey and excess food—estimated by Hitchcock to be fifteen million dollars annually—would fund charitable and missionary work at a level thirty times that presently available.[40] Thoroughgoing as this moral hygiene was, though, it would be surpassed by health reform theorists who saw an even deeper intimacy between physiology and Christianity.

The fusion of science and religion was a broad cultural phenomenon, of course, stimulated by the ascendance of rationalism in the new religion. William Ellery Channing, the leader of American Unitarianism, was so bold as to declare that were Christianity not "a rational religion, . . . I should be ashamed to profess it." Not all voiced their feelings so bluntly, perhaps, but there was by the 1830s a general consensus that religious truth was rational, and that it necessarily agreed with any other truth discovered by reason, meaning specifically scientific truth. Most scientists of the day were, in fact, active champions of natural theology, the belief that the study of God's natural creation was the surest demonstration of His existence and infinite intelligence: "The marks of design are too strong to be gotten over. Design must have had a designer. That designer must have been a person. That person is God."[41] That bond between science and religion, forged in the seventeenth century, had been strengthened during the Enlightenment, but then chal-

---

[40] Edward Hitchcock, *Dyspepsy, Forestalled and Resisted,* Amherst, Mass., 1830, pp. 59, 209–212.

[41] William Kitchiner, *The Art of Invigorating and Prolonging Life,* London, 1824, p. 285. For a good condensed discussion of the early nineteenth-century crisis in natural theology, see John Greene, "Science and Religion," in Gaustad (n. 5), pp. 50–69.

lenged early in the nineteenth century by discoveries in geology and paleontology which raised doubts about the reliability of the book of Genesis. Thus pious (i.e, nearly all) Jacksonian scientists and physicians felt charged with a historic task, that of salvaging the unity of science and religion. They were guided in that project by a necessary set of assumptions: the Bible and nature are the work of God, and therefore cannot possibly contradict one another; any seeming contradiction is only apparent, a temporary embarrassment caused by misinterpretation of either the Book of Revelation or the book of nature. The actual practice of natural theology, therefore, involved much revised interpretation of Scripture to bring it into line with developing science (or, in the case of those committed to a fundamentalist reading of the Bible, as was true of most health reformers, it was science that had to be reinterpreted). The zeal with which the accommodation of science with religion was prosecuted is suggested by another work of Edward Hitchcock, a man who was a minister of the gospel and Massachusetts state geologist, as well as a professor of chemistry and natural history. *The Religion of Geology* (1851) was one of the most ambitious volumes in its class, guided throughout by the belief, stated in the title of the concluding chapter, that "Scientific Truth, Rightly Understood, Is Religious Truth." The lengths to which Hitchcock would go to develop right understanding can be appreciated by considering his determination to reconcile modern chemistry with the doctrine of the eventual resurrection of the body. Skeptics had ridiculed the dogma because the dead body decomposes into its chemical elements, which reenter the environment and could hardly be expected to be available for reassembly at Judgment Day. Hitchcock offered what he considered the first effective response to this objection, pointing out that chemistry had recently provided a new understanding of bodily identity:

The identity of the body consists, not in a sameness of particles, but in the same kinds of elementary matter, combined in the same proportions, and having the same form and structure. Hence it is not necessary that the resurrection body should contain a single particle of the matter laid in the grave, in order to be the same body; which it will be if it consist of the same kinds of matter combined in the same proportions, and has the same form and structure. For the particles of our bodies are often totally changed during our lives; yet no one imagines that the old man has not the same body as in infancy. What but the principles of science could have thus vindicated a precious doctrine of revelation?[42]

What indeed!

Religious enthusiasm was common in a more elemental sense as well. The ultimate expression of the faith in human worth and power, and the promise of universal salvation, was the evangelical fever gripping the first half of the nineteenth century. Mass revivalism, complete with prolonged camp meetings, impassioned oratory, paroxysmal worship, and ecstatic conversions, inflamed the nation and brought on delirious visions of an approaching millennium. Some believers, the premillennialists, expected the millennium would occur only after the advent of Christ, and would be established by divine, cataclysmic action. But more appealing was the postmillennialist inclination toward a millennium to precede the Second Advent, and to be brought about by human improvement. Representative of the latter was the master of all evangelists, Charles Grandison Finney, who formulated a doctrine of Christian Perfectionism affirming the possibility that every human being could achieve a sin-free state of existence in this life. The quest for the kingdom of God on earth (identified by Niebuhr as the distinguishing feature of American Christianity) gained new impetus and confidence, and though Finney's estimate that the millenium could be as near as three years away was

[42] Edward Hitchcock, *The Religion of Geology and its Connected Sciences,* Boston, 1857, pp. 8–9.

a bit too optimistic for many, there was a widely shared expectation that the thousand years of holiness and peace were imminent, or at least attainable.[43]

In the meantime, there was work to be done. An essential part of the perfectionist creed was the responsibility to help others toward sinlessness by purging society of corrupting influences. Christian activism thus flowed readily into numerous social reform campaigns in the mid-1800s. Abolitionism stood at the front of radical, or "ultra," crusades, but there were also vigorous movements to improve conditions in schools, factories, and mental asylums, liberate women from "domestic slavery," restructure the economic system, and annihilate demon rum.

When Emerson wrote Carlyle in 1840 that "we are all a little wild here with numberless projects of social reform," he added that there was "not a reading man but has a draft of a new Community in his waistcoat pocket."[44] Those new, generally socialist, communities were another manifestation of perfectionist passion. Utopias bloomed (and soon faded) in astonishing variety. Merely the ventures in revised Christianity spanned the distance between the Shaker colonies where celibacy was worshipped to the Oneida Community where free love, dressed up as "complex marriage," was enforced. Some settlements were responses to the surging Romantic enchantment with the primitive and natural, others, such as the Fourierist Phalanxes that popped up throughout the country, were the experimental tests of radical socioeconomic theories.

The unifying creed of these multifarious projects—confi-

---

[43] W. R. Cross, *The Burned-Over District. The Social and Intellectual History of Enthusiastic Religion in Western New York, 1800–50*, Ithaca, N.Y., 1950; Timothy L. Smith, *Revivalism and Social Reform in Mid-Nineteenth Century America*, New York, 1959; William McLoughlin, *Modern Revivalism*, New York, 1959; H. R. Niebuhr, *The Kingdom of God in America*, Hamden, Conn., 1956.

[44] Ralph Waldo Emerson to Thomas Carlyle, October 30, 1840, in *The Correspondence of Emerson and Carlyle*, ed. John Slater, New York, 1964, p. 283.

dence that a free, egalitarian society allowed innate human goodness to be fully unfolded—was also the faith of the public at large. The 1830s and 1840s were above all the age of "Jacksonian democracy," of uninhibited celebration of the virtues of common folk and the exalting power of democratic institutions. There was a political perfectionism paralleling the Christian variety, and indeed often merging with it so tightly as to be inseparable. The two appealed to the same audience, the "common people" who, though they had not been born with wealth or privilege, could raise themselves almost indefinitely through equality of opportunity before man and God, and the exercise of common sense and piety.[45]

Self-conscious egalitarianism affected thinking on health matters also. Since common folk distrusted intellectuals and regarded "book-larnin' " as an affectation, they could be rather cynical about the qualifications of educated physicians. Doctors' use of arcane medical terms beyond the grasp of common intellect even made them appear to be milking the public as greedily as lawyers, and more viciously, for they drew blood and life in addition to money. "The application of some dashing, unmeaning, foreign, difficult name to a simple medicine, or to a simple, common disease, is calculated to strike an unlettered person speechless," charged a Thomsonian practitioner, and thus give the doctor a "despotic sway."[46]

That technical education also gave physicians a medical monopoly. By the early 1800s, most states had adopted medical licensing legislation that required applicants for practice to present a medical degree or pass an examination. Such recognition of book-larnin' offended Jacksonian sensitivities, however. It not only granted a favor on the basis of a false distinction, it interfered with the freedom of the individual to pursue a chosen career or to select the kind of medicine he wanted to receive. Licensing laws even implied his

[45] Arthur Schlesinger, Jr., *The Age of Jackson*, New York, 1945.
[46] Benjamin Colby, *A Guide to Health*, Colby, N.H., 1846, p. 8.

vaunted common sense was inadequate to distinguish good medicine from bad. The calls for medical democracy that this state of affairs provoked soon resounded through the halls of state legislatures: "A people accustomed to govern themselves, and boasting of their intelligence, are impatient of restraint. They want no protection but freedom of inquiry and freedom of action."[47] The calls were answered with votes for repeal of medical legislation; by 1845, only three state statute books still held licensing laws.

Thomsonians, self-appointed champions of the common man's medical interests, led the assault on the licensing system. Their encouragement of medical independence did not stop with the destruction of the medical monopoly, though. Thomson's easy-to-understand botanic practice was actually marketed as a system of self-treatment. With the protection of a federal patent, he peddled "Family Right Certificates" to citizens eager to enjoy medical emancipation by practicing on themselves. And though he fell somewhat short of making every man his own physician, by 1839 Thomson could claim to have sold one hundred thousand of his certificates.[48] At twenty dollars apiece, those sales bespeak a public mood hostile to established medicine, one only too receptive to proposals of medical self-help and a fig for the doctors!

[47] Quoted by Richard Shryock, *Medicine and Society in America: 1660–1860*, Ithaca, N.Y., 1960, p. 149.

[48] James Harvey Young, *The Toadstool Millionaires*, Princeton, N.J., 1961, p. 54.

CHAPTER TWO
CHRISTIAN PHYSIOLOGY

EARLY IN THEIR SECOND VOLUME, THE EDITORS OF THE *Journal of Health* paused to proffer brief thanks to a Reverend Graham for his staunch efforts in the battle against alcohol. They had to apologize for insufficient space to do justice to "his zeal and abilities," but consoled readers with the reflection there should be future opportunities to return to the subject.[1] Had they had any inkling how numerous those opportunities would be, the congratulations might well have been less hearty, for Reverend Graham's zeal and abilities were already mounting an offensive against all the enemies of health (not just rum), an offensive beside which the *Journal's* would seem timid and ineffectual. Indeed, the *Journal* would not survive its fourth year and would become defunct while Graham's star was still climbing.

It has become customary to introduce Sylvester Graham as the creator of the Graham cracker, and to bemoan facetiously the cruel destiny that has memorialized his life with so trivial a monument. However unfortunate, or amusing, his fate, it is one that might have been expected, for life never treated Graham with much consideration. The seventeenth child of a septuagenarian father, he entered the world in 1794, in Connecticut, already cursed with a frail constitution.[2] His father passed away within two years, his mother soon became deranged, and the sickly Graham was consigned to years of being bounced back and forth between relatives. At the age of sixteen he began to show signs of

---

[1] *J. Health, 2,* 113–114 (1830–31).

[2] Mildred Naylor, "Sylvester Graham, 1794–1851," *Ann. Med. Hist., 4,* 236–240 (1942).

pulmonary tuberculosis, consumption—the standard self-diagnosed condition among the debilitated of his day—but recovered what with him passed for health, only to suffer a nervous breakdown thirteen years later. These trials of the body must have steeled the soul, however, for in his early thirties he became a Presbyterian minister and began preaching in New Jersey. His clerical career lasted less than two years. Unable to find a parish of his own, he turned in 1830 from guest preaching to lecturing for the Pennsylvania Temperance Society. The course of his life was at last set.

The already well-advanced temperance movement was to a great extent a microcosm of what health reform or "Grahamism" would become. Warriors for sobriety attributed much physical injury to alcohol: it was presumed to weaken the body and undermine its resistance to disease, especially tuberculosis and, after 1832, cholera; to fray the nerves until delirium tremens and insanity came on; and even to dehydrate the tissues and make drunkards susceptible to spontaneous combustion. When Edward Hitchcock penned an allegorical *History of a Zoological Temperance Convention,* he had Africa's animals adopt a resolution to drink only water themselves, but encourage men to drink alcoholic beverages so that the world would soon be rid of the creatures' enemy. A riddle posed by the owl delegate, however, displayed the dominant theme of temperance philosophy: "If Satan should lose his tail, where must he go to get a new one?" The answer—"where they Re-tail spirits"—playfully expressed the grave concern that alcohol was a tool of the devil.[3] It was moral pathology that truly occupied and activated temperance campaigners. The drunkard was lazy and unproductive, abused (or at best neglected) his family, and was given to licentiousness and crime. The utter sinfulness of drinking, the impossibility of the millennium coming

[3] Edward Hitchcock, *History of a Zoological Temperance Convention Held in Central Africa in 1847,* New York, 1849, pp. 53, 84, 146. A good general history of the temperance crusade is J. C. Furnas, *The Life and Times of the Late Demon Rum,* New York, 1965.

while sots still walked the earth, made temperance an ideal vehicle for revivalism. Temperance lecturers such as Graham were in reality evangelical preachers mixing rum with brimstone and demanding total abstinence from alcohol as a prerequisite for Christian perfection.[4]

Graham carried all that temperance baggage with him into health reform. He did, to be sure, reverse the temperance emphases, giving much more attention to the physical effects of bad hygiene. But his heart was still dominated by moral anxiety, and his horror of spiritual sickness dictated his reasoning about physical health, pushing him to imagine the most dire bodily punishments for moral transgressions and to suppose moral rectitude must be essential for perfect health. As with the teetotallers, his hygienic temperance usually meant abstinence.

But the natural theologian's certainty that morality is validated by science led Graham to seek a physiological rationale for self-denial. His account books from the late 1820s, while he was still a minister in a small New Jersey settlement, date the dawning of his awareness of physiology's significance. He purchased a number of texts of anatomy, physiology, and nutrition during that period, and seems to have studied them diligently.[5] He was particularly taken by the writings of Francois J. V. Broussais, a Parisian practitioner who drew a large and devoted following in France during the 1820s. His *Treatise on Physiology applied to Pathology* was translated and published in Philadelphia just at the time Graham was beginning his self-education in that field. This coincidence, and the fact that French medical thought generally had been given much publicity by the Philadelphia medical community in recent years, may account for Graham's purchase of the volume. His embracing of its principles, though, resulted from more profound con-

---

[4] Perry Miller, *The Life of the Mind in America*, New York, 1965, pp. 85–86.

[5] Naylor (n. 2), p. 238.

siderations.[6] Broussais was among the numerous biological scientists at the beginning of the nineteenth century who reacted against the mechanistic reductionism of eighteenth-century Newtonian physiology. Extreme attempts to reduce all functions of the living organism to physical-chemical explanations, capped by La Mettrie's *L'homme machine,* had sparked a resurgence of vitalism, the belief that life transcends the simple inorganic sciences and can be understood only as a manifestation of unique physiological or vital forces.[7] More impressed by the differences between the living and nonliving, than by the similarities, vitalists tended to isolate one or another distinct vital activity as the basic expression of the life force. One of the most striking vital powers has always been the ability of organisms to respond to stimulation from the environment, and in Broussais' day, with the recent elucidation that had been given the nervous system, the power of response was particularly arresting. Broussais assumed that the response to stimulation was directed by a vital force acting through a special *chimie vivante.* Concentrated in the fibers of the body's organs, this living chemistry produced a contraction whenever the fibers were stimulated. The theory, of course, was much more elaborate, but it had certain simple pathological implications that caught Graham's attention. When local fibers con-

[6] An excellent detailed analysis of Graham's ideas has been done by Stephen Nissenbaum, *Sex, Diet, and Debility in Jacksonian America. Sylvester Graham and Health Reform,* Westport, Conn., 1980. In the next three chapters, a number of points already made in that book will necessarily be repeated, though often in a somewhat different context. There will be specific footnote references for each of Nissenbaum's points, but it seems appropriate at the outset to cite his work *in toto* as an engrossing introduction to the health reform movement and a valuable aid in my own study. Broussais' influence on Graham is discussed by Nissenbaum on pp. 57–60. For discussions of Broussais himself, see Thomas Hall, *Ideas of Life and Matter,* 2 vols., Chicago, 1969; 2: 241–245; J. D. Rolleston, "F. J. V. Broussais (1772–1838): His Life and Doctrines," *Proc. Roy. Soc. Med., 32,* p. 1, 405–413 (1939).

[7] Hall (n. 6), 2: 5–30, offers a thorough exploration of vitalist thought in the nineteenth century.

tracted, Broussais proposed, the excited tissue drew in fluid and increased its temperature, assuming a state of "vital erection." Normally, the tissue erection subsided with the removal of stimulation, but repeated stimulation might cause an overexcitation producing irritation, and eventually inflammation. And since the nerves feeding all organs were also contractile, localized inflammation might be transmitted to any part of the body via the nervous system.[8] To condense his theories even further, Broussais concluded that all disease stems from overstimulation of the body's tissues, especially those of the gastrointestinal tract. Irritation of the stomach or gut could radiate outward along nerves to affect other organs; it could also be induced when other overstimulated tissues passed along their condition through the nervous system. In the end, gastroenteritis, or enteric inflammation, was declared to be the source of virtually all illness.

The practical applications of the theory, incidentally, made illness a double ordeal for patients. Since cure required removal of blood from the inflamed fibers, standard therapy involved the application of two to four dozen (or more) leeches to the patient's abdomen. So numerous were Broussais' supporters for a period, that France had to import twenty to forty million leeches a year by the early 1830s to satisfy the demand.[9]

One might think that Graham, opposed to heroic therapy on principle, would have refused any influence from Broussais. But he found the gastroenteritis theory so compelling, he forgave its author his therapeutic extravagance. It was not just that a theory focussing on the stomach necessarily singled out food and drink as potential inflammatory agents, while also implying that nerve irritants (alcohol, tobacco) might have the same effect (Broussais, it should be noted,

---

[8] Francois Broussais, *A Treatise on Physiology*, trans. J. Bell and R. LaRoche, Philadelphia, 1826, pp. 43–46.

[9] Erwin Ackerknecht, *Medicine at the Paris Hospital, 1794–1848*, Baltimore, 1967, p. 62.

insisted on a bland diet for his patients, and abjured heroic emetics, purgatives, and mercury, as well as alcohol, because of their irritating effects on the stomach). Nor was the attraction completed by its medical plausibility: intestinal distress, after all, was one of the most common complaints in this period of lavishly polluted water supplies, and postmortems often turned up intestinal lesions. Graham's interest went deeper—Broussais' ideas had a truly visceral appeal for him, because they concentrated on overstimulation as the mechanism of physiological injury. Stimulation was a loaded word in Graham's time, one which was used at least as frequently in a moral as a physiological context. The determination to promote godliness by suppressing animal appetites and passions, the Victorian antipleasure principle, was sufficiently far advanced as to have branded overstimulation, or nervous and mental excitation, as morally evil, the first step of a gradual descent into drunkenness and debauchery. Graham's was as Victorian a soul as the nineteenth century would produce; he was of the same mind as Sir James Stephen, the Evangelical who "once smoked a cigar, and found it so delicious that he never smoked again."[10] Graham was thus overjoyed with the logic of Broussais. Stimulation, so threatening to the spirit, was now seen to be equally dangerous for the body: what a splendid lesson in natural theology! Thus armed with the minister's end of Christian perfection and the amateur physiologist's understanding of the means, Graham sallied forth to tilt with any unchristian dissipation that dared show itself.

The foregoing version of Graham's formative years is not the one he conveyed to his public. He neglected to acknowledge any debt to Broussais or other writers, swore that his hygienic conclusions were the unpremeditated results of purely objective trial and error and physiological reasoning, and claimed to have been pressed into the service of health

[10] Eric Trudgill, *Madonnas and Magdalens. The Origins and Development of Victorian Sexual Attitudes*, New York, 1976, pp. 13–19.

reform. When he resigned his post with the Pennsylvania Temperance Society after six months, Graham stated, he had no intention of continuing as a public lecturer. But he was soon prevailed upon to deliver a course of talks on physiology and regimen in Philadelphia, and before that task had been completed he was tendered "an urgent invitation" to offer the same enlightenment in New York. In the latter city, "pressing invitations from every quarter" got him so deeply involved in hygienic instruction he finally accepted that as his life's work. Perhaps he was a reluctant crusader, though the image does not square with the belligerence and imperiousness he displayed once mounted. And the assertion that his radical hygienic opinions were derived "purely by my physiological investigations" fails to recognize that in his mind pure physiology was Christian physiology; he simply could not accept that any conclusion about natural law might be valid if it conflicted with his understanding of Christian morality. As one of his correspondents realized, "What is now called Grahamism . . . is in fact Bibleism."[11]

The presupposition that physiology—that is, nature—must be Christian forced Graham and fellow health reformers to perform some tricky mental acrobatics. For in recoiling from the spontaneous expression of appetites and passions, they seemed to be showing distrust of the very nature they professed to worship. The only way out they could find was to deny the naturalness of appetites in the present age by arguing that the pure instincts of original man had been defiled by wrong use of free will and reason. In other paragraphs, however, they make it clear that vitiated appetites could not be subdued except by the exertion of that same slippery will; and natural physiology could be rediscovered only by the exercise of that same unreliable reason. As Twain joked of Christian Science, "It looks inconsistent."[12]

[11] Sylvester Graham, *Lectures on the Science of Human Life,* 2 vols., Boston, 1839, 1: vi–vii; *Graham J. Health and Longevity, 1,* 5 (1837).

[12] Samuel Clemens, *Christian Science; with Notes Containing Corrections to Date,* New York, 1907, p. 38.

But if the qualities of free will and reason were routinely altered to meet the ideological demands of the moment, there was a consistent attitude toward stimulation: it was always bad. As the mechanism of both physical and spiritual pathology, it made the union of physiology and religion possible, and governed Graham's "physiological investigations" from the start. The *Journal of Health*'s account of his temperance lectures, though brief, does report that his argument ran from the accepted view of alcohol as a stimulant, through charges that as a stimulant it must produce "heat and irritation of the stomach first," cause that organ to become "inflamed," and eventually spread its irritation throughout the frame.[13] And since even a single molecule possessed that stimulating property, no quantity of alcohol was safe. True moderation, by this physiological analysis, consisted of abstention.

That line of thought naturally carried Graham to the consideration of other stimulating indulgences, and by the spring of 1831 he was offering a series of lectures covering a broad range of hygienic behavior. The maturing of what he was already calling "the Science of Human Life" was stimulated further by that "urgent invitation" to New York, for it was during his stay in that city that the dreaded cholera finally appeared in America. Weeks before the first cases were reported, in fact, public fear of the new infection had risen to a height sufficient to inspire Graham to add a lecture on cholera to his repertory. As he well realized, the disease presented an ideal opportunity to promote his Broussaisist scheme of health. The symptoms of profuse diarrhea and abdominal cramps stamped it as a gastrointestinal irritation. All medical advice on prevention gave first place to careful diet for the maintenance of resistance, though exactly what constituted care in eating was a matter of much dispute. There was general agreement too that all other forms of intemperance, including sexual excess, increased susceptibil-

---

[13] *J. Health, 2,* 113–114 (1830–31).

ity. Attitudes were tinged with moral judgments as well. It was a striking fact that cholera usually first appeared and most terribly prospered in the filthy slums packed with profane, licentious drunkards. The early consensus of polite society was that cholera was God's way of cleansing the earth of its human scum.[14]

Graham agreed to a point, but he spoke in terms of physiological sin and saw it affecting all levels of society, the high almost as much as the low. Cholera was a particularly acute manifestation of overstimulation of the stomach, he admitted, but it was basically no different from all other disease and debility. The race had long been deteriorating physically, he explained, falling from generation to generation as habits of overstimulation continued. The drinking of stimulating beverages was one such habit, the eating of spices and condiments and meat were others (Graham's insistence on water as the only suitable beverage was, of course, unfortunate in an epidemic of cholera, for the disease was being spread most effectively through contaminated water supplies; cheap, germicidal bourbon would have been a far safer drink). Sexual excitation, through its effects on the nervous system, could also inflame the stomach, and general inattention to exercise, rest, clothing, the emotions, and other non-naturals weakened the vital powers and made it easier for inflammation to be established. It was cholera at the moment, but next year it would be something else, and afterwards still another problem; the real epidemic was not cholera, but overstimulation and improper hygiene. The lecture on cholera was thus actually just another lecture on the Science of Human Life in disguise.[15]

The outline of that science included a final entry that has to be considered in any discussion of Graham. As one might expect of a man so impressed by the wisdom of God as ex-

[14] Charles Rosenberg, *The Cholera Years*, Chicago, 1962, pp. 13–54.
[15] Sylvester Graham, *A Lecture on Epidemic Diseases Generally, and Particularly the Spasmodic Cholera*, New York, 1833.

pressed in nature, he was automatically suspicious of any food altered from its natural condition. Bread made of light flour from which the coarser bran had been removed by bolting had become more popular during the early 1800s, and was perhaps affecting health since it had replaced whole meal bread in many working-class families in which bread was the main food (commercial bread was also commonly adulterated with flour substitutes such as chalk and plaster of Paris). Graham knew nothing about the vitamin and mineral deficiencies of white flour, but he nevertheless regarded it as the crowning touch to humanity's descent from nature to artificial civilization. When he finally published his *Lectures on the Science of Human Life* in 1839, he devoted a long section in the second of the two hefty volumes to the subject of the preparation of bread. That section opened with a disgusted reference to mankind's readiness "to put asunder what God has joined together," and though it progressed through a physiological explanation of the stupidity of such presumption, it kept a resonant undertone of religious and Romantic hatred of any debasement of nature. "Well-made" bread, Graham disclosed, that which "is most highly conducive to the welfare of [humanity's] bodies and souls," must contain "all the natural properties of the wheat." His respect for the natural embraced also an ideal of natural society. Our forefathers, he felt, had been happier as well as healthier because their culture was simply ordered and anchored in the family, the natural Christian social unit. In the 1830s, many families purchased their bread from public bakers, or had it made by domestics, and in those circumstances, even if natural ingredients were used, the finished product would not be natural. When he thought of "those blessed days of New England's prosperity and happiness, when our good mothers used to make the family bread" (the kind of life he had been denied as a child), Graham drifted into a revery displaying the moral underpinnings of his physiological construct. "Who shall make Bread?," he asked:

It is the wife, the mother only—she who loves her husband and her children as woman ought to love, and who rightly perceives the relations between the dietetic habits and physical and moral condition of her loved ones, and justly appreciates the importance of good bread to their physical and moral welfare. . . . could wives and mothers fully comprehend the importance of good bread, in relation to all the bodily and intellectual and moral interests of their husbands and children, and in relation to the domestic and social and civil welfare of mankind, and to their religious prosperity, both for time and eternity, they would estimate the art and duty of bread-making far, very far more highly than they now do.[16]

But even mother's love could not perfect grain that had been stripped of natural ingredients, and there was a physiological reason. Graham believed the vital economy of digestion involved a system of waste and repair: food stimulated digestive organs to activity, in which process they suffered an expenditure of vital force and waste of substance proportional to the intensity and duration of the stimulation. On a healthful diet the loss of force and substance could be quickly replaced by the absorbed nourishment, but if food were too stimulating, the withdrawal of vitality from the system would exceed subsequent deposits and lead to irritation. Hence the "proper alimentary substances" were those "whose stimulating power is barely sufficient to excite a full and healthy performance of the functions of the digestive organs." All the "substances in nature, designed for human aliment," Graham continued, were composed of a mixture of nutritious (stimulating) and innutritious matter in such proportions as to stimulate the stomach to action without exhausting it. When man tampered with God's design and separated bran from wheat, or concentrated the nutritive

[16] Graham, *Lectures* (n. 11), 2: 448, 455–456. Nissenbaum (n. 6) relates this pining for a happy home with a bread-baking mother to Graham's own insecure and unhappy youth, pp. 8–9.

substance of any other food, he ended with a product that was too nutritious and would excite a rapid deterioration of vitality. Also a practical man, Graham added that inclusion of bran in the flour used for bread (and for his immortal crackers) was the best antidote for the costiveness suffered by those who ate so many other unnatural foods.[17]

That argument was already prepared at the time of his New York cholera lectures, and made Graham the man who conferred on unbolted flour its status as a health food.[18] But it was not until he carried his message to Boston, in the winter of 1835, that Graham became nationally known as the prophet of bran bread—though, unhappily for a man of his ego, when he arrived in Boston, he found that much of his gospel of hygiene was already being preached by one William Andrus Alcott. Alcott's customary introduction is as the cousin of the famous Transcendentalist Bronson Alcott (who himself is often introduced through his daughter Louisa May). And in his day and since Alcott the health reformer has been overshadowed by Graham. "Grahamism," usually an epithet, was commonly applied to Alcott's work as well. But in point of fact, Alcott was as busy a lecturer as Graham, a much more prolific and somewhat more readable author, and was the one who actually served, for years, as an officer and an editor of health reform projects (after 1837, Graham pretty much kept to the sidelines). Alcott maintained, as well, a broader perspective on the content of hygiene (true Grahamism came increasingly during the later 1830s to mean only a bran bread and antiflesh diet). Graham was the titular leader of health reform, but Alcott was the one who assumed the lead in elaborating and popularizing a complete and balanced hygienic philosophy.

Alcott was also an easier person to get along with than

[17] *Lectures,* 1: 539–543; 2: 427–429. Earlier hygienic writers had recommended whole wheat bread as superior, though with less elaborate arguments. Thomas Graham, *Sure Methods of Improving Health and Prolonging Life,* London, 1828, p. 29, is an example.

[18] Graham, *Lecture on Epidemic Disease* (n. 15), pp. 54–58.

Graham. The latter confessed to having an acidic personality, and acquaintances were free in confirming his assessment. He was "obtusive," his vanity was "excessive," and he "wore everybody out who listened to him."[19] Alcott was hardly flawless, and could be outrageously self-righteous at times: although in his youth he once consented, for social reasons, to eat screech owl, after he became a vegetarian, he refused to visit his parents for Thanksgiving and even published a letter to his father in which he lectured him that the Thanksgiving feast was, "in point of health, one of the worst meals eaten during the whole year." His portrait shows an extraordinarily earnest man (Figure 1), but his writings generally have a tone of kindliness and cheerfulness, qualities also remembered by his friends and associates. A neighbor's recollection of the elderly Alcott as a man "you would most any day find working in his garden, bareheaded and barefooted, always ready for a chat," betokens a good-naturedness not easily found in Graham.[20]

But, as with Graham, it was seriousness—purposiveness—that ruled his personality. Another native of Connecticut, Alcott demonstrated an inclination for literary endeavors at an early age. Cousin Bronson remembered him as a youth "fired with the love of letters." William and Bronson formed their own "Juvenile Library," corresponded in stilted letters that each delivered to the other's door, and "one even aspired to authorship." By the time he died in 1859, that one, William, had realized his aspirations to the degree of more than one hundred volumes of books and journals on self-improvement. His anonymous claim, toward the end of his life, that he had "probably attempted to guide a greater number of erring young men during the last half

[19] "Sylvester Graham," *Boston Med. Surg. J., 45,* 316–317 (1852). This is admittedly not a sympathetic obituary, but its sentiments seem to have been common among those with no axe to grind as well: see Nissenbaum (n. 6), p. 14.

[20] *Moral Reformer, 2,* 366 (1836); quoted in Donald Winslow, "A Lasell Neighbor a Century Ago," *Lasell Leaves, 79,* 5 (1954).

century that any living individual in this country" was actually modest. He really should have included young women, children, and older people as well.[21]

His "how to live" manuals appear to be classifiable into three categories—health, religion, and education—but, as was the case with Graham, these were merely different faces of a single entity. The molding of that triune began in 1816 in the stultifying environment of the Connecticut schoolhouse Alcott had been persuaded to direct. Though a callow eighteen, he soon came to recognize that the physical and pedagogical arrangements of traditional education encouraged boredom, discomfort, even illness in students. School rooms were typically equipped with poor heating, ventilation, and lighting. The hard benches were too low for some students, too high for others, and had backs for none. Playgrounds were rarely provided and exercise was not part of the scholarly schedule. As Alcott's teaching career advanced, he became occupied increasingly with the reform of such conditions, in his own school and in others. He was regularly contributing to educational journals by the late 1820s, and soon moved to Boston to take a place among the leaders of America's great educational awakening of the 1830s. An innovative teacher and critic, his 1832 *Essay on the Construction of Schoolhouses* was awarded first prize in a competition organized by the American Institute of Instruction. That essay was distinguished, it should be noted, by its attention to the effects of school-building structure on students' health, as well as their ability to learn. And in developing his case for health, Alcott employed a strategy that

[21] Bronson Alcott, *New Connecticut. An Autobiographical Poem*, ed. F. B. Sanbourn, Boston, 1887, pp. 36, 151–152; William Alcott, *The Physiology of Marriage*, Boston, 1855, p. vi. *Barnard's Am. J. Ed.*, 4, 629–656 (1857) is the most detailed biography of Alcott. Others include H. Thoms, "William Andrus Alcott: Physician, Educator, Writer," *Bull. Soc. Med. Hist. Chicago*, 4, 123–130 (1928); and L. Salomon, "The Least-Remembered Alcott," *New England Q.*, 24, 87–93 (1961). Also see James Whorton, " 'Christian Physiology': William Alcott's Prescription for the Millennium," *Bull. Hist. Med.*, 49, 466–481 (1975).

was to be a critical component of the medical profession's public health campaign in later decades—he emphasized the economic cost of preventible illness. He had in mind here something more than the sort of calculation Hitchcock had made (though at other times he speculated on the millions of Bibles that could be purchased and distributed with the money now wasted on gluttony). As a Christian physiologist, Alcott kept one eye on heaven, but the other always took a hard, practical view of terrestrial affairs, and he appreciated most people were more interested in getting money back than in seeing it transferred to a Bible fund. His exhortations to live healthfully because that is God's law were thus followed with reminders that health saves dollars as well as souls. "It is a most mistaken economy," his *Essay* explained, to stint on the construction of school facilities, only to incur much greater medical expenses for pupils physically ruined by impure air and inactivity. An ounce of prevention, he was saying, costs much less than a pound of cure.[22]

During this educational phase of his career, Alcott was also an assistant to William Channing Woodbridge, editor of the *American Annals of Education* and the most successful popularizer of Pestalozzi in this country. Johann Pestalozzi was the Swiss educator of the early nineteenth century who advocated a structured implementation of Rousseau's theory of education. Providing an education in accord with the child's nature, he maintained, required understanding child psychology and devising activities, including play and physical exercise, which would appeal to the child's natural inclinations.[23] The Pestalozzian emphases on the cultivation of reasoning power above memory, on

[22] William Alcott, *Essay on the Construction of Schoolhouses*, Boston, 1832, p. 4. Also see *Library of Health*, 4, 334–335 (1840); and *ibid.*, 5, 78–79 (1841).

[23] Will Monroe, *History of the Pestalozzian Movement in the U.S.*, Syracuse, 1907; E. E. Bayles and B. L. Hood, *Growth of American Educational Thought and Practice*, New York, 1966, p. 106.

the management of children with friendly understanding rather than rigid discipline, and particularly on the harmonious development of all the individual's faculties, the physical and moral as well as the intellectual, appealed to Alcott, and also struck him as something more than a revolutionary method for inculcating the three R's. The new education, used to impart an understanding of the structure and functioning of the human body and a reverence for the full realization of human potential, was to be an essential element in his strategy of hygienic reform.

That strategy was not evolving purely from his teaching experiences however. In the mid-1820s his classroom duties had brought on a physical decline that he had interpreted as a consumptive condition, and to save himself he had taken up the study of medicine. In an unintentionally wry observation on the quality of medical education in his day, Alcott noted that "a course of medical lectures which I heard in 1825–6 [at Yale], left me . . . in about as bad a state of health as school keeping formerly had done." His thesis for the medical degree, though, was on the subject of the prevention of pulmonary tuberculosis, and it indicated the direction both his health and his career would take. He treated himself with drugs for a period, including three daily doses of opium, but soon found better results with a temperate diet and abstinence from alcohol. The culmination of his return to health was a dramatic declaration of "medical independence," an affirmation of nature as the only true physician and a denial of human medical art. He turned his back on medicine as a personal career too, though, it might be mentioned parenthetically, it had been an ill-fated professional choice anyway; on his very first day of practice, Alcott had fallen from his horse in front of his fellow townsmen.[24]

By 1830, then, the doctor-educator possessed energetic health, some formal training in anatomy and physiology, a

[24] William Alcott, *Forty Years in the Wilderness of Pills and Powders*, Boston, 1859, pp. 72–73, 80, 193.

faith born of experience that medicine was useless and careful hygiene nature's method of restoring and preserving health, and excitement at being on the cutting edge of a revolution in education which could transform American society. The product of this fusion of abilities and convictions was what he liked to call "Physical Education": "What a mighty work for this fallen world education has yet to achieve; especially Physical Education! This ... let me say once for all, this physical education, under the guidance of Christianity, whose handmaid all true science should be, and to whose development and application all true religion should be directed, is our chief dependence. It is the lever by which we are to raise the world."[25]

As the oratory insists, the cement holding the various components of Physical Education together was Christianity. And although Graham was the ordained pastor, Dr. Alcott was the one set on presenting health reform as a project of redemption. His special cause was the liberation of the public mind from that fatalism which took disease as it came, accepting it as an unpredictable act of Providence beyond human control. He repeatedly stigmatized resignation as Islamic, as a state of mind unworthy of a Christian whose God had endowed him with free will and responsibility for his own salvation. That physical salvation was won by work, not luck, and poor health was a voluntary condition—slow suicide—became, with Alcott's pushing, one of the dominant themes of health reform literature.

> "Give us this day our daily bread,"
> And pies and cakes besides,
> To load the stomach, pain the head,
> And choke the vital tides.
> And if too soon a friend decays,
> Or dies in agony—
> We'll talk of "God's mysterious ways,"
> And lay it all to thee.

[25] *ibid.*, p. 132.

After five similar stanzas, "The Fashionable Lady's Prayer" drew to a close:

> And if defying nature's laws,
> Dyspeptic we must be,—
> We scorn to search for human cause,
> But lay it all to thee.[26]

The search for human cause, Physical Education, was embraced by Alcott as his ministry. Indeed, so overwhelming was his assurance that his work was opening the way to "the good time coming," this usually modest, even self-deprecating, man could not resist assuming a messianic posture. He regularly referred to himself as a medical missionary, and celebrated his deliverance from the "wilderness" of pills and powders. He even presented potential believers with a garishly melodramatic account of having literally gone up on a mountain to receive the commandments of health.[27]

But most of Alcott's physiological education came from hard work rather than revelation. He attempted to keep stride with physiological literature, and did succeed in reading it if not always in understanding it. He did not, as a rule, present his interpretations in the technical detail Graham did, but he held basically the same "stimulation theory." And that library physiology, so modern and seemingly complete, could transport him back to the mountaintop. "In the present blaze of physiological light," he once exulted, "we can, in ways and processes almost innumerable, manufacture human health to an extent not formerly dreamed of." He even had the audacity to suggest that Christ had drunk real wine, but would have taken only water had he had the benefit of modern physiological knowledge. For the dream of health to be realized, however, physiological knowledge had to be publicized. The science had not yet been pro-

[26] *Water Cure J.*, *4*, 351 (1847).
[27] Alcott, *Forty Years* (n. 24), p. 75.

ductive of human good because it had been "locked up in the dead languages of the medical man's library."[28] An interpreter was needed, someone with at least a physician's understanding of physiology and an educator's ability to simplify complex ideas: someone like Alcott.

Graham's arrival in Boston was thus not an entirely welcome event. The newcomer was at once a comrade and a challenger, and while Alcott was willing to collaborate, he was careful to remind the public of his own originality and independence. He had, after all, been offering hygienic instruction for some time too. Letters to the *Boston Medical and Surgical Journal,* essays in educational magazines, a heavily didactic *Young Man's Guide,* and an engaging anatomy-physiology manual for juvenile readers—*The House I Live In*—had all flowed from his pen in the early 1830s. In 1835, with the *Journal of Health* now extinct, Alcott launched only the second popular health periodical in the country, his *Moral Reformer and Teacher on the Human Constitution* (whose purpose was to show "the almost inseparable connection of health and morals"). So he was less than pleased to be repeatedly asked if he were a Grahamite. Initially he claimed to "not exactly know what is meant by a Grahamite"; once that excuse became untenable, he generously conceded that though he was not guilty "of suffering Mr. G. . . . to think for us, . . . no other individual has aided us more." But as Grahamism continued as the common designation for all health reform, Alcott became testy. When a Boston doctor dismissed him as a Grahamite, he snapped back that he had abstained from meat and alcohol and had publicized his system of health for two years before he knew "there was such a man in the world as Mr. G." That same month (May, 1837), he took umbrage at the first issue of the *Graham Journal of Health and Longevity* for not giving credit for the work already accomplished by his journal; he

[28] William Alcott, *Lectures of Life and Health; or, the Laws and Means of Physical Culture,* Boston, 1853, pp. 32, 43; *American Vegetarian, 2,* 9 (1852).

wished the new project well, but scolded "we are hardly willing to be thus undervalued."[29]

The oversight rankled all the more because Graham's success in Boston was so much greater than in Philadelphia or New York, and was due at least partly to Alcott's having already prepared the soil. Yet despite the internal friction, Grahamism or physical education (call it what they would) rolled forward, albeit over a very rocky road. Graham and his doctrine were showered with contempt by the unregenerate. A Boston paper offered the opinion, for example, that "a greater humbug or a more disgusting writer never lived." Venom flowed as freely through the medical press, particularly in the pages of the *Boston Medical and Surgical Journal*, where the possibility that Grahamism caused insanity was just one of the ideas entertained. Professional bakers, understandably miffed at Graham's charges that their business was injurious to health, attempted to disrupt his lectures, and though Christian physiologists tried to turn the other cheek, at least once they retaliated by dousing their tormentors with slaked lime.[30]

The refusal to be bullied is all the more remarkable for coming from a group of such apparently puny specimens. Those attracted to Graham's lectures, obviously, were the ones who needed help most desperately. Alcott described the membership of the American Physiological Society, an organization established in 1837 by 124 male and 39 female converts to health reform, thusly: "Most of these individuals were more or less feeble, and a very large proportion of them were actually suffering from chronic disease when they became members of the society. Not a few joined it, indeed, as a last resort, after having tried everything else, as drowning men are said to catch at straws."[31]

[29] *Moral Reformer, 1,* 42 (1835); *ibid., 2,* 34 (1836); *Library of Health, 1,* 165, 168 (1837).

[30] William Walker, "The Health Reform Movement in the United States, 1830–1870," doctoral dissertation, Johns Hopkins University, 1955, p. 56; *Boston Med. Surg. J., 14,* 38–46 (1836); Naylor (n. 2), p. 239.

[31] Quoted in Hebbel Hoff and John Fulton, "The Centenary of the

If one is to believe the wags of the day, participation in the society did little to help these decrepit creatures. Their physical appearance, as a result of belonging to "the bran bread and sawdust pathological society," was the subject of countless jests: Alcott's followers were "gaunt, wry-faced, lantern-jawed, ghostly-looking invalids"; among Graham's "lean-visaged cadaverous disciples," "the gentlemen resemble busts cut in chalk," the ladies "mummies preserved in saffron"; the opinion that "emasculation is the first fruit of Grahamism" was corroborated by another observer who colloquially described a Grahamite he had met as looking "like a full-blown bladder arter some of the air had leaked out, kinder wrinkled and rumpled like, and his eyes as dim as a lamp that's living on a small allowance of ile. He puts me in mind of a pair of kitchen tongs, all legs, shaft and head, and no belly, a real gander gutted looking creature, as hollow as a bamboo walking cane, and twice as yaller."[32]

The ridicule was surely a bit exaggerated, for not only did the membership rolls of the society steadily grow (to 251 in less than a year and a half), but the energy with which the members carried out their multiple projects suggests they were living on more than a small allowance of "ile." They had, after all, a heroic self-image. They were the new *philosophes,* using science and education to smash the chains of religious superstition. In this instance, the superstition was that disease was inevitable, a willful act of God which man could not avert. Destruction of that myth, and the liberation of humanity to dignity and power, was the ultimate object of the society. Led by Alcott, their president, the young physiologists collected a library of more than fifty volumes. They

---

First American Physiological Society Founded at Boston by William A. Alcott and Sylvester Graham," *Bull. Hist. Med., 5,* 696 (1937).

[32] *Graham J. Health Long., 3,* 116 (1839); *Boston Med. Surg. J., 19,* 221 (1838–39); *ibid., 14,* 169 (1836); "Dietetic Charlatanry; or the New Ethics of Eating," *New York Rev., 1,* 339, 341 (1837); *Water Cure J., 8,* 93 (1849).

organized the nation's first health food store to supply Graham bread and fresh fruits and vegetables grown in virgin, unfertilized soil. They supported the establishment of "Physiological Boarding Houses," so that members without families, as well as transient Grahamites, might live in a natural style (skeptics imagined "one of the rarest spectacles in the world" must be a Graham House at the dinner hour, as the inmates gathered around a board groaning with "straggling radishes, . . . a soggy bunch of asparagus, . . . corpses of potatoes, . . . a thin segment of bran bread," and a "tumbler of cold water."). They also planned a "Physiological Infirmary" to help dyspeptics and other sickly comrades back to a level of health that would permit residence in a boarding house, though the project never reached fruition.[33] They supported health publications; the *Graham Journal of Health and Longevity,* primarily a medium for testimonials of physical salvation—advertisements that Grahamites were not gander-gutted creatures—lasted only three years (1837–39) before being absorbed by a satisfied Alcott's journal. But the latter continued prosperous for some time, though under changing names—*Moral Reformer and Teacher on the Human Constitution* (1835–36), *Library of Health and Teacher on the Human Constitution* (1837–42), and *Teacher of Health and Laws of the Human Constitution* (1843). Most of all, the members of the American Physiological Society attended meetings, listened to lectures, and adopted resolutions.

Through all their works runs the thread of Christian physiology. A simple recitation of some of their innumerable resolutions is an exposition of the philosophy of health as an obligation to, and promoter of, Christian society:

> *Resolved,* That life, health, and all the physical interests of the human body are established upon precise and determinate principles, and that the highest welfare of

[33] "Dietetic Charlatanry" (n. 32), pp. 337–338; Hoff and Fulton (n. 31), give detailed attention to the society's history and projects.

man as an organic and animal being depends on the fulfilment of the constitutional laws of his nature.

Resolved, That a thorough knowledge of the anatomy and physiology of the human system is essential to the highest intellectual development; and that the greatest mental activity and power cannot be secured without a correct observance of physiological law.

Resolved, That the true principles of political economy are founded on the physiological laws of human nature and that the best interests of man in his social, civil and political capacities require that legislators and rulers should act with a just regard to those laws.

Resolved, That it is a duty morally binding upon man, to study the principles of health, and to understand and obey those laws which God has established for the perpetuation of his existence.

Resolved, That the practice and advocacy of physiological reform is a duty which we owe to ourselves, to the community, to posterity, and to God our Maker and Redeemer.

Resolved, That the highest moral and religious interests of man require a strict conformity in his dietetic and other voluntary habits to all the physiological laws of his nature.

Resolved, That the millennium, the near approach of which is by many so confidently predicted, can never reasonably be expected to arrive until those laws which God has implanted in the *physical* nature of man, are, equally with his moral laws, universally known and obeyed.[34]

In what respites from resolution making as there were, the society liked to discuss questions that had not yet been pursued far enough to have their answers anointed with "Resolved." Most were rather innocuous, but one, proposed at

[34] Quoted in Hoff and Fulton (n. 31), pp. 701–706.

an 1838 meeting, was more penetrating than health reformers could appreciate, or if they did appreciate, more embarrassing than they would care to admit: "Is 'a little knowledge' of Physiology 'a dangerous thing?' "[35] If the answer is yes, no better evidence could be offered in support than the health reform version of the physiology of nutrition.

[35] *Graham J. Health Long.*, *2*, 160 (1838).

☆☆☆☆☆☆☆☆☆☆☆☆☆☆☆☆☆☆☆☆☆☆☆☆☆☆☆☆☆☆☆☆☆☆

CHAPTER THREE
TEMPEST IN A FLESH-POT

☆☆☆☆☆☆☆☆☆☆☆☆☆☆☆☆☆☆☆☆☆☆☆☆☆☆☆☆☆☆☆☆☆☆

*In my first voyage from Boston, being becalm'd off Block Is-
land, our people set about catching cod, and hauled up a great
many. Hitherto I had stuck to my resolution of not eating animal food, and on this occasion consider'd . . . the taking every
fish as a kind of unprovoked murder, since none of them had,
or ever could do us any injury that might justify the slaughter. All this seemed very reasonable. But I had formerly been a
great lover of fish, and, when this came hot out of the frying-
pan, it smelt admirably well. I balanc'd some time between
principle and inclination, till I recollected that, when the fish
were opened, I saw smaller fish taken out of their stomachs;
then thought I, "If you eat one another, I don't see why we
mayn't eat you." So I din'd upon cod very heartily, and continued to eat with other people, returning only now and then
occasionally to a vegetable diet. So convenient a thing it is to
be a reasonable creature, since it enables one to find or make a
reason for everything one has a mind to do.*

BENJAMIN FRANKLIN, *His Autobiography.*

AS IF THE PRESIDENTIAL CAMPAIGN OF 1860 WERE NOT MO-
mentous enough, the eminent health reformer Russell Trall
announced to a Philadelphia audience that neither Lincoln,
nor Douglas, nor the other contenders had yet "broached
any subject so vitally important to the voters, as that of beef
versus bread, hog *v.* hominy, mutton *v.* squash, . . . [or]
chicken *v.* whortleberries."[1] From any other assembly, the
charge would have drawn only hoots, but Trall was speaking

---

[1] This chapter is a revised version of an article, " 'Tempest in a Flesh-
pot': The Formulation of a Physiological Rationale for Vegetarianism,"
J. Hist. Med., 32, 115–139 (1977); Russell Trall, *The Scientific Basis of
Vegetarianism*, Philadelphia, 1860, p. 2.

before the American Vegetarian Society. Its members followed the nearly two hour address "with profound attention to the close,"[2] for they knew that true emancipation meant the liberation of all men from the perverted appetite for flesh food.

Their battle against slavery was, of course, an ancient one, but in recent decades a new strategy had been adopted, one which was reflected in the title of Trall's address: "The Scientific Basis of Vegetarianism." Historically, "Pythagoreans" (the nineteenth century's preferred derisive synonym for vegetarians) had relied on philosophical arguments to lead the attack on beef and mutton, with the evidence of science being given a place only in the rear guard, if at all. When the American Vegetarian Society was founded in 1850, however, the list of adopted resolutions, while including religious and humanitarian statements, began with the declaration that "comparative anatomy, human physiology, and ... chemical analysis ... unitedly proclaim ... that not only the human race may, but *should* subsist upon the production of the vegetable kingdom."[3] Vegetarians had "got science" to go with their religion, had been converted by a dazzling vision of modern physiology. "Light—the light of physiology—has flashed in upon my mind," a new believer proclaimed, "sufficient to emancipate me from the dreadful thralldom I so long endured.[4]

The light and the science came, of course, from the health reform movement, which placed food (the most frequent stimulant of the gastrointestinal tract) at the heart of its philosophy. The second volume of Graham's *Lectures on the Science of Human Life*, the volume dealing with the practical aspects of hygiene, gave 610 pages to the discussion of food and drink, and only 50 to the other non-naturals. And not one of those pages (nor any other written by a health re-

[2] *Water Cure J., 30,* 73, (1860).

[3] *American Vegetarian, 1,* 6 (1851).

[4] *Lib. Health, 2,* 241 (1838).

former) had a kind word for meat. Flesh food was ruined by the double-tainting that Christian physiology ascribed to all hygienic evils: it was immoral (the cruelty of the slaughter-house could never be condoned), and it was stimulating (its stimulating quality, in fact, was the reason carnivorous fools gave for eating it). But the health reform's determination to found all its principles on a solid scientific base required a much more extensive physiological refutation than an un-qualified charge of "stimulant." To be legitimized by health reform standards, the most moral diet had to be thoroughly demonstrated to be the most healthful, or the most physio-logical, as well. It was not, predictably, a demonstration dis-tinguished by scientific sophistication or objectivity. Health reformers saw themselves not as active scientists, but as educators interpreting science to the public. Their investi-gations were conducted not in the laboratory, but in the li-brary, where they combed the literature of physiology for experiments and theories relevant to practical hygiene and defined that relevance within the context of Christian physi-ology. This use of science as grist for an ideological mill, by people generally short on formal scientific training, natu-rally stirred the wrath of many physiologists and physi-cians. The result was a series of exchanges aptly character-ized by one participant (of *nom de plume* Emancipated) as "a tempest in a flesh-pot!"[5] As was unintentionally implied, the tempest does not constitute a major chapter in the his-tory of physiology, but its examination does serve to eluci-date further the character of the health reform movement. Nowhere is the determination to have the new science ratify the New Testament clearer than in the early formulation of a physiological rationale for vegetarianism. And the persis-tence, to the present, of a vegetable diet as a central compo-nent of hygienic ideology, as well as the continuing reliance on science to validate vegetarian philosophy, require that the tempest be examined in some detail.

[5] *Graham J. Health Long.*, *1*, 274 (1837).

It would be easy to overstate the impact of Grahamism on vegetarianism, as there is a strong temptation to say that before the 1830s the concern of vegetarians was to save animals, and that afterward it was to save people. There was indeed a reordering of priorities, but it was less abrupt and well-defined than the generalization would suggest. The health reformers inherited (and preserved) quite a mixed set of claims for the desirability of vegetable diet, of which the immorality of the shambles was but the most compelling. From the ancients (from Pythagoras and Porphyry in particular) came the idea that the killing and eating of beasts contaminated and brutalized the human soul. The original direction of vegetarianism had been metaphysical, toward the goal of an exalted state where "the eye of the soul will become free, and will be established as in a port beyond the smoke and the waves of the corporeal nature." This ideal was to be frequently repeated throughout the nineteenth century, though less insistently than its opposite—that animal food arouses animal passions. By Graham's day it was a truism among vegetarians that a flesh diet twisted the personality and made it as ferocious as a tiger's, and history was finely combed for evidence that the most murderous and bloodthirsty races had been meat eaters.[6]

Savagery could be manifested not only by inhumanity to man, but by cruelty toward animals as well. Ancient writers such as Ovid and Plutarch had deplored the killing of innocent creatures, but it was primarily the impulse of that humane sentiment that flowered in late eighteenth-century England that moved this argument to the front. A new genre of vegetarian literature appeared, one whose outlook was capsulized by the title of its first major work, John Oswald's *The Cry of Nature; or, An Appeal to Mercy and to Justice, on Behalf of the Persecuted Animals* (London,

[6] E. Wynne-Tyson, ed., *Porphyry on Abstinence from Animal Food*, London, 1965, p. 53.

1791). Through references to scripture and the classics, and appeals to common sense and conscience, such works strove to prove that meat eating was a crime against nature, both because humanity was never intended for a flesh diet, and because that diet required excrutiating tortures of lower, yet sentient, fellow beings. Naturally, Romantic sentiment gushed through these demonstrations. Oswald's frontispiece portrayed a wounded fawn spilling its blood upon the earth while its hovering mother tearfully called on it to rise. Nearby an unclothed child of nature hid her face in shame. Yet behind the oft-times maudlin paragraphs that followed, there stood a conviction that the repulsiveness of such scenes was proof of man's physical incapacity for flesh food. "But come," Oswald invited,

> approach and examine with attention this dead body. It was late a playful fawn, which, skipping and bounding . . . , awoke, in the soul of the feeling observer, a thousand tender emotions. But the butcher's knife hath laid low the delight of a fond dam, and the darling of nature is now stretched in gore upon the ground. Approach, I say, . . . and tell me, tell me, does this ghastly spectacle whet your appetite? Delights your eyes the sight of blood? Is the steam of gore grateful to your nostrils, or pleasing to the touch, the icy ribs of death? . . . or with a species of rhetoric, pitiful as it is perverse, will you still persist in your endeavour to persuade us, that to murder an innocent animal, is not cruel nor unjust; and that to feed upon a corpse, is neither filthy nor unfit?

Contrast such carnage to the sight of trees "overcharged with fruit; the bending branches seem to supplicate for relief; . . . the ripe apple, the mellow peach invoke thee . . . to save them from falling to the ground." Vegetarians of the health reform period were to suggest more explicitly that the horror of the slaughter and the beauty of the harvest were physiological responses indicating humankind's proper diet (though this humanitarian feeling was absent from Graham's writings, it was common among other health reformers).[7]

As heavy a debt as health reform vegetarianism owed to Romantic humanitarianism, its moral content derived more directly from Christianity, from both the letter and the spirit of holy writ. It seemed inconsistent with the character of God and Christ that animals should suffer that man might live:

> It cannot be that God has so designed,
> That we, by shedding blood, our food should find.

Furthermore, Genesis 1:29 clearly stated that the original diet appointed for man by God did not include flesh. The meaning of this and other dietary passages of the Bible had already been exhaustively debated, and another distinct group of vegetarians had evolved from this religious discussion. The Bible Christian Church, established in the early 1800s by the Manchester minister William Cowherd and brought to America in 1817 by William Metcalfe, held to vegetable diet as its principle tenet. Metcalfe, in addition, is supposed to have influenced Graham to adopt a vegetable diet, though of greater significance is the reciprocal influence Graham, and Alcott, exerted on Metcalfe. Under their tutelage, he came to place nearly as much weight on the physical, as on the spiritual, wickedness of flesh food. In advanced years he even completed a homeopathic medical education to gain expertise in the physiology of diet.[8]

---

[7] John Oswald, *The Cry of Nature,* London, 1791, pp. 22–23, 36–38. Other works in this class include George Nicholson, *On the Primeval Diet of Man . . . on Man's Conduct to Animals,* Poughnill, England, 1801, and Joseph Ritson, *An Essay on Abstinence from Animal Food, as a Moral Duty,* London, 1802. The American Vegetarian Society naturally adopted a resolution to the effect that the repulsiveness of gore was proof of the unphysiological nature of animal food: *American Vegetarian, 1,* 7 (1851).

[8] *American Vegetarian, 2,* 44 (1852); James MacKenzie, *The History of Health and the Art of Preserving It,* Edinburgh, 1759, pp. 44–50 summarizes the debate over Bible dietetics. John Metcalfe, *Memoir of the*

Metcalfe's progress symbolizes the transformation of vegetarianism from a moral to a physical preoccupation, but the process began much earlier. The great outpouring of popular literature on hygiene in the eighteenth and early nineteenth centuries may have concentrated on quantitative considerations, urging control of the amount of food, but there were occasional attempts to draw qualitative distinctions favorable to a vegetable diet. Two figures did particular service in this line. The first, London physician George Cheyne, turned to vegetarianism in the 1720s in order to reduce his thirty-two stone frame. Through subsequent observations on "my own crazy Carcase," as well as on patients, Cheyne was led to recommend a vegetable diet for all, whether overweight or not. Overindulgence in flesh, he came to feel, "*inflames* the *Passions,* and *shortens* Life, begets *chronical* Distempers, and a *decrepid* Age," injuries never inflicted by vegetable food. Meat, he decided by a vague Newtonian analysis, was less digestible and more stimulating than vegetables, and the implication that any quantity could be dangerous was quite clear. Finally, meat was responsible for a discomfort normally blamed on vegetables, which were commonly thought to be so "windy" as to provoke "insupportable *Hurricanes* and Convulsions in the Stomach and *Bowels* of some *Persons.*" In fact, Cheyne maintained, all food contains wind, and flatulence is simply the result of an excess of air freed by faulty digestion, itself due to inflammation of the stomach by too much meat. On a vegetable diet, the inflammation would subside and the chronic flatulence would, as it were, pass. Even before this complete recovery, though, the dieter would find the pains of vegetable wind much milder than those of animal origin, the difference being that "as is between a freezing *Northeast Wind,* and a warm *Western Breeze.*"[9]

Reverend William Metcalfe, M. D., Philadelphia, 1866, pp. 22–25. Also see *Library Health, 4,* 69 (1840), for information on Metcalfe's conversion to physiology.

[9] George Cheyne, *An Essay on Health and Long Life,* London, 1834,

The second major advocate of vegetarianism on physiological grounds was another London physician, William Lambe (Providence showed a Dickensian flair in giving leading vegetarians herbivorous names—Lambe, Metcalfe, Cowherd). In 1806, Lambe cured himself of long-standing illness by removing meat from his diet, then went on to cure others by the same methods. Word of these cures of pimples, consumption, and virtually all ailments in between was widely distributed by his several publications, which asserted that vegetables were best for those in health as well. Repeatedly describing animal food as an "habitual irritation," Lambe blamed it for corpulency, early aging, and decreased intellectual power. That it had never been intended for human consumption was evident from human anatomy, which was herbivorous (man's lack of the carnivore's claws, teeth, and short intestinal tract had already been frequently noted by anatomists, including the master, Cuvier; but the meaning of these differences, it will be seen, could be variously interpreted). His patients had shown animal food was not necessary for maintenance of life, and "we may safely conclude . . . that what is not necessary cannot be natural: it is easy to go one step further; and say, what is not natural cannot be useful." Most physicians balked at taking even the first step (Lambe claimed the contempt shown his ideas by many doctors was "immeasurable"), but reservations about flesh food, mostly about its consumption in excess, did appear in several popular works of hygiene written by doctors.[10]

More visible, however, was the wake stirred up by Lambe

---

pp. xvi, 94; Cheyne, *The Natural Method of Cureing the Diseases of the Body,* London, 1742, pp. 70–71, 218–219. The opinion that vegetable flatulence is more common and painful ultimately triumphed, of course, and is still pointed out in nutrition texts: H. Sinclair and D. Hollingsworth, *Hutchinson's Food and the Principles of Nutrition,* London, 1969, p. 420.

[10] William Lambe, *Additional Reports on the Effects of a Peculiar Regimen,* London, 1815, pp. 90, 127, 131, 147, 172. B. Hill, "Vegetables and Distilled Water. William Lambe, M. D. (1765–1847)," *Practitioner, 194,* 285 (1965).

outside the medical profession. His early writings influenced John Frank Newton to cure his invalidism with vegetable diet, and to then write *The Return to Nature*, an exposition of vegetarianism that combined the humane, Romantic, and religious approaches with physiology. Newton's style was too pedestrian to attract much attention, but it did somehow catch the eye of Shelley, and from his conversion there followed the most impassioned, and comprehensive, presentation of the case for vegetarianism to predate the health reform era. The exuberance of *A Vindication of Natural Diet* (1813) was chiefly for the diet's moral virtues (that the recent bloody excesses of French society were due to that country's consumption of flesh, was but one of Shelley's revelations). Comparative anatomy, chemistry, and medical experience were also called upon for support, however, and the poet concluded with a typically Romantic illustration of the physical benefits of vegetarianism: "Above all, he [the vegetarian] will acquire an easiness of breathing ... with a remarkable exemption from that powerful and difficult panting now felt by almost everyone after hastily climbing an ordinary mountain."[11]

Realistically, the uphill battle had to be fought by vegetarians, for Cheyne, Lambe, even Shelley notwithstanding, the overwhelming force of medical belief was on the side of a flesh diet. It was general opinion among orthodox hygienists that the stimulus of meat was essential for strength and endurance, that animal food was more easily digested than vegetable, and that food already "animalized," hence closer in nature to human flesh, could be more easily assimilated.[12] In the minds of nearly all writers on health, the danger of meat seemed only to be not to assimilate too much of it. Gluttony,

[11] Percy Shelley, *A Vindication of Natural Diet*, London, 1884; reprint of the Vegetarian Society, pp. 16–17, 27.

[12] See, for example, Anthony Willich, *Lectures on Diet and Regimen*, New York, 1801, pp. 209–222; William Lawrence, *Lectures on Physiology, Zoology, and the Natural History of Man*, Salem, Mass., 1828, p. 187; and MacKenzie (n. 8), p. 18.

no matter what the food, seemed the great abuse, and though too much meat was recognized as injurious because of its tendency to produce plethora and internal putrefaction, the total elimination of meat seemed unphilosophical extremism. Dietitians, quite simply, were inclined to join with the wit who jeered,

> "Abstain from flesh!" ... Pythagorean,
> Feed *thou* on *pulse—roast-beef* feed *we* on.[13]

Clearly, however strong a case one might build against flesh eating on metaphysical, religious, or humanitarian grounds, so long as physiology indicated that meat was required for health, vegetarianism could not be conscientiously supported or even seriously considered. And while this burden of proof had been recognized before the 1830s, no vegetarians had shouldered it so eagerly or made it so central an element of strategy as the health reformers were to do. Hitherto, it had been asserted only that it was possible for adequate vitality to be maintained on a meatless diet, and a few liberal physiologists had even agreed. But the logic of health reform required its proponents to demonstrate more than the physiological equality of a vegetable with a mixed diet. God would not compromise in His creation, and if a fleshless regimen was morally best, it must be physically best. Could humankind be healthfully omnivorous? "Indeed, strange that the Creator ... should have so signally failed to adapt the organization of his creatures to the purposes of his *wisdom* as displayed in his word." Could, indeed, a meat eater be Christian? "How," came the reply, "can a man serve God with a stomach full of grease?"[14] The religious need to establish vegetarianism as physiologically superior to a meat diet is what spurred health reformers to their dietetic exaggerations and peculiar readings of

[13] Quoted by William Wadd, *Comments on Corpulency*, London, 1829, p. 142.

[14] William Metcalfe, "Bible Doctrine," *Library Health, 4,* 159 (1840); *Graham J. Health Long., 2,* 317 (1838).

physiology, and what made their disagreements with physiologists a tempest instead of a more reasoned scientific debate.

Rationality was strained further by the seeming refusal of most physiologists to examine vegetarian arguments seriously. The dietetic system, it appeared, was being judged by the eccentricities of its practitioners rather than by its scientific merits. And exasperation was heated to anger by the personal insults common to those judgments: the snide remarks about cadaverousness and emasculation, or the suggestions that vegetarians were embittered ascetics who secretly longed for the good life. "Some men seem to 'seek to merit *heaven,* by making earth a *hell,*'" snickered Oliver Wendell Holmes, "and we can readily conceive how a dyspeptic in his closet, might look a little enviously upon his sleek and oily neighbor, who sleeps well, eats well, and perchance smokes his cigar."[15]

Pythagoreans tried to give as good as they got, pointing out that they appeared emaciated only because flesh eaters were plethoric, "portly gentlemen, with forms that might have shamed Jack Falstaff, and visages which would provoke the envy of a turkey-cock." In one of the impracticable thought experiments of which he was so fond, Graham submitted that "if a very fat man, in the enjoyment of what is ordinarily considered good health, and a lean man in good health" be confined and left to starve, "the lean man will lose in weight much more slowly, and live several days longer than the fat man." The hope of vengeance behind this "experiment" was but thinly veiled; elsewhere the need to retaliate for meat eaters' calumnies found unrestrained expression. A list of the kinds of people who ought to use animal food included not just "those who wish to become corpulent," and "those who wish to have their fluids continually in a half-putrid state," but also "idiots" and "those who wish to become stupid, like idiots."[16] If dietary dogmatism was al-

[15] Oliver Wendell Holmes, *Boston Courier,* Dec. 12, 1840.
[16] *Graham J. Health Long., 1,* 258 (1837); Sylvester Graham, *Lectures on the Science of Human Life,* Boston, 1839, 1: 340; William Alcott, "Eating Animal Food," *Lib. Health, 5,* 120 (1841).

most unavoidable given the rigidity of the health reformers'
guidelines for theorizing, it was made inevitable by their desire for personal vindication.

This combination of physiology and pique was evident
from the opening of hostilities between the two groups of dietitians. In 1835, the Boylston Medical Committee's prize
was awarded to a New Hampshire physician, Luther Bell,
for his essay discussing, "What diet can be selected which
will ensure the greatest probable health and strength to the
laborer in the climate of New England?" At the outset, Bell
admitted he was writing to counter the "schemes of Pythagorean or Utopian dreamers," and at the conclusion proposed that the mixed diet of most New England laborers was
quite healthful, containing "no grand errors" and requiring
"no radical change."[17] In reaching these standard judgments, however, Bell had deviated from the usual justification for a diet including meat. The traditional argument was
that while human teeth and alimentary organs were closer
in structure to those of vegetable eaters than those of flesh
eaters, they were nevertheless identical to neither; man
"preserves a medium between the complicated apparatus of
herbivorous, and the simple apparatus of carnivorous animals, and is, therefore, *omnivorous.*"[18] Bell regarded this as
quibbling on one point while missing a more significant one.
Human anatomy was too close to that of frugivorous animals
to allow classification as intermediate, "but the only conclusion which ought to be drawn from this similarity," he concluded, "is that he is designed to have his food in about the
same state of mechanical cohesion, requiring about the same
energy of masticatory organs as if it consisted of fruits, etc.
alone." Anatomy, in other words, indicated what it was pos-

[17] Luther Bell, "Dr. Bell's Prize Dissertation on Diet," *Boston Med.
Surg. J., 13,* 303 (1836). Bell did suggest that the proportion of animal
food in the New England diet was often too large, and should be reduced,
but he was strongly opposed to elimination of meat.

[18] Francois Magendie, *A Summary of Physiology,* Baltimore, 1824, p.
178.

sible to eat, not what was necessary, and for humankind the
possibilities were almost limitless. The distinction overlooked by vegetarians comparing human anatomy to animal
was that man was more than an animal. He possessed the
faculty of reason, bestowed by God to be used. And by the
application of reason to cookery, many kinds of foods, animal as well as vegetable, could be rendered masticable by
frugivorous teeth. Thus the natural diet of man consisted of
any food that his reason could adapt to his body, and he
must indeed be considered omnivorous.[19]

As high as was their regard for human reason, vegetarianism's protagonists could not accept such a conclusion.
Reason was the gift of God, but so was free will, so reason
could be abused. Underlying reason was a basic set of laws
and instincts of self-preservation that defined humankind's
fundamental nature; and reason, to be natural, must be used
in accord with these laws and instincts. The Romantic vegetarians of the beginning of the nineteenth century had
argued from a similar feeling when maintaining that since
the sight and smell of raw flesh were repulsive to man, they
were not natural for him. The health reformers would only
have added that to make the flesh more appealing through
cookery was to set reason against instinct, to use it unnaturally. A general statement of the health reform understanding of the relation of reason to human nature was offered by Graham in a quick reply to Bell's essay: "We
possess, to some extent, the physiological *capability* of
adapting ourselves to conditions and things to which we
are not *naturally* adapted; and we possess the rational and
voluntary powers of adapting many things to our *use*, which
are not *naturally* fitted for us; nevertheless all departure
from the constitutional laws of our nature, in the exercise
of these *capabilities,* is always, and necessarily, attended
with commensurate injury to our physiological interests."
And there was much evidence in addition to anatomy to

[19] Bell (n. 17), pp. 248–249.

demonstrate that man was *"naturally* a fruit and vegetable eating animal."[20]

The anatomy lesson alone, of course, sufficed for proof, and at the risk of belaboring the point it must be stressed that the anatomical (and other) evidence was never separated from a scriptural context. "What was an orang, a chimpanzee, or a gorilla made for?," Reuben Mussey pondered: "In reply it may be asked, for what more probably than to present to man a standing attestation to the truth and the value of the dietetic lesson given him in Paradise; to demonstrate to him than an animal with an organization like his own in relation to food may subsist exclusively on the eatables granted to himself in Eden, and yet enjoy enduring health and an adequate amount of activity and strength."[21] Imitation of the orang was thus a natural use of reason, one in accord with God-given instinct. An example of an unnatural use would be the phenomenon so frequently pointed to by physiologists as proof of human omnivorousness. Bell cited with approval the common argument that since humanity covered the globe and thrived on a nearly infinite variety of animal and vegetable products, it must have been "designed by infinite wisdom" to subsist on a mixed diet.[22] On the contrary, vegetarians responded, since flesh was never intended for food by infinite wisdom, inhabitants of the Arctic and other barren regions where flesh was the only available food must be there by choice (not divine design), and must have used their reason wrongly. As Alcott moralized, "Man has no right to reside in northern regions till he can carry the climate ... along with him [i.e., carry along the agriculture of

[20] Sylvester Graham, "Remarks on Dr. Bell's Prize Essay," *Boston Med. Surg. J., 13,* 332 (1835–36).

[21] Reuben Mussey, *Health: Its Friends and Foes,* Boston, 1862, p. 175.

[22] Jonathan Pereira, *A Treatise on Food and Diet,* New York, 1847, p. 286. Any number of other references could be listed to demonstrate the wide acceptance of this position.

temperate climes].[23] Ultimately these arguments were but insoluble wranglings over nature versus nurture, though Bell's essay is important for drawing out the contrasting attitudes toward the nature of man which lay behind the dietetic dispute. Bell also raised the intensity of the more strictly physiological debate over vegetarianism, and the *Boston Medical and Surgical Journal* was kept busy for months printing the angry exchanges between Bell, Graham, and their supporters. Even after the *Journal*'s editor tired of the battle and barred further sniping from his pages, the conflict raged on other fronts, with health reformers keeping constant watch for signs of unnatural reasoning by physiologists.

Their own reasoning was done within an up-to-date scheme of atomistic biology that was nevertheless malleable enough to meet moral demands. They were in complete agreement with the orthodox view that nutrition was the result of "all parts of the human body undergo[ing] an internal motion, which has the double effect of expelling the molecules which are no longer needed as components of the organs, and of replacing them by new molecules."[24] Two aspects of this perennial renovation of the body were seen by vegetarians as having fundamental importance for health: the quality of the particles supplied by the food and the rate of molecular turnover. Since meat products decomposed more rapidly than vegetables, and meat chyle was quicker than vegetable chyle to putrefy, it was clear which foods supplied the best particles—vegetables must have "greater purity and a more perfect vitality." Further, as animal systems carried waste molecules from their own tissue renovations—molecules that had "become worn out, effete, dead

[23] William Alcott, "Vegetarianism in Ohio," *American Vegetarian, 2,* 35, (1852). Also see Alcott, "The Arctic Regions," *Lib. Health, 2,* 260 (1838).

[24] Francois Magendie, quoted by Joseph Fruton, *Molecules and Life: Historical Essays on the Interplay of Chemistry and Biology,* New York, 1972, p. 401.

and putrid"—flesh foods actually contained particles of poison.[25]

The resistance of its particles to decay also suggested a second virtue of vegetable food, the slowness of replacement of its atoms. In health reform thought, strict obedience to all the laws of hygiene would be rewarded not just with perfect health at all ages, but by a greatly protracted life span. Antediluvian longevity was assumed to be the norm from which humanity had degenerated, and if it was to be regained, each stage of development of the body (infancy, childhood, etc.) would have to be retarded. Only when the child took a hundred years to become a man could ideal health be claimed, and since maturing was but a process of molecular exchange, the slower this exchange, the healthier and longer-lived the individual. The mechanics of life were simple: "A man may not inaptly be compared with a watch—the *faster it goes the sooner it will run down.*"[26]

This fear of fast living directed the response to one of the longest standing nutritional assumptions of conventional physiology, and the misconception that most frustrated vegetarians. The opinion that meat was required for strength and stamina was a standard item in texts on diet. The Grahamite riposte was to offer countless examples of vigorous vegetable eaters, and even an argument to support the claim of the herbivorous rhinoceros to the title of "king of the jungle." But a more telling strategy was their effort to show that flesh, as unnatural food, actually brought on debility rather than imparting strength. Declarations to this effect were rarely substantiated, but here the reasoning is more significant than the statement. Again one sees the informing of physiology by Christian morality, with flesh eating being condemned in the process. Meat had long been regarded as more "stimulating" than vegetables because of its high spe-

[25] William Alcott, *Vegetable Diet: as Sanctioned by Medical Men and by Experience in all Ages,* Boston, 1838, p. 230; O. May, "Is Meat Poisonous," *Water Cure J., 22,* 102 (1856). Also see Trall (n. 1), p. 10.

[26] *Graham J. Health Long., 1,* 291 (1837).

cific dynamic action (the specific dynamic action of protein
is its effect, during digestion, of stimulating the production
of considerable heat over and above that released by the
basal metabolism). The term "digestive fever" was actually
employed by orthodox dietitians to designate the feeling of
warmth following a meal rich in protein. This stimulating
power of flesh was regarded by physicians as both its contribution and its danger to health: a certain degree of stimulation was required, but, as the authority John Ayrton Paris
warned, "a diet of animal food cannot . . . be exclusively employed. It is too highly stimulant; the springs of life are
urged on too fast; and disease necessarily follows."[27]

But an acceptable amount of stimulation for an ordinary
physiologist could seem unacceptable to a health reform
physiologist, particularly if the stimulant offended moral
sensitivity too. In fact, even though life was impossible
without some degree of stimulation, vegetarians almost
never described the phenomenon except as a pathological
process: "Those effects which are called *stimulant, tonic,* etc.,
are in reality the evidences of the *resistance* which the vital
powers make to the injurious or impure substance, and not,
as is commonly supposed, the action of the article on the system. The *feeling* of *strength* is increased, for the reason that
the energies of the system are roused into unnatural intensity of action to defend the vital machinery; and the reason
that a depression of power is always experienced afterwards,
is because the vital energy has been expended, uselessly
wasted, in the struggle."[28] The excessive stimulation of meat,
furthermore, accelerated the body's molecular transformations and thereby shortened life, or, as Alcott phrased it,
"The system . . . is inevitably worn into a premature dissolu-
tion, by the violent and unnatural heat of an over-stimu-
lated and precipitate circulation."[29]

[27] Graham, *Lectures* (n. 16), 2: 186; John Ayrton Paris, *A Treatise on
Diet,* London, 1837, p. 133.
[28] Russell Trall, footnote in John Smith, *Fruits and Farinacea. The
Proper Food of Man,* New York, 1854, p. 171.
[29] *Lib. Health,* 4, 221 (1840).

In the sentence immediately following, Alcott added that the cool vegetable diet "has a tendency to temper the passions," thus announcing again the oneness of morality and physiology. If immoral behavior was the product of depraved, uncontrollable appetites, then any stimulus to the passions must be removed. Mussey was being somewhat restrained when he advised that "every degree of unnecessary excitation of the organic actions must be regarded as a departure from the highest health, and the increased irritability of the nerves dependent on disease will give rise to peevishness, despondency, and selfishness." The same consideration of "excitation" moved Trall to a more typical charge, that "there is no delusion on earth so widespread as this, which confuses stimulation with nutrition. It is the very parent source of that awful ... multitude of errors, which are leading the nations of the earth into all manner of riotous living, and urging them on in the road to swift destruction. This terrible mistake is the primal cause of all the gluttony, all the drunkenness, all the dissipation, all the debauchery in the world—I had almost said, of all the vice and crime also." The moral need to suppress stimulation made the condemnation of flesh food on physiological grounds imperative—this was the *double entendre* of references to meat as the "brandy of diet."[30]

Unnatural stimulation was also at the basis of the attack on what vegetarians recognized as a second misconception about their diet, the belief that it was less digestible than animal food. The traditional assumption that similarity of composition made the transformation of meat into human flesh relatively easy, still held sway. This common-sense argument had been recently reinforced, furthermore, by the extensive experimentation of William Beaumont, the American army physician who studied gastric digestion *in vivo* on a subject with a permanent gastric fistula (an opening from the abdomen into the stomach) caused by a gunshot wound.

[30] Mussey, *Health* (n. 21), p. 232; Trall, *The Scientific Basis* (n. 1), p. 10; William Metcalfe, "Reasons for Being a Vegetarian," *American Vegetarian, 1,* 74 (1851).

Beaumont's experiments, performed throughout the 1820s, included measurements of the digestion times required by various foods. Food samples tied to a string were introduced into the stomach and retrieved for hourly inspections. Beaumont's conclusion from numerous observations on his unfortunate "patent digester" was that "generally speaking, vegetable aliment requires more time, and probably greater powers of the gastric organs, than animal."[31] Bell had cited this conclusion of Beaumont's in his Boylston essay defending a mixed diet, so the question of digestibility was not one that the Grahamites could ignore. The experiments might be simply dismissed out of hand as inapplicable, since they had been performed on a diseased, rather than normal stomach.[32] But to do that would be to pass up a golden occasion to demonstrate the conflict between flesh and physiology. Thus the very first issue of the *Graham Journal of Health and Longevity* carried the opening installment of a long series of extracts of Beaumont's book, extracts designed to "prepare the reader's mind for the reviewer's notes." In the meantime, the American Physiological Society was corresponding with Beaumont, "to see on what terms St. Martin [Beaumont's subject] would come to Boston and submit to further and perhaps more perfect investigations." The effort to obtain St. Martin came to naught, but the language of the request betrayed the vegetarian attitude toward the work already done by Beaumont. It was by implication imperfect, and when the long promised review by Graham appeared, it explained why Beaumont was not a "truly scientific physiologist."[33]

By Graham's analysis, Beaumont's great failing was to

[31] William Beaumont, *Experiments and Observations on the Gastric Juice, and the Physiology of Digestion,* Plattsburgh, N.Y., 1833, p. 36. This opinion was repeated on pp. 46–47, 144, and 275, and was adopted by other physiologists, e.g., Andrew Combe, *The Physiology of Digestion,* Edinburgh, 1842, pp. 138, 143–144.

[32] *Moral Reformer, 2,* 260 (1836).

[33] *Graham J. Health Long., 1,* 187, 225, 264 (1837).

think that physiology could be reduced to chemistry, and to treat chymification (stomach digestion) as a chemical, rather than a vital process. Graham was a vitalist in the mold of the early nineteenth-century French physician Xavier Bichat; he admitted that the body was composed of the same atoms as inorganic matter, but asserted unique laws governed the arrangement of the atoms. He regarded life as a "forced state" of constant conflict between the vital power and the more primitive affinities of unorganized matter. And he despised the presumption of modern chemists who tried to quantify the variable phenomena of life. If physiology were subject to chemistry, then indeed Beaumont's tables of chymification times could serve as an accurate guide, and the foods "which passed through the stomach in the shortest time, . . . whether it be soused tripe, pig's feet, or whatever else" could be regarded as the most easily digested. But in fact, digestion was accomplished by vital force, which acted against, not through, chemical force. The digestibility of an item, therefore, was to be measured not by the time, but by the energy expended in dissolving it. If experience showed the body to be weakened more by flesh food than by vegetables, then flesh could hardly be considered more digestible, no matter how quickly it passed through the stomach. And what was the "digestive fever" (the greater heat of protein digestion), if not a sign of the abnormal exertion of vital force in the digestion of meat? For that very reason, "they who subsist principally on animal food . . . always feel more stupid and dull during gastric digestion, and feel a much greater degree of exhaustion." Again stimulation was identified as pathological, and in such a way as to turn Beaumont's data against him: "It may [therefore] be regarded as a general law, that those kinds of food, appropriate for man, which naturally pass slowly through the stomach, are digested with the least vital expense and . . . are most conducive to the general welfare of the system." Digestibility, Graham thus suggested (with a curious quantification of vitality) is directly, not inversely, proportional to the time of digestion. Other health reformers followed Graham's lead, and the principle of "slow digestion is good digestion" became an axiom of vegetarianism.[34]

Digestibility dovetailed with nutritiveness in the vegetarian construct, for if vegetables took longer to pass through the digestive tract, it must be because they contained a greater quantity of nutritive matter to be absorbed. This was a congenial conclusion apparently validated by analytical chemistry. Virtually every presentation of vegetarianism during the health reform period included a table, derived "from the works of Percy, Vaquelin [sic; Vauquelin] and other distinguished analytical chimests," which demonstrated many vegetables to be much more concentrated nourishment than meat. Accepting the ancient belief in a single nutritive substance, "aliment," and using analyses of the water content of various uncooked foods, vegetarians were able to suppose that wheat, 15 percent by weight of water, contained 85 "nutritive parts" per 100. Rice was thus 90 percent aliment, lentils 94 percent, sugar 95 percent, and tapioca 98 percent. "Butcher's meat (average)" held an enfeebling 35 nutritive parts per 100, and milk only 20 parts. The prevalent idea that meat was highly nutritious, therefore, was fallacious, an error caused by mistaking stimulation for nutrition. The higher nutritive value of vegetables, moreover, reinforced the demand for moderation at the table; in this sense, vegetable gluttony could be even more injurious than flesh gluttony, and the quantity eaten had to be carefully restricted.[35]

Insistence on the higher nutritional content of vegetables, at first glance an effective tactic, nevertheless led vegetarians into a clumsy situation. It directly conflicted with another cherished belief, that of the innutritiousness of vegeta-

[34] *ibid.*, p. 270. The best presentation of his vitalism is in Graham's *Lectures* (n. 16), 1: 62–83, 291–294, and 2: pp. 110–112. *Graham J. Health Long.*, *1*, 270 (1837); *ibid.*, *3*, 77 (1839).

[35] *American Vegetarian*, *1*, 43 (1851); *Graham J. Health Long.*, *2*, 159 (1838); *ibid.*, *3*, 77 (1839).

ble diet discussed in the preceding chapter. The advantage of Graham flour over white, it will be remembered, was that its nourishment was diluted by nonnourishing (nonstimu-lating) matter. The necessity of the latter was argued on the-oretical grounds by Graham, but he and his dietary compa-triots also took note of experimental work. One of the first questions to activate the fledgling animal chemistry of the early nineteenth century was that of the origin of the large quantities of nitrogen (in protein) in animal tissue. Particu-larly with regard to herbivores, whose foods contained rela-tively small proportions of the element, there was much speculation as to whether the diet could supply all the nitro-gen needed (and what internal processes of "animalization" might transform nonnitrogenous food into flesh), or whether some amount might be absorbed from the atmosphere.[36]

The 1816 experiments of Francois Magendie were in-tended to settle the dispute. Feeding dogs on diets of sugar and water, olive oil and water, and butter and water—all ni-trogen-free rations—he found that the animals invariably sickened and died. Magendie's conclusion that "the nitrogen which is found in the animal economy is in great part ex-tracted from the food" erred only in using the words "in great part," but it was not fully demonstrable at the time. Pure fibrine, albumen, or gelatin—all proteins and high in nitrogen—also failed to maintain life, so that Magendie's work could be given at least a second interpretation. Several reputable physiologists, in fact, argued that the experiments "merely prove that an animal cannot be supported by highly-concentrated aliment." Vegetarians welcomed this interpretation, as it made the bulkiness of vegetable diet more healthful than concentrated animal food, and for the most part they ignored the question raised by their concur-rent use of analytical tables showing vegetable foods to be

[36] Frederic Holmes, "Elementary Analysis and the Origins of Physio-logical Chemistry," *Isis, 54,* 61–63, 71–72 (1963), places this problem within the context of the growth of analytical organic chemistry. Also see Fruton (n. 24), pp. 398–399.

more than twice as nourishing as meat. When they did address it, the conflict was easily resolved by maintaining that highly nutritious foods like bread must be tempered by low nutrition foods (potatoes, beets, turnips).[37] But the usual presentation of these ideas as separate from one another— the claim in one article that the virtue of vegetables is in their concentrated nutrition, and in another article that it resides in their dilute nutrition—suggests an attempt to get the most out of diverse chemical and physiological data with the hope that neophytes would not detect the contradiction.

The deceit soon became unnecessary, however, for the remarkable sophistication that animal chemistry acquired in the 1840s made the tables of nutritive parts per hundred obsolete, and also presented new challenges to vegetarians. Associated with the opinion that Magendie had shown nothing more than that concentrated food is inadequate, was the belief that at least some of the nitrogen of the body derived from the atmosphere. The careful experiments performed by Jean-Baptiste Boussingault in the late 1830s and early 1840s, however, refuted this theory and demonstrated all tissue nitrogen, even in herbivorous animals, is obtained from food. The subsequent demand by physiologists that a nourishing diet must contain considerable amounts of nitrogenized foods was intensified by the pronouncement of Justus von Liebig, the most respected authority on animal chemistry, that muscular motion can be produced only by the oxidation of protein.[38] Health reformers thus felt constrained to prove that their relatively low protein diet did in fact supply sufficient nitrogen. Actually there remains good

[37] Francois Magendie, "Memoire sur les proprietes nutritives des substances qui ne contiennent pas d'azote," *Ann. chim. phys.*, *3*, 75 (1816). Paris (n. 27), p. 180, and Beaumont (n. 31), p. 39, were among those who differed with Magendie's interpretation. *Moral Reformer*, *1*, 278 (1835); *ibid.*, *2*, 219 (1836).

[38] Richard Aulie, "Boussingault and the Nitrogen Cycle," *Am. Phil. Soc., Proc.*, *114*, 435–479 (1970); Justus von Liebig, *Animal Chemistry*, Cambridge, Mass., 1842, p. 233.

reason to question whether Grahamites did consume adequate protein. Ignorant of essential amino acids and the mixed vegetable diet necessary to obtain these, and intent on eating sparingly of only one or two dishes per meal, the conscientious health reform vegetarian (if he eschewed milk, as many did) would have been hard put to achieve a proper protein intake.[39] At the time, however, the objection evoked only amused disbelief. "The purely herbivorous animals derive their growth and strength from vegetable food. . . . *their* systems are supplied with azote (nitrogen) without eating animal food; why may not man's system be supplied in the same way?" But if the fact of healthy animal life on a vegetable diet was undeniable, the explanation was less than certain. Several approaches to explaining it were tried, the most direct being to deny the pertinence of the chemical data. Alcott toyed with this, submitting that the argument that since body tissues contain nitrogen, they must be supplied with food containing much nitrogen was akin to the syllogism: "Lime enters into the composition of the bones; mortar contains lime, therefore we must eat mortar." The mystery of how low nitrogen foods could form high nitrogen tissues, however, invited a more frank vitalism, and Graham was the one to dispute most loudly the legitimacy of animal chemistry. In response to Magendie's demand for nitrogen in the diet, Graham offered simply, "It is not in the power of chemistry in the least possible degree, to ascertain what substances the alimentary organs of the living animal body require for the nourishment of the body, nor from what chemical elements the organic elements are formed."[40]

As had occurred among orthodox physiologists, though, the majority of health reformers were turning away from such attempts to shield the science of life entirely from

[39] Some idea of recommended vegetarian meals may be obtained from *Moral Reformer*, 2, 316–317 (1836), and *Lib. Health*, 5, 297–312 (1841).

[40] William Alcott, "Is Animal Food Necessary Because of the Azote it Contains?," *Lib. Health.*, 2, 175–176 (1838); Graham, *Lectures* (n. 16), 1: 542–543.

chemistry. If nitrogen were present in the body, it must have been digested. Those who doubted the ability of vegetables to supply all the required nitrogen continued to argue for absorption of the element from the atmosphere, but from the early 1840s forward, vegetarians preferred to support the position that all body nitrogen was extracted from food, and extracted most efficiently and beneficially from vegetable food. Their inspiration for this point might seem an unlikely one, for Justus von Liebig eventually marketed an extract of beef as a health food. But in his epochmaking *Animal Chemistry* of 1842, Liebig presented information that struck vegetarians as precisely the chemical evidence they needed. The nitrogenized constituents of the food of herbivorous animals—vegetable fibrine, albumen, and caseine—were, he pointed out, "identical in composition with the chief constituents of blood, animal fibrine, and albumen" (the chemical composition and structure of proteins is not nearly so simple, but the crudeness of analytical technique at the time allowed such a generalization). The proteins required by the animal body existed ready made in plants, he continued, and had only to be absorbed. Even carnivores obtained their protein ultimately from vegetable sources, and one might even see "the animal organism [as] a higher kind of vegetable." But when considered as food, the animal was not a better kind of vegetable. If plant protein was already adequate, what purpose was served by subjecting it to a contaminating, and expensive, passage through the animal body? "Do we not take materials fresh from nature when we wish to build a substantial, beautiful and durable mansion, instead of taking down some other edifice to build from its rubbish? So also in vital architecture, let us build up our earthly tabernacles by materials taken freshly from nature, and then we shall find ourselves possessed of sound and durable bodies."[41]

[41] Smith, *Fruits* (n. 28), pp. 136–137; Liebig, *Animal Chemistry* (n. 38), pp. 47–48; *American Vegetarian, 1,* 23 (1851).

Vegetarians found ways to turn other Liebig theories to their advantage as well. He attempted to simplify metabolism, for example, by assigning the basic foodstuffs to two categories: plastic and respiratory, or blood-forming (proteins) and heat-forming (fats and carbohydrates). Maintenance of tissue structure and temperature accordingly demanded a diet composed of the right proportions of each type of food. It was hardly a challenge to health reform ingenuity to fashion arguments that celebrated the superior balance of plastic and respiratory components in vegetable foods; details need not be given.[42]

Thrilling though such flights of theory were, the most impressive aspect of the vegetarian campaign was its solid, down-to-earth demonstration by cases. The proof of the theory was in the state of health of those who practiced it, and history could offer robust vegetarians aplenty in evidence. The first to be recognized, predictably, were the antediluvians, those original men whose simple diet kept them vigorous and kindly all the way to the end of their nine hundred years. "Can we suppose that the delicate hands of Eve took the quivering flesh of the young fawn, and prepared it for the coals, . . . then sat down and chewed it as a sweet morsel between her teeth? Can we suppose she talked of nausea, of headaches, of a palpitating heart, or agitated nerves?"[43]

Other scriptural figures of extraordinary beauty, courage, and vitality were used (Daniel, 1:8–16 was a favorite passage), but pagans could serve Christian physiology as well. Surprisingly, it was pagan soldiers who were held up as paragons of hygiene, especially those of the Roman army, who had marched to their greatest victories on plain vegetable rations. The incongruity of the diet of gentleness and benevolence providing the strength for battlefield slaughter was missed by the health reformers in their excitement over the physical glory of the vegetarians of antiquity. Subsis-

---

[42] William Alcott, "Is There Carbon in Flesh-meat?," *American Vegetarian, 1,* 214 (1851).

[43] *Lib. Health, 1,* 212 (1837).

tence on vegetable food, according to an agitated Graham, was "true of all those ancient armies whose success depended more on bodily strength and personal prowess, in wielding warclubs and in grappling man with man in the fierce exercise of muscular power, and dashing each other furiously to the earth, mangled and crushed and killed."[44] More recent, less brutal examples were more convincing and appropriate. Alcott allotted nearly two hundred pages of a book on *Vegetable Diet* to the presentation of testimonials he had actively solicited, and received by the score. They included some accounts of prodigious vitality. The amazing Amos Townsend, for example, was a graminivorous bank cashier who could "dictate a letter, count money, and hold conversation with an individual, all at the same time, with no embarrassment." Not surprisingly, vegetarians' zeal for collecting such evidence of the physical advantages of their diet made them incredibly gullible at times. In 1850 the *American Vegetarian* published a history, which even its editors considered remarkable, of a man who starved away his dyspepsia on a diet of three Graham crackers and a gill of water a day. After steadily losing weight for two months, he claimed to have begun to gain, adding as much as half a pound a day, "or nearly three times as much as the whole weight of my food; . . . though I never in my life, came to the table with a better appetite, I was never better satisfied with my meals, when they were finished."[45]

Even dismissing this hoax, it is valid to say that testimonial evaluation was so uncritical as to make anecdotes admissible as proof. But when their opponents showed the same laxity, vegetarians pounced on the blunder. Did consumptives sent to the Rocky Mountains recover on an all flesh diet? That was because the patients "were also compelled to be almost continually in the open air, enduring healthful and invigorating exercise . . . had they added to

[44] Graham, *Lectures* (n. 16), 2: 188.
[45] Alcott, *Vegetable Diet* (n. 25), pp. 75–76; *American Vegetarian, 1,* 154 (1851).

these a pure and well-regulated vegetable diet their recovery would have been rendered more certain and complete." The first point, at least, was fairly taken, but what of the many cases of flesh eaters who also indulged in spirits, or tobacco, or opium, or all of these, and still lived to advanced years? "If here and there one of them lasts till old age, it is by virtue of an iron constitution." The prejudice of health reformers is perhaps never clearer than in such statements, and in their corollaries, the apologies for vegetarians who died young. To note merely the most prominent example, the announcement of the death of Graham in 1851, at the relatively early age of fifty-six, was prefaced with the assurance that "there is nothing, when we take into view his whole history, his peculiar constitution and habits which militates against . . . the superior healthfulness of a well-selected vegetable diet." Graham had inherited a weak frame, and had occasionally strayed from his own teachings; he had even turned to meat and whiskey in his last days in a frantic effort to stimulate his vital forces.[46] The "weak frame" excuse could be made for any vegetarian who expired too soon. The health reformers could thus have their cake and eat it too, and did so with hypocritical intemperance. There was no limit to the number of times vegetables were absolved of blame by a frail constitution, and flesh forbidden credit by an iron one.

An identical style marked the analysis through cultural comparisons. One of the pillars of the physiological argument against meat eating was the contrast between the vigorous vegetarian races of the world and the puny flesh eaters. Time and again, the Eskimo and Laplander were humiliated by being lined up against the natives of the South Seas and of central Africa, the peasantry of Ireland, Spain, and Russia, even the slaves of the American South, whose "bodily powers are well-known." Were there some races living primarily on flesh who nevertheless displayed vigor?

[46] *Graham J. Health Long.*, *2*, 56 (1838); *Lib. Health*, *1*, 342 (1837); *American Vegetarian*, *1*, 187 (1851); Stephen Nissenbaum, *Sex, Diet, and Debility in Jacksonian America. Sylvester Graham and Health Reform*, Westport, Conn., 1980, p. 15.

Certainly, but the American Indians were highly susceptible to smallpox and measles, and the Tartars were vicious
people whose very "forms and features have become coarse,
brutal and revolting." And were there no vegetarian cul-
tures in which poor health prevailed? Unfortunately, yes,
but their condition could be explained. The apology made
for the Hindus, frequent butts of flesh eaters' ridicule, could
serve for all degraded vegetarian societies. The inhabitants
of India were admittedly "feeble, effeminate, indolent, and
stupid," but their physical depravity was not due to the absence of meat from their diet, but rather to the inclusion of
irritating spices, the use of opium and alcohol, the licentiousness that drove them into marriage as early as age ten,
and their barbaric socioreligious systems.[47] Freed from
these, the Hindus could gradually become as fine a race
physically as any in the world. The compulsion to manufacture such defenses is an index of the transition in vegetarian
emphasis from morality to physiology. Oswald's *The Cry of
Nature*, an example of the older humane appeal, both began
and ended with a reverent presentation of the philosophy of
"the merciful Hindoo." His physical condition had not been
considered pertinent.[48]

There is no purpose in continuing down the list of vegetarian stalwarts—not only is it interminable, but the moral
never changes. From Asian ricksha men to the Graham-
boarding inmates of the Albany Orphan Asylum, the planet
was teeming with meat-hating models of health, "and if the
civilized world will not learn wisdom from it, then is the
perverseness of the human heart exceedingly incorrige-
able."[49] Incorrigible it was, but health reformers could still

---

[47] Alcott, *Vegetable Diet* (n. 25), p. 265; Larkin Coles, *Philosophy of
Health*, Boston, 1857, pp. 69–70; Graham, *Lectures* (n. 16), 2; p. 194.

[48] Oswald, *The Cry of Nature* (n. 7), pp. 1–10, 78–82.

[49] *Graham J. Health Long.*, 2, 261–262 (1838). For a full account of the
health of the children of the Albany Orphan Asylum, a subject that
roused considerable debate in the late 1830s, see *Moral Reformer*, 2,
344–340 (1836).

take solace in the knowledge that their duty had been done.
Whether or not the world cared to listen yet, they had uncovered the scientific basis of the only Christian diet, and made
enlightenment available for future ages:

Nature's Dietetic Laws lay hid in the Night,
Let Vegetarians be to give us light.
Or in other words,
Mankind in the dark ages were mostly Carnivorous,
But now the light shines, let us all be Frugivorous.[50]

[50] *American Vegetarian, 4,* 131 (1854).

CHAPTER FOUR
PHYSICAL EDUCATION

IT MIGHT EASILY HAVE BEEN A HEALTH REFORM APHORISM that he who is frugivorous will never be lascivious. That meat excited libido was a truism, and only compounded the flesh diet's murderousness, since sexual appetite was presumed to be as dangerous to the body as the soul. Indeed, so violent seemed the agitation of the nervous system during venereal excitement, even moral, marital sex was suspect. Fortunately, physical intercourse was the divinely appointed means for propagating the race, or health reformers would have outlawed figurative flesh as completely as they did the literal kind. As it happened, only the tiniest portion of venery could be allowed by those who appreciated what Nissenbaum has called "the pathology of desire." His fascinating exposition of Graham's doctrine of "careful love" explores that pathology in much more depth than will be attempted here. What Nissenbaum demonstrates is that Graham did essentially the same thing for virginity that he did for vegetarianism; he revealed that an ideal previously exalted by moral-religious assertions was actually rooted in the physical nature of man.[1]

The danger of sexual stimulation had been recognized by Graham and made a part of his lectures by 1833. The following year his conclusions were given wider circulation by the publication of his *Lecture to Young Men on Chastity*, a work which enjoyed brisk sales and several editions. No doubt many young men, as well as parents and guardians to whom the book was also directed, were taken aback by the content,

---

[1] Stephen Nissenbaum, *Sex, Diet, and Debility in Jacksonian America. Sylvester Graham and Health Reform*, Westport, Conn., 1980, pp. 105–121.

for it not only substituted a physiological for the time-honored moral approach to the issue, it also concentrated on new abuses. Chastity literature had previously been occupied with adultery and fornication, and, to a much lesser degree, masturbation. Graham was hardly ready to ignore the former sins, but he demoted those "social vices" to a position well below the "solitary vice," and added to them a vice that had hitherto been a virtue—marital sex. It was standard in pre-Grahamite days to actually prescribe marriage as the cure for masturbatory and libertine tendencies, and even to hint that liberal doses of marital pleasure would do no harm to soul or body.

But earlier writers had not been aware of the physiological turmoil caused by sexual excitement. "The convulsive paroxysms attending venereal indulgence," an aroused Graham warned,

are connected with the most intense excitement, and cause the most powerful agitation to the whole system that it is ever subject to. The brain, stomach, heart, lungs, liver, skin, and the other organs, feel it sweeping over them with the tremendous violence of a tornado. The powerfully excited and convulsed heart drives the blood, in fearful congestion, to the principal viscera—producing depression, irritation, debility, rupture, inflammation, and sometimes disorganization: and this violent paroxysm is generally succeeded by great exhaustion, relaxation, lassitude, and even prostration.[2]

Because those nervous paroxysms preceded the sexual climax, orgasm did not have to occur for injury to result (contemporary opinion held that debility was caused by the loss of the vital semen, one ounce of which was equivalent to forty ounces of blood according to a popular rule of thumb; health reform ideology blamed instead the nervous turbulence causing the expulsion of the semen). For that matter,

[2] I used a later edition of Graham's book, *Chastity, in a Course of Lectures to Young Men*, New York, 1857, p. 5.

physical contact was not even required, for excitation was the product of mere desire. Lusting in the heart could be physiologically equated with lusting in the flesh, though since the fleshly variety was more stimulating, there was more to be feared from real contact. A certain amount of contact, completed by orgasm, was necessary for procreation, but that physiological stimulation would become pathological, in Graham's view, if enjoyed more than once a month. And that licentious frequency was permissible only for the young and robust; older and more delicate lovers would have to get by on less if they wished to maintain physiological integrity.

The appalling catalogue of ills that Graham listed as nature's punishment for those who transgressed these bounds—who practiced "marital excess"—ran from languor to apoplexy, and of course included "disorders of the genital organs." His Victorian mind defined "disorder" in extraordinary terms, though. Earlier authorities on sexual hygiene had assumed that genuine excess, as well as masturbation, should decrease sexual power, bringing on impotency, frigidity, sterility, or the weakness of *ejaculatio praecox*. Graham, however, troubled in spirit and mind by the awesome power of stimulation, saw an increased sexual strength as the likely consequence of excess. He warned in fact, of a diseased state in which the genital organs would be "far more susceptible of excitement."[3]

The moralistic backdrop showing through here is even more noticeable in his discussion of the other categories of sexual abuse—pre- and extra-marital sex and masturbation. Anyone could see that marital excess, social vice, and the solitary vice were morally ranked in that order, but it took a Graham to demonstrate an identical physiological ranking: the more immoral an indulgence, the more injurious it must be. The correlation escapes detection at first glance, for it would seem an orgasm is an orgasm, whether experienced

[3] *ibid.*, pp. 14–15, 20.

with a spouse, a paramour, a prostitute, or alone. But when examined through the Broussais-Graham lens that makes nervous stimulation a cause of degenerative inflammation, the different grades of injury can be differentiated clearly. Illicit sex is more exciting by virtue of being forbidden; as the rendezvous requires planning, it entails an erotic antici-pation that inflames the brain (and hence the nerves) even before the meeting takes place; and once the liaison is con-summated, the partner's unfamiliar body generates a ner-vous frenzy never experienced in the bed of one's spouse. There is logic no critic past puberty can refute, given the va-lidity of the stimulation-breeds-disease premise. And there is equally unassailable reasoning behind the condemnation of the morally disgusting habit of masturbation as even more injurious than libertinism. Self-pollution can be started ear-lier in life; as a secret vice requiring no second's cooperation, it can be practiced with greater frequency; and as a solitary vice involving no stimulating partner, it requires a vi-gorously lewd imagination. Masturbatory fantasy, Graham feared, inflamed the brain more than "natural" arousal, and was the reason why insanity was so often the end of de-praved young men. He was not the sole source of the mas-turbation phobia that possessed the medical profession to the end of the century and made masturbatory idiocy an ac-ceptable diagnosis, but the rationale outlined in his *Lecture on Chastity* clearly affected medical thinking. Many physi-cians honored his formula for sexual frequency, and other ideas on sexual hygiene. They were as vulnerable as the public to the emotional force of Graham's preface statement that his work "proved . . . that the Bible doctrine of marriage and sexual continence and purity, is founded on the physio-logical principles established in the constitutional nature of man."[4]

[4] *ibid.,* pp. v, 12–13, 60–20, 25–26. Similar concern for masturbation had been approached occasionally in earlier hygiene guides—e.g., An-thony Willich, *Lectures on Diet and Regimen,* New York, 1801, p. 374. For analyses of nineteenth-century physicians' fear of masturbation, see

Graham's was not the only health reform voice raised against the physiological iniquity of improper sex. Alcott's *Young Man's Guide*, which preceded the *Lecture on Chastity* by a year, ended with a solitary vice chapter, though it was so delicate and diffuse in its language that only a devoted habitué could have understood what was being condemned. The words of warning were more explicit: *"Beware,"* Alcott admonished young men already embarked on "an unhappy course of solitary vice," for he saw them threatened "by the severest penalties earth or heaven can impose" (at least two readers are known to have stopped their pernicious habits on the *Guide*'s urging).[5]

Alcott incorporated this, and other facets of sexual hygiene, into his lectures and articles, and continued to make observations and inquiries that allowed him to expand his teaching, until after two decades he felt ready to publish one of the more comprehensive sex guides of the nineteenth century. *The Physiology of Marriage* (1855), sent forth initially under anonymous authorship, covered far more ground (from courtship through lactation) than Graham's *Lecture*, and did it with the common sense and humanity that always distinguished Alcott from Graham. That is not to say dire punishments were no longer meted out to sexual transgressors—"most dreadful idiocy" was still the sentence for masturbation—but Alcott recognized men, and women, had natural sexual appetites which should be enjoyed. Graham's recognition of that had been grudging, and he usually described orgasm with the imagery of suffering—"tension,"

E. H. Hare, "Masturbatory insanity: the history of an idea," *J. Mental Sci., 108,* 2–25 (1962); R. MacDonald, "The frightful consequences of onanism: notes on the history of a delusion," *J. Hist. Ideas, 28,* 423–432 (1967); H. Tristram Englehardt, Jr., "The disease of masturbation: values and the concept of disease," *Bull. Hist. Med., 48,* 234–248 (1974); and A. N. Gilbert, "Doctor, Patient and Onanist Diseases in the 19th Century," *J. Hist. Med., 30,* 217–234 (1975).

[5] William Alcott, *The Young Man's Guide,* Boston, 1835, p. 345; *Moral Reformer, 1,* 130 (1835).

"convulsion," "paroxsym," "the tremendous violence of a tornado." Alcott, on the other hand, while agreeing that once-monthly intercourse was the physiologically correct schedule, justified the recommendation with the assurance that "the pleasures of love, no less than the strength of the orgasm, are enhanced by their infrequency." That was a frustrating calculus of pleasure, perhaps, but it did evidence a respect for human sexuality alien to Graham. That respect was shown again in Alcott's identification of impotence, rather than heightened virility, as the sexual penalty for masturbation.[6]

Alcott's work improved upon Graham's in other ways. It was less technical, abandoning the *Lecture*'s discourse on spinal marrow, ganglions, and plexuses in favor of generalizations about *"wear* and *tear* of the vital powers," and "great agitation of the nervous system." It dropped Graham's contrived rationale for the greater injuriousness of solitary vice and replaced it with the simple reminder that any abuse, including tobacco and whiskey as well as sex, is likely to be more damaging *"when begun before maturity."* Graham had only hinted that young girls might be guilty of self-pollution, and had hoped that only European ones were: "For ever may the females of our blessed country remain pure." Alcott knew that women possessed sexual urges, that they practiced masturbation often, and feared that with their "finer wrought, more susceptible" constitutions they would suffer even greater injury than males.[7]

The most significant advance made by *The Physiology of Marriage*, though, was its integration of heredity with sexual hygiene. Prehealth reform authors, it has been seen, suggested the transmissability of the parents' general state of health to their offspring. The inheritance of acquired characteristics was, in fact, virtually unchallenged among physi-

[6] William Alcott, *The Physiology of Marriage*, Boston, 1866, pp. 77–78, 119.
[7] *ibid.*, pp. 52, 73, 86; Graham, *Chastity* (n. 2), p. vii.

cians throughout the nineteenth century, and was commonly supposed to apply to the physical and emotional condition of parents at the exact time of the child's conception. Alcott was thus well within conventional wisdom in taking six pages to build up his recommendation that mates engage in sexual intercourse early in the day, while still fresh and fully invigorated. The fundamental error of child propagation, he insisted, was the saving of sex for the evening, when the body's vital energies were at ebb tide.[8]

While that may seem an absurdly precise application of the theory, the broader interpretation that the general state of health during the period of conception was hereditary, was potentially a very valuable tool for promoting health reform. It not only made possible a gradual perfecting of the human race, it allowed the compelling argument that to live healthfully was not just an individual choice, but a solemn responsibility to one's children and their children. It offered parents reassurance they could have some control of their offspring and endow them with the strength to succeed in a changing, unstable world. Graham, however, gave heredity only passing attention in his *Lecture*, noting that the children of feeble parents would themselves be feeble, and leaving readers to imagine the implications. Alcott, on the other hand, devoted an entire chapter of his *Physiology* to the importance of hygiene for posterity, maintaining with passion that while a person's destruction of his own health might be merely foolish, the mortgaging of his innocent child's life is criminal:

> Is it not true that every young person who abuses his own system ... robs his child of a measure of that vitality which God ... designed for him? Fortunate, indeed, is he, if his transgressions do not prove the means of the abso-

---

[8] Alcott, *Physiology* (n. 6), pp. 131–136. See Charles Rosenberg, "The Bitter Fruit: Heredity, Disease and Social Thought in Nineteenth-Century America," *Perspect. Amer. Hist., 8,* 189–235 (1974), for a thorough discussion of the influence of the idea of the inheritance of acquired characteristics on hereditarian thought.

lute destruction of his child! ... We think, sometimes, and speak of Eve—and her mighty work of declension. We speak of her fallen posterity.... Now, every young head of a family ... may one day have been the progenitor of more millions than Eve yet has. And is not this a solemn thought? ... Whose heart does not beat high at the bare possibility of becoming the progenitor of a world, as it were, of pure, holy, healthy, and greatly elevated beings—a race worthy of emerging from the fall—and of enstamping on it a species of immortality?[9]

If Alcott here sounds like Graham, he also exhibited a decidedly pragmatic side that might be even more appealing to his materialistic countrymen. As noted earlier, he knew that the man who was unmoved by moral obligation might be deeply touched by pecuniary considerations. And at times he could be positively crass in bringing those considerations up. He thus reminded male readers that they would not want to spend "days and nights, perhaps in harvest time," nursing sick children, nor to waste their earnings on physicians and, "perchance, ... coffins, and grave-diggers." Reinforcing his point some pages later, he asked the reader to "suppose you have in your family a drivelling idiot. To support him by your hard earnings might be borne.... But to bear with his weakness and folly; to be subjected day after day, and year after year, to all the physical, intellectual, moral, and social trials to which his condition must inevitably subject you ... how could your heart endure it?"[10] Alcott's own heart was less given to this economic argument than to the moral one, but both gave the injunction to be healthy for the sake of posterity a standing within hygienic ideology which it would hold into the twentieth century.

If sex was the immediate means of passing poor health to the next generation, it was only one of the abuses that caused debility in the present generation. Alcott's, and other

[9] Alcott, *Physiology* (n. 6), pp. 95–96; Graham, *Chastity* (n. 2), p. 12.
[10] Alcott, *Physiology* (n. 6), pp. 90, 141.

reformers', advice on how to become healthier, for self, children, race, and God, entailed much more than sexual restraint, vegetarianism, and teetotalism. That toxic nerve stimulant tobacco was next on most lists, and was made to appear so reprehensible that just one of Graham's lectures was reported to have inspired more than a dozen men to "eschew . . . the vile weed." Condiments, spices, confectionary, coffee, tea, and all medicines were equally condemned as stimulating. The body's need to continually renew and purify itself was strenuously affirmed by recommendations for fresh air (to maintain a full supply of oxygen); regular exercise (moderate recreations such as walking, sailing, fencing, calisthenics, and gardening accelerated respiration and circulation, and assisted the elimination of impurities); and daily cold bathing (keeping the skin soft, pliable, and clean improved capillary circulation and insured free, purifying perspiration). Crude biochemical justifications were provided for all these practices, but supplemental moral arguments were never far away. Bathing, for instance, was advised as an act of Christian kindness—a person who loved his neighbor as himself would not subject the neighbor to his body odor reminiscent of "garlic [or] woodchuck." The remaining standard non-natural advice on sleep and rest, the passions, and so forth, was updated by commentary on a thousand modern incidentals, from feather beds and night caps to nostrums and novels, and even the breath of cats and dogs.[11]

Finally, there was the matter of female health, a subject that assumed a special place in health reform ideology. Women had distinctive problems—they might not chew tobacco or swill rum, but they were guilty of enough other sins to make them a godsend to an overpopulated medical profession. "Were it not for the diseases produced by the practices and customs of fashion," a New York doctor calculated,

[11] *Moral Reformer,* 1, 21, (1835); *ibid., 2,* 162 (1836); *Lib. Health, 3,* 200–228, 232–255, 265–287 (1839); *Teacher of Health, 1,* 156–158 (1843).

"the great proportion of medical men would have nothing to live on and perhaps nothing to do. A nervous and irritable lady ... may be worth from one to five hundred dollars a year."[12] Semi-invalids of such value naturally enjoyed an international reputation for debility. A British physician struck by the weakness of American womanhood dismissed the customary excuse that the extreme climate was to blame, and submitted instead that improper habits were at fault: "They rarely walk abroad for the sake of fresh air and exercise. In general, they live and sleep in ill-aired apartments. Their duties press constantly on their minds, and they do not give sufficient effect to the maxim, that cheerful amusement and variety of occupation are greatly conducive to health. They do not properly regulate their diet; pies, pastry and animal food are consumed in quantities too abundant for a sedentary life, and baths and ablutions are too rarely used.[13]

But this depressingly familiar catalogue of neglect left out the specifically female form of abuse that health reformers—and orthodox physicians as well—believed to be far the greatest threat to women's health. The sway of fashion over female behavior was an ancient subject for jest:

> False rumps, false teeth, false hair, false faces,
> Alas! poor men! how hard thy case is;
> Instead of WOMAN—heavenly woman's charms,
> To clasp cork, gum, wool, whalebone in his arms.[14]

But the whalebone, particularly, was not really a laughing matter. The literature of hygiene for decades past had bemoaned the determination of fashion-conscious ladies to restyle their figures into hourglasses by wearing tightly laced, whalebone-braced corsets. Doctors had warned that ailments of the lungs, stomach, and reproductive organs,

[12] Edward Dixon, *Scenes in the Practice of a New York Surgeon*, New York, 1855, p. 64.
[13] Quoted in *Lib. Health*, 6, 186 (1842).
[14] Quoted in *Graham J. Health Long.*, 3, 387 (1839).

and even breast cancer, could be induced by the continued pressure of the rigid stays used to squeeze the waistline toward the ideal nineteen-inch circumference. Health reformers, though, were still more pessimistic. Alcott devised a fable about the extinction of the human race due to persistent bad hygiene, which featured the corset as chief villain. After the race had existed for about fifty-seven hundred years (he accepted the Biblical calculation of the date of creation), "it so happened that . . . the females . . . undertook to *improve* their structure." Within a century, the corset habit had become universal, and had incited an epidemic of labored breathing, pale complexion, bad digestion, consumption, as well as nervousness, feeble minds, and "cold affections towards their fellows, and their Creator." The decline continued through generations, until

> by the year 6200, the last of this beautiful and originally noble race of men—a solitary idiot—sank down with age and its decrepitude at thirty, and rose no more. The other races of men continued a little longer. The latest race to expire was the noble, but unfortunate Africans. . . . At last, the only remaining individual of their number, . . . a feeble individual, not more than three feet in height, and differing from a wasp only in size, having breathed out her uncomfortable spirit on this spot—became a prey to a few wretched, famished dogs and vultures; for there were none to bury her.[15]

The basis for such extraordinary fear of the corset was partly revealed in the section of the tale relating that during the second century of corset wearing, "not only the one sex, but the other began to be slender and wasp-shaped." The acquired characteristic of the wasp waist, in other words, was

---

[15] Shadrach Ricketson, *Means of Preserving Health and Preventing Diseases,* New York, 1806, p. 81; *J. Health, 1,* 369 (1829–30). For the history of the corset, see James Laver, *The Concise History of Costume and Fashion,* New York, 1969, and Carrie Hall, *From Hoopskirts to Nudity,* Caldwell, Idaho, 1938. *Moral Reformer, 1,* 53–59 (1835).

being passed by heredity, so that noncorseted men suffered as much as women. It was, predictably, the reproductive capacity of woman that made her an object of special interest to health reformers. Both parents influenced heredity, to be sure, but women seemed likely to exert a more profound effect. They carried the child for months within their generative organs, and if those organs had been damaged by imprudent habits, a fetus with an excellent endowment from its father could be warped and ruined. Since the corset put so much pressure on the lower viscera, and undoubtedly did contribute to the blight of *prolapsus uteri* that many doctors believed was ravaging the land, it was inevitably singled out as the major insult to female reproductive health. Much of the obloquy was deserved, but the fear of inherited debility allowed the menace of the corset to be exaggerated. Women's health writer Catherine Beecher, by no means a hygienic extremist, somehow discovered that tight lacing "has operated so, from parent to child, that a large portion of the female children now born have a deformed thorax, that has room only for imperfectly formed lungs."[16]

The vitality of women was a dominant issue for health reformers for a second reason. The Victorian ideal of womanhood included a belief in the moral and spiritual genius of the female that fitted her to train children in purity and uprightness, manage the home, excel in works of charity, and ultimately point the way to a better, more Christian society. The constitution of the American Physiological Society recognized this talent, making special provision for the admission of women to membership because, "to no individuals, after all, is this subject [physiology] of more immediate importance than to mothers and housewives. In the education of a household, it is indispensable; and cannot be useless in the preparation of our food, especially bread." The point was explained more fully in yet another of the society's resolu-

[16] *Moral Reformer, 1,* 59 (1835). Catherine Beecher, *Letters to the People on Health and Happiness,* New York, 1855, pp. 93–94.

tions: *"Resolved,* that woman in her character as wife and mother is only second to the Deity in the influence that she exerts on the physical, the intellectual and the moral interests of the human race, and that her education should be adapted to qualify her in the highest degree to cherish those interests in the wisest and best manner."[17]

As the resolution suggests, physiological education was seen as a weapon for a conservative kind of female liberation. Alcott, particularly, hoped to use it to emancipate women from "domestic slavery." His books of advice to young married people encouraged the wife to recognize her moral and intellectual equality with her mate, and disdained the treatment she typically received with an indignation worthy of Elizabeth Cady Stanton. *The Young Husband,* for instance, contained a chapter on "Conjugal Servitude" that compared most wives to negroes and horses, decried their subjection to "that round of duties amid pots and kettles ... which ... stints, dwarfs, diseases, and gradually destroys the soul," and denounced the husband as the "devourer of her individuality, if not of her personal identity." He concluded with a profession of surprise that, woman's plight being so onerous, there had not been more Wollstonecrafts or Wrights.[18]

But when he described those renowned feminists' labors as "erratic," Alcott ran up his true colors. Female freedom, to his mind, meant freedom from oppression within the home, freedom to exercise intellect and spirit to their full power in the education of children and elevation of the husband. His comments to *The Young Wife* included an expression of dis-

---

[17] Quoted by Hebbel Hoff and John Fulton, "The Centenary of the First American Physiological Society Founded at Boston by William A. Alcott and Sylvester Graham," *Bull. Hist. Med.,* 5, 701, 729 (1937). The resolution is also quoted by Regina Markell Morantz, "Nineteenth Century Health Reform and Women: a Program of Self-help," in *Medicine Without Doctors,* ed. Guenter Risse *et al.,* New York, 1977, p. 78. This is an excellent discussion of the response of women to the health reform movement.

[18] William Alcott, *The Young Husband,* Boston, 1846, pp. 345–350.

may at the recent encouragement of women to seek literary or political stature, a trend that must "indirectly . . . disparage woman, as a wife and as a mother." "The truth," as Alcott saw it, "is, that these characters [literary and political women], however valuable to the world they may be, would be more valuable if more devoted to their appropriate sphere. But has not the custom of lauding to the skies such individuals, while thousands in useful domestic life have been overlooked and forgotten, been one reason why so many young females of the present day have such aversion to the kitchen, and gravely tell us they would almost as soon die as have their hands employed in dish-water?"[19]

Yet even when the true nobility of her domestic role was rediscovered, a woman would be inadequate to fulfill her mission unless she possessed the energy, strength, and optimism of health. Physiology was the key to genuine female liberation, and, as Morantz has argued, health reform did in fact contribute in its quiet way to woman's rise to equality. Those women who became involved in the movement were encouraged to assume more authority and new duties within the family, and even in organizations outside the home, and to expect that the strength to be brought by new health would allow still more activity.[20]

All agreed that no real activity was possible until restrictive dress was eliminated. But when Graham, Alcott, and other health reformers attempted to delineate the evils of tight corsets for their female disciples, they found themselves equally constricted by the stays of popular moral prejudice. As the *Boston Medical and Surgical Journal* editorialized on the subject of "popular lectures on tight lacing," it was one thing to explore "the mysterious anatomy of

[19] William Alcott, *The Young Wife*, Boston, 1838, pp. 359–360.

[20] Morantz (n. 17), pp. 89–90. Also see Martha Verbrugge, "The Social Meaning of Personal Health: The Ladies' Physiological Institute of Boston and Vicinity in the 1850s," in *Health Care in America. Essays in Social History,* ed. Susan Reverby and David Rosner, Philadelphia, 1979, pp. 45–66.

the chest" in the form of a book a lady might read in private, but quite another to present that, and other anatomy, in public discourse: "This newly broached plan of collecting [women] by the hundreds into churches and town halls— misses, maids and matrons ... —is so revolting to any one not lost to a sense of delicacy and common propriety, that ... we hope there will never be a repetition.... The essential evils to which the [corseted] female is predisposed ... cannot be mentioned—no, nor even adverted to by a well-bred professional gentleman, without forfeiting all claims to modesty, and offending those for whom he pretends to be laboring."[21]

Women were caught in the same dilemma that would confound them again when they attempted to gain admission to medical schools in the 1840s and 1850s. The corset apparently injured health, especially the health of the female organs. Going to a male physician to have such problems treated was a humiliating ordeal, compromising as it did that most cherished of Victorian virtues, female modesty (the desire to preserve modesty by having female doctors available to treat gynecological and obstetrical problems was a major force pushing women to seek medical training). Understanding the way the corset pressured the womb and inhibited the respiratory movement of the chest was thus a step toward the preservation of modesty—discarding the corset would save women from having to endure examinations by male doctors. But the only way women could acquire that understanding was to absorb instruction in the anatomy and physiology of the thorax and reproductive tract, instruction before which the face of delicacy would blush, if not contort, in outright horror. Women were shamed if they did, and shamed if they didn't—at least as long as physiological lectures were delivered by men.

That the world had here a problem "from which nothing

[21] "Popular Lectures on Tight Lacing," *Boston Med. Surg. J., 12,* 336–337 (1835).

but female instruction and female philanthropy could extricate it" was self-evident, and the ideal female philanthropist was soon found. Mary Neal Gove, born in New Hampshire in 1810, had become interested in medical and health topics at an early age. She did not come across the works of Graham until 1837, though, when she and her tyrannical lout of a husband moved to Lynn, Massachusetts. Quickly won over by the Graham gospel, she began preaching the wonders of bran and water to the pupils in her school and to a female lyceum in the town. Soon she had her school charges boarding on the Graham system, so when the summons was issued for a lady lecturer on physiology, she was well prepared to present "physiological facts, of a delicate nature and which many ladies would not bring themselves to hear from a gentleman." (That ladies needed to hear physiological facts from someone is indicated by the remark of a female correspondent of the *Graham Journal,* who supposed a friend was sick because she had a spine in her backbone.) Gove's first course was given in Boston in the autumn of 1838 and drew audiences estimated at four to five hundred. According to reports, the lecture on tight lacing attracted two thousand, and when she carried her message on to Providence and New York, standing room only was the rule. But even those who had to stand received full value for their money, if Gove's climactic comments on corsets are representative of her style: "Shall we torture and distort our forms, render our muscles paralytic, obliterate the air cells in our lungs, stop partially or entirely the course of the crimson current that flows in our veins, thus bringing disease and anguish and unutterable misery upon body and mind, which is followed by death long before we should have been laid down in the grave?"[22]

[22] Mary Gove Nichols, "Mrs. Gove's Experience in Water Cure," *Water Cure, J.,* 7, 40–41, 68–70, 103–105 (1849); John Blake, "Mary Gove Nichols, Prophetess of Health," *Proc. Am. Phil. Soc.,* 106, 219–234 (1962); *Graham J. Health Long.,* 2, 304, 339 (1838); *Lib. Health,* 2, 248, 272 (1838).

One would think such an oratorical barrage would have obliterated the corset for all time, but, as Samuel Johnson observed, few enterprises are so hopeless as a contest with fashion. Physiologically conscientious ladies took heed, but the majority of women from the comfortable classes clung to their laces for another half century, making dress reform one of the most protracted hygienic crusades of the 1800s, for the medical profession as well as lay health reformers.

Gove's own health cracked under the strain of lecturing and travelling, and late in that first year, she suffered, in midlecture, a pulmonary hemorrhage (consumption again!). She recovered to offer lectures on masturbation the next year, and to edit a new health journal the year following. Her journal survived less than twelve months, and before long she had wandered into hydropathy and activities that would take her well beyond strict health reform. Along the way, however, she had kindled an unprecedented interest in female health. Dozens of bold ladies, including future feminist leaders such as Paulina Wright Davis, followed her to the lecture platform, to edify the hundreds of women who joined the female physiological societies and anticorset associations that sprouted all over the northeast and, though less thickly, in other parts of the country. Many of the women who were won to physiological living came to espouse the kind of aggressive feminism that Alcott considered so improper, and though they eventually subordinated physiology to political and sociological topics, most feminists appreciated, as Morantz has shown, "the importance of good health as a prerequisite for woman's place in the world."[23] The corsetless Bloomer costume was a true physical, as well as symbolic, liberation.

The early women doctors were among the most vocal advocates of improving female hygiene, and their words often carried the brand of health reform ideology. Elizabeth Blackwell, who in 1849 was awarded the first medical degree

[23] Nichols (n. 22), p. 40; Morantz (n. 17), p. 81.

ever granted a woman, published her first book three years later, on *The Laws of Life*. Taken from lectures she had "delivered to a class of ladies," it taught a system of hygiene that, it is true, was not Grahamite—it concentrated on exercise and said nary a word about vegetarianism. But its motivating philosophy was still Christian physiology. Beginning with a hymn to the "primeval grandeur of the human race," Dr. Blackwell asked, "Who ever imagined Adam suffering from dyspepsia, or Eve in a fit of hysterics?" In exhorting readers to commit themselves to regain that physical glory, and strive for millennial perfection, she directed their eyes almost entirely toward Eve, but the book was dedicated, after all, "to American Women."[24]

Except for that feminist bias, doctors like Blackwell represented what health reformers hoped would be the next stage of evolution for medicine. The traditional therapeutic orientation of the profession was despised, not merely because of the obvious dangers of bleeding and calomel, but basically because any medicine was, by definition, a stimulant—it would not be called a medicinal agent unless it provoked some exaggerated or abnormal response from the body. The same point was to be stressed by the therapeutic skeptics within medicine. Oliver Wendell Holmes, the most eloquent of their number, proposed in his "nature-trusting heresy" address, that "a medicine should always be presumed to be hurtful. It always is *directly* hurtful; it may sometimes be indirectly beneficial." Health reformers would merely have deleted Holmes' last clause and demanded complete trust in nature. They were aware of the work of Louis and others of the Paris School, and frequently debated the merits of nature versus art. The outcome was always the same: natural function was healthy function, and even though that function might be deranged by bad hygiene, it would return to normal if correct hygiene were restored and

[24]Elizabeth Blackwell, *The Laws of Life*, New York, 1852, pp. 10, 16–17.

no unnatuural stimulants such as medicines allowed to interfere. "The *vis medicatrix* which I contend for," Graham explained, "is none other than the renovating and conservative power of nature's own vital economy."[25]

Since it was also contended that the *vis medicatrix* must reward physiological propriety with invulnerability to disease, it might appear there would be absolutely no need for a medical profession in the golden days to come. But in reality the design for the millennium placed a heavier load on physicians than on women. They would have to be reformed physicians—the constitution of the American Physiological Society proclaimed that " 'prevention is better than cure,' is our favorite motto"—and Alcott's inaugural address to the society concluded with a challenge to transform medical practice into a system that paid the doctor for preventing, rather than curing, illness. The holistic movement of recent years has revived the idea of training doctors to be "wellness counselors," but there is still no fuller description of such a counselor's duties than Alcott's. "The right use of physicians," as he styled it, required first of all making the doctor a good nurse, a man determined to "follow nature" in any illness he had to treat. Secondly, he should teach nature, or God's natural laws of health, while delivering care, and as he did, the demand for therapy would drop. His teaching should be extended to the lecture hall, the school, the factory, and even the jail; he should become "a missionary of health," regarding his work in the same light as that of the minister. He must present a holistic gospel, not just tailoring his advice on life-style to the individual client's needs, but analyzing his client's environment for wholesomeness: is his home properly constructed and ventilated? are there poisons or mechanical dangers associated with his employment? is there lead in his water pipes? are there toxic metals lining her pots and pans? Above all, the preventive physician must

[25] Oliver Wendell Holmes, *Medical Essays*, Boston, 1891, p. 202; *Lib. Health, 3,* 195–196 (1839); *Graham J. Health Long., 1,* 117 (1837).

impress upon the public the realization that illness is sin; it comes only from transgression of divine laws.

And success on his mission would not make the doctor obsolete. Actual disease might be eradicated, but there would continue to be potential disease as long as there were people. Even though given sound advice on how to live, humans would err, sometimes unwittingly, and their errors would have to be detected and corrected. There would always be a need for expert diagnosticians. The final right use of physicians was their administering of regular physical examinations to all "patients"—a Well Adult Program, if you will—to discover the signs of physiological abuse before serious damage occurred, and reform faulty habits.[26]

But where, Alcott asked rhetorically, shall the reform begin? The medical profession cvould not be expected to reform itself—doctors had always been paid in proportion to the amount of disease they treated, not prevented, and the public was accustomed to, and, in their ignorance, satisfied with that system. "If medical men will not move to enlighten the public mind, and that mind, being unenlightened, will not move, . . . must [we] sit down in despair?" The answer to the dilemma, of course, was Alcott's original love—Physical Education! In all his wanderings through medical school, editorial offices, and lecture halls, Alcott never really left the common school classroom. Adults habituated to medicines and set in their unphysiological ways would be next to impossible to reform, he knew, but if the science of healthy living could be impressed on young minds while they were still forming, and taught with as much rigor as reading and arithmetic, a new public consciousness could be created. People demanding health would be a market for the new medicine, and doctors would no longer find their healing mission in conflict with their economic interests. They would

[26] Hoff and Fulton (n. 17), pp. 698, 727; William Alcott, "The Right Use of Physicians," *Lib. Health, 5,* 41–57, 75–88 (1841); Alcott, *Lectures on Life and Health,* Boston, 1853; pp. 444–478.

be paid in proportion to the health, not the sickness, of society. In Alcott's vision, the future physician would contract with one hundred families, at twenty dollars per family, to provide care for a year:

> Is it not obvious that, having made such an engagement, it would be for his pecuniary advantage to do all in his power to keep my family in health? . . . If by four quarterly visits, and judicious instruction as to the best means of promoting and preserving health, the physician can prevent disease at all, he will get his twenty dollars comparatively easy. But if, by his neglect, some of the family get sick, and he is obliged to make one or two hundred visits in the course of the year, his case will be a sad one indeed. Against this, however, self-interest, you may depend upon it, will lead him to look out in the best manner possible.[27]

The realization of that scheme hinged, in its entirety, on the success of physical education, and Alcott was an indefatigable campaigner for the adoption of hygiene into the common school curriculum. The fruition of that campaign, however, was due more to the labors of Horace Mann, the developer with Henry Barnard of the system of public elementary education in America. A temperance activist who moved to Boston in 1833, Mann was undoubtedly aware of Alcott as both health reformer and educator. In his first report for the Massachusetts Board of Education, presented in 1838, he discussed the subject of the construction of schoolhouses in much the same way Alcott had, and in fact admitted the latter's prize essay of 1832 had been valuable to him.

---

[27] Alcott, *Lectures* (n. 26), pp. 476–478; Alcott, *The Young Husband* (n. 18), p. 373. This same idea of the physician as an advisor on preventive medicine was also forwarded, later, by leaders of the orthodox public health movement: John Griscom, *The Sanitary Condition of the Laboring Population of New York*, New York, 1845, p. 55; Lemuel Shattuck, *Report of the Sanitary Commission of Massachusetts, 1850*, Cambridge, Mass., 1948, pp. 228–229.

Alcott's broader concern for the introduction of physiological instruction was taken up by Mann several years later, in
his 1842 report for the board. He had used it that year to
compile statistics on the number of students in Massachusetts schools being taught different subjects. American history led the list, being given to more than 10,000 pupils. Al-
gebra had more than 2000, bookkeeping almost 1500, but
human physiology a mere 416, ahead of only logic, survey-
ing, and Greek. "In the entire list above given," Mann asked,

> is there one which can claim rightful precedence of that
> which stands almost the lowest in it?—I mean human
> physiology, or an exposition of the laws of health and life.
> After a competent acquaintance with the common
> branches, is there a single department in the vast range of
> secular knowledge more fundamental, more useful for in-
> creasing our ability to perform the arduous duties and to
> bear the inevitable burdens of life, more astonishing for
> the wonders it reveals, or better fitted to enforce upon us a
> lively conviction of the wisdom and goodness of God, than
> a study of our physical frame, its beautiful adaptations
> and arrangements, the marvelous powers and properties
> with which it is endowed, and the conditions indispen-
> sable to its preservation in a state of vigor, usefulness, and
> enjoyment?

Alcott himself would have been taxed to state the health reform faith any better; he in fact reprinted lengthy extracts
of the report in his journal, and intimated Mann's attention
gave him cause to rejoice and to almost feel triumphant.[28]

Mann returned to his theme in subsequent annual reports,
and gradually gathered support. Lemuel Shattuck, for instance, in his monumental 1850 survey of the sanitary conditions and public health of Massachusetts, included among

---

[28] Mary Tyler Mann, *Life of Horace Mann,* Boston, 1888; Mann, *The
Life and Works of Horace Mann,* 5 vols., Boston, 1868, 2:456, 3:130;
Teacher of Health, 1, 297–312 (1843).

his recommendations the implementation of Mann's proposal "as soon as persons can be found qualified to teach it." Action came quickly, for in April of the same year the state legislature enacted a law requiring the teaching of "physiology and hygiene" in the state's schools, and the examination of all teachers on their ability to give instruction in those subjects. Other states responded with less eagerness, but a commitment to physiology teaching did slowly take hold, only to be perverted toward the end of the century by the Women's Christian Temperance Union's determination to make hygiene synonymous with the "scientific" repudiation of alcohol.[29]

The health reformers' concerns that individuals be educated in the laws of life by schoolteachers and physicians, and that they assume responsibility for using that education to build their own health, were reflections of the democratic spirit that pervaded their movement as thoroughly as any Jacksonian reform effort. Previous health instruction had been an elitist enterprise, valuable only to those with the education to understand it, and the wealth and leisure to apply it. True, the audience had been enlarged during the 1700s to include the bourgeosie, but even then it comprised only a privileged minority. Not until the 1830s were the doors of hygiene opened to all. Americans' pride in their free political system and unmatched resources, their sense of destiny, and above all their reverence for the rights of the common man, combined to make physiological education and health appear to be opportunities that must be made available to all, and even patriotic responsibilities to be accepted by all. The literature of health reform rang with the rhetoric of democracy. The American Physiological Society's constitution virtually began by chastizing medical men for

[29] Mann, *Life and Works* (n. 28), 3:651–662; Shattuck, *Report* (n. 27), p. 178. For followup on the law, see *Boston Med. Surg. J., 43,* 59–62, 133–134, 151–153 (1851). On the efficacy of the law, see Edward Hartwell, "Physical Training in American Colleges and Universities," U.S. Bureau of Education, *Circulars of Information,* 1885, no. 5, p. 150.

monopolizing the knowledge of physiology (this was at the same time as Thomsonians were denouncing the medical monopoly on treatment). The constitution went on to emphasize that the body's structure and function were comprehensible by "common observation" made by any person of good "common sense." Alcott was even more self-conscious about Jacksonian values. At the outset of his hygiene career, when he realized the necessity of making a break with drugs and stimulating diet, he struggled to reach his "declaration of independence" on July 4. Disappointed at being unable to free himself completely until July 5, Alcott seems to have done penance by ever after castigating gluttony as "unrepublican."[30]

The republican way was for every man to become his own hygienist, an act in which he would fulfill his part in the perfecting of the nation. His *Young Man's Guide*, Alcott stated, was intended specifically for American youth:

> *American!* did I say? This word, alone, ought to call forth all your energies, and if there be a slumbering faculty within you, arouse it to action. Never, since the creation, were the youth of any age or country so imperiously called upon to exert themselves, as those whom I now address. Never before were there so many important interests at stake. Never were such immense results depending upon a generation of men, as upon that which is now approaching the stage of action. These rising millions are destined, according to all human probability, to form by far the greatest nation that ever constituted an entire community of free men, since the world began. To form the character of these millions involves a greater amount of responsibility, individual and collective, than any other work to which

---

[30] William Coleman, "Health and Hygiene in the Encyclopedie: a Medical Doctrine for the Bourgeosie," *J. Hist. Med.*, *29*, 417 (1974); Hoff and Fulton (n. 17), pp. 723–724; Alcott, *Forty Years in the Wilderness of Pills and Powders*, Boston, 1859, pp. 72–73; *Moral Reformer*, *1*, 22 (1835); *ibid.*, *2*, 368–369 (1836).

humanity has ever been called. ... Now it is for you, my
young friends, to determine whether these weighty responsibilities shall be fulfilled. It is for you to decide
whether this *greatest* of free nations shall, at the same
time, be the *best*. And as every nation is made up of individuals, you are each, in reality, called upon daily, to settle this question: "Shall the United States, possessing the
most ample means of instruction within the reach of
nearly all her citizens, the happiest government, the
healthiest of climates, the greatest abundance of the best
and most wholesome nutriment, with every other possible
means for developing all the powers of human nature, be
peopled with the most vigorous, powerful, and happy race
of human beings which the world has ever known?"

To answer that question yes, and follow the answer with action, he declaimed on another occasion, was one of "the responsibilities of a Christian nation."[31]

This fervid individualism, so cherished by most of his contemporaries, put Alcott at odds with the numerous communitarian experimenters of the 1840s who believed that social
reorganization, the establishment of an ideal community
structure, was prerequisite to the regeneration of pure
human nature. Christian physiology presumed the ability of
the individual to perfect himself privately, provided he had
sufficient understanding of religion and science. And ac-
quiring that understanding did not necessitate drastic social
remodelling. His objection to all the associations, communities, and phalanxes, Alcott explained, was "that it is
hardly worth while to multiply associations. God, has, from
the first, established two, the *family* and the *church.*"[32]

Those may sound like impossibly stodgy sentiments from
a man who considered himself an ultra, but health reform
ideology did allow for nearly boundless individual improvement within an unchanging (because divinely ordained) so-

[31] Alcott, *Young Man's Guide* (n. 5), pp. 32–33; *American Vegetarian,*
4, 176 (1854).
[32] *Teacher of Health, 1,* 104 (1843).

cial framework. The individual renovations accomplished by physical education, furthermore, would, to reverse the communitarians' argument, put right the social organization. Despite family and church, serious social abuses had arisen in America, and Alcott was eager to see them remedied. But individual physiology had to come first. He consistently spoke out against the enslavement of the African race, against the domestic enslavement of women, and against the economic enslavement of laborers. But the "slavery of bad physical habits" was to Alcott "still more shocking," and was the root from which the others grew. Until that slavery was abolished, all other reforms would be futile, and once it was abolished, other reforms would be needless. Men restructured by Christian physiology would not want to own other men, oppress women, or work their employees long hours in dirty factories for starvation wages. Socially, Alcott's utopia was a composite of Jacksonian reform ideals.[33]

Its distinguishing feature, however, was contributed by health reform philosophy specifically: the truly Christian society would be a hygienic millennium. There had long been scriptural authority for such a hope in Isaiah's prophecy of the day when "the child shall die a hundred years old." Now there was physiological evidence of the physical perfectibility of man. If the particles making up the body's organs were constantly changing as old ones were worn away and replaced by new ones from the food and atmosphere, one might find a kind of salvation in carefully regulated metabolism. If nurtured by pure diet and pure air, "what ... is to hinder an organ," Alcott wondered, "from becoming, in process of time, comparatively perfect?" And if the individual could accomplish so much by "the perpetual renovation of his system, ... in his own little life time, how much can be done in a series of generations for the improvement and elevation of the human race?"[34]

[33] *Moral Reformer,* 1, 77, 91, 335 (1835); *ibid.,* 2, 212–215 (1836); *Lib. Health,* 1, 160 (1837).
[34] *Lib. Health,* 3, 95 (1839).

How much physical improvement might there be? Certainly a species of physical beauty unrivalled since Adam and Eve should become ordinary. The total eradication of disease might also be expected, for "how could a person in perfect health, and obeying, to an iota, all the laws of health—how could he contract disease? What would there be in his system which could furnish a nidus for its reception?" The life span should be greatly lengthened, and not simply because of the negative factor of the absence of disease, but more significantly because of the positive influence of hygienically improved body functioning. Patriarchal longevity was Alcott's hope, and at the least he could "see no reason why life may not be lengthened . . . to several hundred years, and the value of each year be doubled or tripled." The final clause was added to forestall the objection that several centuries of old age would be more a burden than a blessing. In the first place, by improving either his "infantile particles" or his "octagenarian [sic] particles," a person would be much more vigorous at any age. He would enjoy what is today being extolled as "high level wellness"; Alcott suggested more poetically that one would feel like it was "morning all day." Secondly, the replacement of the present artificially stimulated "hot-house" development of the body by a natural hygienic maturing should so retard the rate of growth that a person "may be thirty, or fifty, or a hundred years, in attaining to maturity." And, finally, that maturity would be moral as well as physical. By the divinely wrought sympathy of soul with body, physical purity necessarily promoted moral purity. Had he been a man of lighter humor, Alcott might have proposed that "pretty does as pretty is." In any event, he saw a properly governed body as "a means of lifting us toward the Eden whence we came."[35]

[35] Alcott, *The Young Husband* (n. 18), p. 27; Alcott, *Vegetable Diet as Sanctioned by Medical Men and by Experience in all Ages,* Boston, 1838, pp. 242–243; Alcott, *Gift Book for Young Men,* New York, 1856, p. 17; Alcott, *The Laws of Health,* Boston, 1859, pp. 2, 17, 187; *Lib. H., 2,* 189 (1838).

His longing for Eden, so frequently expressed, should not be interpreted as a desire to return to the state of nature. Alcott shared his period's uneasiness about the rapid changes accompanying industrialization. He lamented the passing of the agrarian economy because it had necessitated the living of a relatively hygienic life. The unnatural, confined employments of urban society forced people to violate health laws in order to make a living. Industrialism had diverted mind and energy into a degrading and debilitating competition for money, while churning out products that widened the gap between man and nature. But the proper solution was to redirect industry, not reject it. When carefully used, Alcott believed, "art improves Nature, and finally becomes a part of Nature herself." Art's "plastic hand" could transform the earth, produce better food to support a larger population, design health-enhancing manufactures instead of softening luxuries. His return to nature was thus actually "a gradual ascent to nature. Man's nature is intended, most certainly, to include art, and to be affected and modified by science. But in making our ascent up the mount whence we have fallen, it is by no means necessary that we should return to barbarism."[36] What Alcott envisioned, though only vaguely, was a Christian civilization, a society combining the moral and physical vigor of Biblical days with the scientific knowledge of the modern era.

It is impossible to know exactly how many Americans shared that vision, though it is certain that only a very small percentage of the American public held it for any length of time. In 1837, when the national population was about fifteen million, Alcott seemed proud to announce his *Library of Health* subscription list was approaching two thousand. Four years later, with health reform as robust as it would get, he estimated the New England following as at most "a

---

[36] Alcott, *Lectures* (n. 26), pp. 226, 280–281; *Lib. Health, 5,* 82 (1841); *ibid. 6,* 121 (1842); *American Vegetarian, 4,* 175 (1854).

few thousands." And by the latter date, the American Physiological Society had been dissolved. Members' interest began to lag after the first round of physiological study, testimonial collection, and resolution passing was completed. Repetitiveness was made worse, in Alcott's opinion, by narrowness. The society tended toward Grahamism, and became a "mere anti-flesh-eating" association, to the neglect of exercise, dress, and other matters essential to full physical education. Though still its president, Alcott divorced himself from the organization in 1840, and no later record of the American Physiological Society survives.[37]

The philosophy for which it had been founded, however, continued to show strong signs of life through the 1840s. Indeed, it could not easily have died as long as the spirit of perfectionism coursed so forcefully through society at large. Ultras bent on reshaping the world by whatever means had to find Alcott's philosophy attractive, if not almost irresistible. They were drawn by reflex, of course, by the autonomic readiness of the reformer to endorse all other good causes (how often today does one meet a natural foods enthusiast who favors the construction of nuclear power plants?). But the attraction had substance, too, for physical education concentrated on matters that were undeniably fundamental to any work of reform. Whichever formula for human perfection one preferred to follow, human strength, endurance, energy, passion, and morality were ingredients that could not be overlooked. The French "positive" school of social planning, foreseeing a society where priests would be replaced by scientists, had already identified physiology as the indispensable science for understanding human nature and social interactions. The Saint-Simonians especially had built from a cornerstone of physiology, and their leader had even voiced maxims that might just as easily have come from the lips of Alcott: "The moralist who is not a physiologist can

[37] *Lib. Health, 1,* 9 (1837); *ibid., 5,* 91 (1841); Hoff and Fulton (n. 17), p. 711.

only demonstrate the reward of virtue in another world."[38] That was widsom reflecting the inherent sympathy between all programs of social reorganization and the ideology of health reform, a sympathy that guaranteed the ideology a hearing, and some degree of acceptance, wherever the work of human liberation was attempted.

Its associations with educational reform and the feminist movement have been noted. It might be added that the unpredictable wanderings of radical minds could carry health reform into some strange intellectual territory. Mary Gove, for example, the first female physiology lecturer, became a maid-of-all-reforms during the 1840s (while also escaping her brutish first husband, taking a succession of lovers, and finally marrying the equally versatile reformer Thomas Low Nichols). Both her feminist involvement and private experience sensitized her to the issue of sexual self-government for women, so when the free love movement burst into the open in the early 1850s, Mary Gove Nichols was its ranking female representative. But her free love notions, scandalous as they were to her contemporaries, shock the historian still more for having been conceived by such improbable bedfellows as sensuality and Grahamism. Personal liberation had given Nichols an appreciation of the intense physical and emotional pleasure of sex, and the right of women to its uninhibited enjoyment. She had not, however, forgotten her initiation in physiology, or her own lectures on the dangers of sexual excess. In marriage, a woman was a slave to her husband's appetite, an appetite that usually demanded much more than the once-monthly indulgence allowed by physiology. To her mind, therefore, free love meant not just the freedom to enhance quality, but also, and of equal importance, the freedom to regulate quantity. While agreeing with Alcott that quality and quantity were related in-

[38] Frank Manuel, *The New World of Henri Saint-Simon*, Cambridge, Mass., 1956, p. 135. Also see Manuel, *The Prophets of Paris*, Cambridge, Mass., 1962, pp. 113-129.

versely, Nichols differed with him on the effect of marriage on sexual health. Thus was sexuality turned against the very Christian institution that health reformers had used it to defend.[39]

Since her own husband could be trusted, Mary Gove Nichols remained married. The couple in fact continued to publicize conventional health reform doctrine as well, and even planned to dispense it from a health institute to be opened at Modern Times, the notorious anarchist, free love colony on Long Island. That project never materialized, but Grahamite practices did find a place at other communitarian settlements in America. It has to be admitted, of course, that the Romantic utopian temperament, already slanted toward simple, unaffected living, had a predilection for vegetarianism independent of any health reform inspiration. Bronson Alcott surely acquired specific ideas on diet from cousin William, but was also, as he said, a vegetarian "by instinct." Fruitlands, his abortive "New Eden," was guided by the principle that "outward abstinence is a sign of inward fulness," and would have been a meatless paradise even if attempted two decades earlier.[40]

But Fruitlands was a community founded on primitive diet. At settlements with different philosophical bases, where religion or political economy dominated table conversation, food seemed of less consequence and some leeway in eating was generally allowed. Many of their residents had an innate inclination for simple food, but it might not have been hardened to resolve without the radical peer pressure of health reform. That there was some pride to be taken in tempering one's utopianism with Grahamism is evidenced by the popularity of Graham tables at the Fourierist Phalanxes that came and went in such profusion in the 1840s. It

---

[39] *Lib. Health, 2,* 156–158 (1842). Nissenbaum (n. 1) explores Nichols' sexual radicalism in detail, pp. 159–170. Also see Taylor Stoehr, *Free Love in America. A Documentary History,* New York, 1979, pp. 9–22.

[40] Odell Shepard, *Pedlar's Progress. The Life of Bronson Alcott,* Boston, 1937, p. 440; Clara Sears ed., *Bronson Alcott's Fruitlands,* Boston, 1915, p. 52.

is not easy to imagine the sensualist Fourier approving of the ascetic Graham diet, but his philosophy, after all, was one of restructuring society so as to accommodate man's natural physical passions, and therefore had an ear bent toward physiology—and in America, utopian physiology meant health reform. The Nicholses were ardent Fourierists, and a number of associations had meatless tables. The Trumball Phalanx, in fact, was described as "a glorious resort for the Grahamites." The Skaneateles Community also included Grahamites, as did Modern Times and many Shaker settlements. And the Oneida Community at least flirted with vegetarianism. Even if colonies were driven to fleshless diet by so mundane a consideration as economic hardship, the move was not uninfluenced by health reform. When Brook Farm fell upon hard times one winter, and retrenchment took the form of culinary restraint, Marianne Dwight supposed that by living on turnips and squashes, "we shall have fewer headaches, etc."[41]

The appeal of health reform extended even to those most militant of ultras, the abolitionists. The first Graham boarding house was opened in New York City in 1833, ostensibly to shelter those who liked rising at four in the morning, retiring at ten in the evening, and filling the hours between with coarse bread, a cold bath, and walking "with an occasional leap, run, hop, etc." But according to a young Amherst tutor who stayed there briefly during its first year, the house's inmates were even more eccentric: "The Boarders in this establishment are not only Grahamites, but Garrisonites—not only reformers in diet, but radicals in Politics. Such a knot of abolitionists I never before fell in with. Slavery, Colonization, etc. constitute the unvarying monotonous theme of their conversations except that they give place to

[41] John Humphrey Noyes, *Strange Cults and Utopias of 19th-Century America*, New York, 1966, pp. 166, 177, 179, 318–319, 338, 431, 477; *American Vegetarian, 3,* 1–3 (1853); Harriet Skinner, *Oneida Community Cooking, or a Dinner Without Meat*, Oneida, N.Y., 1873; Marianne Dwight to Anna Parsons, Dec. 14, 1844, in *Letters From Brook Farm, 1844–1847,* ed. Amy Reed, Poughkeepsie, N.Y., 1928, p. 51.

an occasional comment upon their peculiar style of living."
Tappan, Goodell, and Dennison were the "most prominent
characters," he added, but even William Lloyd Garrison
himself was known to visit. A Graham banquet later in the
decade was graced by the attendance of the almost equally
prominent Gerrit Smith.[42]

At that same feast was Lorenzo Fowler, one of the leading
American popularizers of phrenology, the pseudoscience
holding that the brain was organized into thirty-seven
organs or faculties, each responsible for a specific intellectual or character trait. An individual's personality was presumably determined by the different degrees of development
of his various cerebral organs. A man with a large organ of
acquisitiveness was likely to end up a thief; one blessed with
an exceptional faculty of causality could hope to become a
philosopher. As formulated by its discoverer Gall, phrenological doctrine was rather pessimistic, assuming a person's
fate to be more or less set by his brain's structure. Later
phrenologists took a brighter view, supposing individual
organs might be encouraged to expand or atrophy, and a
more desirable character thus molded for each individual.
But it was in the United States, in the 1830s and 1840s, that
phrenology was given its most optimistic interpretation, and
also democratized, and even vulgarized, being reduced in
many hands to a type of fortune telling accomplished by
feeling the client's skull for protrusions and depressions
caused by over- and under-developed regions of the brain.
But since any faulty development so diagnosed might be
corrected, enthusiasts expected the perfecting power of the
new science to prove boundless; phrenology, one devotee
bubbled, could even improve an oyster.[43]

As a scheme linking physical traits with character, and
directed at individual and social improvement, phrenology

[42] *Moral Reformer*, 1, 250 (1835); Thomas LeDuc, "Grahamites and
Garrisonites," *New York Hist.*, 20, 189–191 (1939). *Graham J. Health
Long.*, 3, 399 (1839).

[43] John Davies, *Phrenology, Fad and Science. A 19th-Century Crusade*, New Haven, Conn., 1955, p. 88.

seemed to duplicate health reform. At least the phrenologists thought so, and many combined Grahamism with their original faith. Lorenzo, and his brother Orson Fowler, published books relating physiology to phrenology, and devising physical mechanisms to bind brain and body. The age-old belief that carnivorous diet begets a carnivorous temperament was given a phrenological-health reform rationale with the argument that meat's stimulating power passes through the nerves to inflame the lower region of the brain: "Animal food constitutionally develops Combativeness and Destructiveness." Even the procuring of food was related to the excitation of phrenological organs. Whereas the hunting of flesh was directed by the propensity of destructiveness, agriculture exercised the intellectual and moral faculties. The Fowlers, with their colleague Samuel Wells, also retailed a set of forty plaster casts of heads of great men, a collection which included Voltaire, Napoleon, Henry Clay—and Sylvester Graham.[44]

Graham returned the compliment by lecturing to phrenological audiences at the Fowlers' auditorium, but neither he nor Alcott could bring himself to wholehearted approval of phrenology. At best, phrenology encompassed only a portion of the physical body, and one which was already handled adequately by health reform theory. The attitudes of the leaders of the broader movement were a blend of tentative support and condescension toward an immature subspecialty of physiology. Alcott once admitted to being "more than half Phrenologists ourselves," but objected its advocates were trying to spread it too soon, before the public had mastered physical education. Several years later, when explaining his model of the physician (physiology teacher) of the future, he punctuated his idealizing with a warning to "mere head feelers [to] stand at a distance."[45]

[44] Orson Fowler, *Physiology, Animal and Mental*, New York, 1847, pp. 64, 95; Davies (n. 43), p. 51.

[45] *Moral Reformer*, 2, 35 (1836); Alcott, *Lectures* (n. 26), p. 459. For Graham's views on phrenology, see *Lectures on the Science of Human Life*, 2 vols., Boston, 1839, 1:378–379.

Allied with phrenology or not, health reform ideology was certain to be debated in a final arena, the college campus. The student "Physiological Society" was an organization of some popularity around the beginning of the 1840s. Some societies were established on strict Grahamite principles, others hesitated to commit themselves to anything but free inquiry. At least one of the former was actually imposed upon students. Oberlin Collegiate Institute was founded in 1832 specifically for the purpose of training teachers and ministers to meet the intellectual and spiritual needs of the growing Mississippi Valley, and was an ultra institution from the start. It was the first coeducational college in the country, the first to admit black students on an equal basis with whites, and even served as a post on the underground railroad. It is not surprising, then, to learn that in 1836 about one hundred of Oberlin's female students organized a society that repudiated corsets and other unhealthful dress, as well as tea, coffee, and condiments. Two years later, under the leadership of Charles Grandison Finney, the prime expositor of Christian perfectionism and an Oberlin executive, an Oberlin Physiological Society was established to include staff and male students. Physiology was made a required course at the same time, and less than two years later, physiological living became demanded of all students. In 1840, Finney imported David Cambell, erstwhile editor of the recently deceased *Graham Journal of Health and Longevity,* to supervise the tables at the school's student commons. Praising the college as "a model institution for the approaching 'Millennial Church,'" Cambell immediately eliminated the elective meat table and required pure Grahamism of all. Revolt was not long in coming. A professor dismissed from the faculty, in part for using pepper at the table, accused the Cambell system of having "physiologically reformed" some students "into eternity," while a yet incompletely reformed student summarized the horrors of the official diet with a threat:

But dread you not, some *famished foe* may rise,
With vengeful arm and beat you to a jelly?
Ye robbers of our vitals best supplies,
Beware! "There is no joking with the belly."
Nor hope the world will in your footsteps follow,
Your *bread* and *doctrine* are too hard to *swallow*.[46]

Cambell's reign of terror was summarily ended in 1841, and a more varied diet restored. But while the Oberlin experiment was a microcosm of the entire health reform movement, the inability of the large majority of Americans to swallow either its bread or doctrine does not mean health reform was inconsequential. Much of the advice given by health reformers was sound, and although these same hygienic rules were also being publicized by more moderate physicians, it cannot be denied that a new awareness of the nature of health and its dependence on personal habits of life was built to a significant degree by the labors of men like Alcott and Graham. Their works were especially valuable for combatting the popular notion that disease was the work of Providence and largely unavoidable and for doing it within a scheme of thought that made sense to a lay audience. That they failed to totally eradicate gluttony and alcohol abuse can be forgiven; physician writers did no better. Human beings are simply not the tractable, perfectible creatures health reformers (and many others of the day) wished them to be.

One has to wonder furthermore how the consciousness of the medical profession was affected by health reform philosophy. The first half of the nineteenth century was a period of remarkable change in the American medical psyche. Grob,

[46] *Graham J. Health Long., 3,* 222 (1839); *Moral Reformer, 2,* 155–157 (1836); Robert Fletcher, "Bread and Doctrine at Oberlin," *Ohio St. Arch. Hist. Q., 49,* 66 (1940). The Oberlin episode is also discussed by William Walker, "The Health Reform Movement in the United States, 1830–1870," doctoral dissertation, Johns Hopkins University, 1955, pp. 134–141, and Nissenbaum (n. 1), p. 143.

in his study of Edward Jarvis, has characterized a new (and small) generation of American medical activists that slowly emerged during the middle third of the century in terms which must now be familiar:

> The younger activists who reached professional maturity in the 1830s and 1840s were, unlike their predecessors, concerned primarily with the maintenance of health. Influenced as much by their moral and religious beliefs as their scientific training, they defined health in terms of a proper and symbiotic relationship between nature, society and the individual. Convinced that a divine power had created a universe governed by immutable natural law, they interpreted disease and social evil as the results of unlawful (or immoral) behavior. Mortality patterns—like crime rates—were the true measure of the moral fibre of a society. The role of the physician was twofold: to discover those individual and social factors governing health and to disseminate those findings among their fellow countrymen in order that they be put to practical use.[47]

This is close to being a portrait of a health reformer, but though it is obvious that reformers and physician-hygienists were created by the same cultural forces, their coming from a common crucible did not prevent one from helping shape the other. Health reform emphases on the dangers of heroic therapy, the superiority of nature to art and of prevention to cure, the hygienic hazards of industrial civilization, the economic cost of illness, and the influence of physical circumstances on individual morality were generally more pronounced in the 1830s than was true for medicine. In the mid-1820s the *Boston Medical Intelligencer,* under the supervision of the unfortunately named Dr. John Coffin, tried to stimulate professional interest in prevention, but failed

---

[47] Gerald Grob, *Edward Jarvis and the Medical World of Nineteenth-Century America,* Knoxville, Tenn., 1978, p. 5.

after little more than a year. The prevention-oriented *Journal of Health* lived more than twice as long, but though it was edited by physicians, it was directed to a lay audience. As late as the mid-1840s, the physician Jarvis could complain without much exaggeration, that "our education has made our calling exclusively a curative ... one, and ... with health, with fullness of unalloyed, unimpaired life, we professionally have nothing to do."[48]

Undoubtedly the medical profession would have eventually come to have more to do with preventive medicine and health maintenance had Alcott, Graham, and their compatriots never been born. But it seems clear the process was accelerated by the health reform challenge. Doctors of the Jacksonian era were being pressed hard by competitors they considered to be incompetent and a public danger. Nostrum vendors, Thomsonians, hydropaths, and homeopaths all had to be refuted, and in all cases their refutation influenced regular doctors' attitudes toward therapy. Homeopathy especially, with its patently inert dilutions, taught physicians lessons about the healing power of nature that they had resisted when presented by their Paris colleagues. The unorthodox preventive medicine of health reform, no less than irregular therapeutic systems, had to be exposed, and in the process doctors were themselves exposed to stronger statements of the power of preventive hygiene than they were accustomed to seeing. The result might have been a discrediting of the ideal of prevention in the reader's mind, but it might also have been a quickening of any preventive impulse already felt. Oliver Wendell Holmes' comment on a phrenology text he read might have characterized more than a few doctors' feelings about health reform literature:

---

[48] John Blake, "Health Reform," in *The Rise of Adventism: Religion and Society in Mid-Nineteenth-Century America,* ed. Edwin Gaustad, New York, 1974, p. 36; Walker (n. 46), pp. 103–104; Wilson Smillie, *Public Health, Its Promise for the Future. A Chronicle of the Development of Public Health in the United States, 1607–1914,* New York, 1955, p. 232.

Holmes enjoyed hearing the author "teach good sense under the disguise of his equivocal system."[49]

At the very least, health reform forced physicians to wrestle with questions of hygiene, and to assume a more aggressive interest in popular health education. Dr. Caleb Ticknor's 1836 *Philosophy of Living*, for example, was almost bellicose in its prefatory declaration that the volume was designed specifically as a remedy for the "epidemic" of "ultraism" which was causing so many of his countrymen to "run into unwarrantable extravagances": "Retrenchment and self-mortification seem to be the order of the day in relation to food and drink; there being no virtue, on the principle of radicalism, which does not consist in going counter to the appetites and instincts of nature.... Such sentiments have been put forth on the subject of diet, and such ultra measures urged, that the very injury is caused which is attempted to be averted—to wit, ill health and consequent unhappiness." Any uncertainty the reader may have had as to the particular radicalism at which Ticknor was aiming his blow was relieved by later sneers at the "bran bread and cold water system" as "ill-timed money-making quackery."[50]

The scorn was returned—Alcott described Ticknor's book as a "crude, contradictory work"; Graham preferred the adjective "contemptible"—but it was an ironic exchange. For if the question of diet is deleted from Ticknor's *Philosophy* (which was firmly antivegetarian), there are few differences between that work's recommendations and those of any standard health reform volume. Ticknor allowed moderate amounts of coffee and tea, but he criticized the corset as the worst error of dress, blasted even ale as a hellish brew, and levelled devastating sarcasm against all forms of tobacco use. Most of the same generalizations could be made about

[49] John Forbes, "Homeopathy, Allopathy and 'Young Physic,'" *Brit. Foreign Med. Rev.*, *21*, 225–265 (1846); Worthington Hooker, Physician and Patient, New York, 1849, pp. 138–142; Davies (n. 43), p. 165.

[50] Caleb Ticknor, *The Philosophy of Living*, New York, 1836, pp. iii, 25, 81.

other hygiene texts authored by Jacksonian physicians. The New York doctor John Griscom, one of America's pioneers in environmental hygiene, even quoted (at length) "Dr. Alcott, of Boston" on the effects of bad air, and prophesied a *"sanatory regeneration* of the human race" to be accomplished by the public being educated: "educated physically, educated morally, educated intellectually, educated religiously, or, in short, *educated physiologically.*"[51]

The parallels between health reform and progressive medical thought were not always that distinct, but even if physician authors did not repeat so much of the health reformers' creed, they were stimulated to teach whatever they did by the need to offset health reform radicalism. With so many self-styled "professors of physiology" roaming the land, doctors could not stand aloof. According to the editor of the *Boston Medical and Surgical Journal,* a number of area physicians had attended some of the popular physiology lectures, and found themselves "listening to stuff that . . . nauseated them." The remedy, as a correspondent of the same periodical explained, was for doctors to respond with "truly scientific lectures." The prescription was not purely altruistic, of course; physicians hoped to benefit themselves by educating the public "to discriminate between the ignorant pretender and the truly scientific practitioner." But the same philanthropy animating health reform was also at work. A people being duped by ignorant pretenders deserved knowledge: doctors "have an important mission to fulfill," William Workman harangued the Massachusetts Medical Society in 1854, "and that is, to *instruct the people* on medical subjects."[52] In other words, physicians should become part-time physical educators! So in reacting against health reform, the medical profession reformed itself, if only partially, along the lines laid out by Alcott.

[51] *Moral Reformer,* 2, 196 (1836); *Graham J. Health Long., 3,* 335 (1836); John Griscom, *The Uses and Abuses of Air,* New York, 1850, p. 143.

[52] *Boston Med. Surg. J., 41,* 202, 206 (1850); Blake (n. 48), p. 44.

CHAPTER FIVE
HYGIENE IN EVOLUTION

☆☆☆☆☆☆☆☆☆☆☆☆☆☆☆☆☆☆☆☆☆☆☆☆☆☆☆☆☆☆☆☆☆☆☆☆

IN 1857, ALCOTT ACCEPTED THE OFFER OF A J. SILAS BROWN, M.D., to become "associate physician" at the Hygeopathic and Dietetic Institute in Boston. Dr. Brown's institute was primarily an infirmary where patients given up by regular doctors as incurable, were immersed in "electrochemical baths" and treated with other "natural" remedies. Alcott's assignment was to assist with the curing of dyspeptics and consumptives, co-edit the institute's journal, *The Hygeist*, lecture on hygiene, and, most importantly, organize "a school or schools for the inculcation of these Divine Laws of Human Health."[1] The school never left the drawing board, however; *The Hygeist* died in its infancy; and the institute failed utterly to drive orthodox medicine from the field. Alcott easily replaced these aborted projects, returning to his life's work of writing self-improvement volumes (his last book, in fact, was published shortly after his death in 1859). But the Brown fiasco had more than temporary significance: its failure was symptomatic of the faltering of health reform generally. The decade that had opened so triumphantly, with the requirement of physiological instruction in Massachusetts public schools, was the decade in which health reform began its slide into obscurity. It was partly the victim of its own success: with so much more attention being given to hygiene by physicians and educators, there was less need for, and less public curiosity about, health reform. The people would have become jaded anyway, without those additional instructors, for there were only so many ways to present the simple truths of Christian physiology. Once

[1] *Hygeist, 1,* 22 (1857).

sparkling insights quickly became banalities through repetition. Most significantly, an ideology directed at such prosaic matters as proper food and clothing was bound to appear trivial to a public now struggling desperately to resolve the problems of human slavery and national unity. And the failure of that struggle, with the shattering disillusionment of civil war, made the antebellum perfectionist spirit appear terribly naive and sentimental. The patronage provided health reform by the optimism and philanthropy of the Jacksonian era was largely swept away by the cynicism and materialism that brought on the Gilded Age. Hygienic ideology did survive the second half of the century, but it was stripped of its earlier dynamism.

There actually were signs of ebbing vitality almost as soon as health reform reached its full strength. By the end of 1843, family pressures were forcing Alcott to give up his journal in favor of more lucrative book writing, and no one stepped forward to preserve this chief medium of communication between his disciples. At the same time, Alcott was undergoing an ironic mental transformation that was sharply narrowing his outlook on physical education. As the movement's growth stalled in the 1840s, he apparently came to feel health reform had attempted too much too soon. At any rate, after having begun the decade by severing his ties with the American Physiological Society because it was confining itself to Grahamism, he ended it by asserting that the society had fallen because "it embraced too much." And he offered that revision of history, wondrous to say, in his inaugural address as president of the American Vegetarian Society! The physical educator who had so often rebuked Graham for his preoccupation with meatless diet had become a Grahamite. Alcott, had, of course, given vegetarianism top rank in his philosophy all along, but it had never been placed very far above the other components of hygiene. As the work of reform dragged, however, he came to feel that the craving for stimulation and nervous excitement which drove men through all the many forms of self-abuse was established in the body by flesh food. It was the major stimulant first and most frequently experienced in life, and thus created an appetite for the other stimulants. Little advance could be made against the host of hygienic evils, therefore, until the dominant enemy—meat—had been routed. The altered strategy of health reform was presented at the new vegetarian society's banquet. As revellers rested between the molded farina course and a light dessert of fruits and nuts, their president rose and lifted his glass of cold water in a toast to the proposition that, "A Vegetable Diet lies at the basis of all Reform, whether Civil, Social, Moral, or Religious." The toast, and the rousing remarks that followed, revived the ghost that had haunted Alcott early in his reform career: they provoked renewed inquiries as to whether he considered himself a Grahamite. His response that he preferred to be known as a hygeist, but would accept the title vegetarian, was, of course, a very roundabout way of answering yes.[2]

Alcott continued to preach the complete message of health reform in his books published in the 1850s, but most of his energy was channelled into vegetarianism. He remained ensconced in the presidential chair of the American Vegetarian Society until his death in 1859, and contributed most of the articles that kept its journal afloat. Yet despite Alcott's leadership, vegetarians soon began to straggle. Society membership was dwindling by the mid-1850s, and there was too little interest to support the organization's journal after 1854. Henceforward, vegetarian news was condensed into a short section in a sympathizing periodical, the *Water Cure Journal and Herald of Reforms*. It was in this forum, in fact, that the total philosophy of health reform—not just vegetarianism—was kept alive. One might even say it was given new life, for a period, for the *Water Cure Journal* was much more widely circulated than any strictly health reform journals had been, and the doctrine was insured more atten-

---

[2] *American Vegetarian, 1,* 25 (1851); *ibid., 3,* 64 (1853).

tion by being placed in a therapeutic context. Paradoxically, the very frame of mind health reformers were trying to destroy, the popular preference for cure over prevention, helped prolong the survival of their system.

A certain therapeutic orientation had been implicit in health reform from its origins. That the same nature preserving the healthy could also restore the sick—if allowed to operate freely—was even openly stated periodically. But there was no attempt at systematic enlargement of the therapeutic side of natural hygiene until the work of Isaac Jennings. An 1812 graduate of Yale's medical school (Alcott's medical alma mater), Jennings came to health reform rather late in life. He practiced conventional medicine for some years, but steadily lost faith in heroic treatments and began substituting bread pills for calomel in many cases. The experiment convinced him of the worthlessness of drugs, and by the 1830s he had discarded even placebos. He also soon found confirmation of his new style of practice in both health reform and the Parisian therapeutic philosophy then entering the country. Jennings' articulate discussions of the questions of nature versus art and self-limited disease show he was better versed than other health reformers in contemporary medicine, but he advanced beyond the Paris line of therapeutic skepticism to the position of complete therapeutic nihilism. Nontherapy was for him a positive action, an action he defined as orthopathy: "From *orthos*, right, true, erect; and pathos, affection. Nature is always upright—moving in the right direction." It was a simple doctrine, a patience and warm flannel faith that nature and nature alone could "restore her damaged machinery and revitalize it."[3] The wise physician simply stayed out of nature's path, except to remove any items (alcohol, tobacco, a corset) he saw obstructing it.

The orthopathic analysis, developed first at Boston, then Oberlin, where Jennings spent the rest of his life, was per-

---

[3] Isaac Jennings, *The Tree of Life,* New York, 1867, pp. 118, 209.

formed within the bounds of standard Grahamite pathology. Drugs were stimulants, and thus wasted vitality and undermined the body's efforts to cure itself. Jennings took infinitely more space than that to present his philosophy, but in the end it was still nothing more than an extension of health reform from the dining room to the sick room. It was, however, carried out with an evangelistic flamboyance that exceeded anything else in its class. Orthopathy was presented with camp-meeting fervor, held up as the only salvation from the satanic plot to ensnare humankind in stimulation. And the millennial glory that would spread from the "Oberlinean 'Paradise Regained' " through the rest of the world in the twenty-first century would be more pure than any yet dreamed. Jennings had an uneasiness about sexuality that was extreme even by Victorian measure; it was "the Devil's stronghold, the very citadel of his empire on earth." Thus orthopathy was nothing if it could not cure the illness of sexual passion. It could, of course, and in the millennium of Jennings' imagining, unavoidable "procreative duty" would be "spotlessly pure and severely appropriate," and would not even compare in pleasure with the joy of "the pursuit of knowledge [in which] there will be no sex."[4]

It was probably not the elimination of sexual pleasure, nor even the communistic organization of his utopia, which prevented Jennings' ideas from capturing the public fancy. Orthopathy was handicapped most of all by not really being "medicine." It offered no drugs, promised no quick recoveries, left the patient almost entirely on his own. The several other antiheroic systems of treatment being promoted by midcentury fit much more smoothly with the popular conceptions of what medicine should do, and orthopathy could never escape from their shadows. Yet one of these more prominent alternatives was also highly compatible with health reform theory. The distinction drawn by Alcott in 1845, shortly after hydropathy had carved its foothold in

[4] *ibid.*, pp. 65, 276.

America, was the critical factor. He had treated himself with cold baths several times since his youth, he reported, and had seen how in many complaints "medicine could be wholly dispensed with ... and cold water could be substituted."[5] Water, to look at it matter of factly, was not medicine, but a natural, physiological substance. It was an element of hygiene, and though European hydropaths had already included other hygienic prescriptions (walking and fresh air) in their practice, it was left to Americans to integrate water cure with the complete health reform program.

Credit for the merger goes not to Alcott, but to Mary Gove. She had read of hydropathy, and even practiced it crudely on herself and daughter, in the early 1830s, before becoming a Grahamite. The latter involvement, however, led her to a more serious association with water cure, for her health reform lecturing and editing, it will be recalled, greatly aggravated her consumptive condition. In the early 1840s, while convalescing from her latest attack of the lungs, Gove's interest in hydropathy was renewed by Henry Wright, a Fruitlands defector, and then by the water cure institutions themselves that began to be opened in the northeast. She recuperated at a hydropathic institution in Vermont in 1844, recovering sufficient strength to offer hygiene lectures to other female patients. She quickly moved on to actually take charge of patients at other water cure establishments and, after marrying Thomas Nichols, to open the first hydropathic medical school in the country and take the lead in other hydropathic projects. The most restless of reformers, the Nicholses jumped next to sexual radicalism, then spiritualism, Catholicism, and as many other isms as they could find time for.[6]

---

[5] *Water Cure J.*, *1*, 21–22 (1845).

[6] For Mary Gove Nichols' hydropathic career, see William Walker, "The Health Reform Movement in the United States, 1830–1870," doctoral dissertation, Johns Hopkins University, 1955, pp. 156–160; and Harry Weiss and Howard Kemble, *The Great American Water-Cure Craze*, Trenton, New Jersey, 1967, pp. 33–35, 72–80.

But the first, Grahamism, was left as Gove Nichols' legacy to hydropathy. From its first issues in 1845, the *Water Cure Journal* advertised health reform principles, and even published excerpts from the works of Alcott and Graham. It became standard practice for American hydropaths to keep a close eye on their patients' diets; some demanded strict vegetarianism, others were more anxious to prevent gluttony. Exercise was given much more attention than in Europe, as was dress (the Bloomer outfit adopted by feminists was most popular at hydropathic institutions). Many water cures were, in effect, Graham boarding houses with elaborate baths, and their overseers took themselves to be physical educators as well as physicians. An 1850 American Hydropathic Convention, for example, announced as its object, "the diffusion of those physiological principles which are usually comprised under the term HYGIENE, and the development of the therapeutic virtues of water to their fullest extent." Hydropathy's advocates even affected that same intimacy with the deity that health reformers had. Water cure literature was rife with poetry whose common theme was that the system was God's own: "Thy maker designed it in wisdom and love," one sang of water, while Mrs. Judson's "Cold Water Song" reverberated with praise to "That bright rich gem from heaven."[7]

The exemplar of the physical educator-hydropath was Russell Thacher Trall. Still another physician who had lost his faith in regular therapy, Trall opened the second water cure establishment in America, in New York City in 1844. Immediately he combined the full Priessnitzian armamentarium of baths with regulation of diet, air, exercise and sleep. He would eventually open and/or direct any number of other hydropathic institutions around the country, as well as edit the *Water Cure Journal, The Hydropathic Review,* and a temperance journal. He authored several books, including popular sex manuals which perpetuated Graham-

[7] *Water Cure J., 10,* 15 (1850); *ibid., 2,* 111 (1846); *ibid., 3,* 125 (1847).

ite precepts into the 1890s, sold Graham crackers and physiology texts at his New York office, was a charter member (and officer) of the American Vegetarian Society, presided over a short-lived World Health Association, and so on. His crowning accomplishment was the Hygeian Home, a "model Health Institution [which] is beautifully situated on the Delaware River between Trenton and Philadelphia." A drawing presents it as a palatial establishment with expansive grounds for walking and riding, facilities for rowing, sailing, and swimming, and even a grove for open air "dancing gymnastics." It was the grandest of water cures, and lived beyond the Civil War period which saw the demise of most hydropathic hospitals. True, Trall had to struggle to keep his head above water during the 1860s, but by the 1870s he had a firm financial footing (being stabilized by tuition fees from the attached Hygeio-Therapeutic College). With Trall's death in 1877, however, the hydropathic phase of health reform passed.[8]

When in 1871 Trall had left New York for good, to attend to the Hygeian Home, his water cure there had been converted into The New Hygienic Institute, where the sick were to be cured "by hygiene agencies alone." One of the coproprietors of the institute was Martin Luther Holbrook, a budding health reformer who had paid his dues to the trade with a decade of illness in his twenties, then recovered sufficiently to earn a medical degree in 1864. Holbrook's institute offered the first Turkish bath in New York (and only the second in the country). He taught hygiene at the New York Medical College for Women (the school organized by Elizabeth Blackwell) for fifteen years. He wrote books to cover the full spectrum of health behavior: *Eating for Strength, Hygiene of the Brain and Nerves and the Cure of Nervousness, Marriage and Parentage,* and others. But Holbrook's greatest service to the cause was as an editor. In 1866 he replaced Trall at the head of the *Herald of Health*, which had descended from the *Water Cure Journal and Herald of Reforms* (1845–1861) by way of the *Hygienic Teacher and Water Cure Journal* (1862). Under Holbrook's direction, the periodical would pass through two more name changes (*Journal of Hygiene and Herald of Health*, 1893–1897, and *Omega*, 1898–1900) before merging with *Physical Culture*.[9]

The journal's significance, though, lay in its content, not its title. Change was the rule there, too. Most of the old wisdom was preserved: Holbrook was a vegetarian teetotaller who despised tobacco and drugs, worshipped bathing and exercise, and hoped to see physicians become teachers of health. As his editorial reign advanced, however, new themes intruded his pages, and scientific and social process made itself felt. During the 1890s especially, Holbrook's journal was stretched and shaped into a veritable bridge over which hygienic radicals could pass from now quaint Jacksonian health reform philosophy to the merging intellectual terrain of Progressivism. The new world's lure was irresistible; the Progressive mentality was vibrant, alive with a lust for restoration that had not been felt since the 1840s. Hygienists, at least, tended to be that florid in their welcoming of the resurgent reform spirit. Progressivism combined confidence in science with an expansive social optimism and sense of progress. It appealed to all the basic instincts of the health-minded, and inevitably drew forth a throng of hygienic utopians.

That that crowd was much more varied and complex in makeup than the Grahamites had been was also in keeping with the new times. Progressive is a fetching label, but it is difficult to identify the typical individual on whom to pin it. Progressivism involved many and varied political orientations and reform interests, and represented a society energized by an array of diverse, sometimes conflicting, concerns

[9] *The National Cyclopedia of American Biography*, vol. 12, New York, 1904. 12:334; Weiss and Kemble (n. 6), pp. 26, 83–84.

and aspirations.[10] And Progressive health reformers were just as eclectic in identifying hygienic problems, proposing remedies, and formulating goals. Yet unity of a sort reigned over these individual differences. Most Progressive hygienists were residents of a tight community of seekers, each with his own plan and often critical of others', but also curious about his coreformers' ideas and willing to borrow and lend with them. There was not a single health reform movement in the Progressive period, but there was a coherent turn of mind that guided the shaping of all individual programs. Holbrook's intellectual career is a case study in the formation of the Progressive hygienic outlook.

Just as Alcott had done, Holbrook counted himself blessed to live in an age of astonishing advance in the sciences of human life. By the century's end, it was the science of nutrition (ever the cornerstone of practical hygiene) that was maturing at the most impressive rate, becoming so sophisticated, in fact, as to draw orthodox scientists into dietary reform activities. Thus when Wilbur Atwater, America's leading developer of the new nutrition, returned from his advanced biochemical studies in Munich, he was already bent on analyzing the composition of all common American foods, determining the nutritional requirements of different types of American workers, and consequently establishing new American eating patterns that would be at once more healthful and more economical. The dietary philosophy he presented in his numerous technical and popular articles was based, unfortunately, on an incomplete science: full nutrition was presumed to require only protein (for growth and tissue repair), fats and carbohydrates (for energy), and minerals. Vitamins were as yet unsuspected, so some of his

[10] For good general coverage of Progressivism, see Richard Hofstadter, *The Progressive Movement, 1900–1915*, Englewood Cliffs, New Jersey, 1963; David Noble, *The Progressive Mind, 1890–1917*, Chicago, 1970; Lewis Gould, ed., *The Progressive Era*, Syracuse, New York, 1974; and George Mowry, *The Era of Theodore Roosevelt*, New York, 1958, pp. 85–105.

advice, such as the recommendation to regard wheat bran and potato skins as "refuse," was unsound. More germane to this context, however, was his dedication to applying nutritional science to practical life. Lay ignorance of protein and energy requirements, he recognized, allowed custom and craving to dictate eating habits, leading people at all social levels to eat too much of the wrong foods, and spend an unnecessarily high proportion of income on food. By heeding Atwater's instruction, though, the public would gain in health by eating fewer sweets and more protein, and in wealth by getting their protein from cheaper cuts of meat and more beans and grain.[11]

Helping the poor through nutritional education was also the mission of the New England Kitchen, a Boston institution opened in 1890 to offer cheap, nutritious food to the city's laboring class. The kitchen did not present formal classes or cooking lessons, but trusted instead in example and exhortation, and did win recognition. Hospitals requested the kitchen's beef broth for their convalescents, and the Boston high schools contracted for the first school lunch program in the country. Similar facilities, furthermore, were spawned in other cities, as far west as Chicago, yet the original object of these kitchens, the urban poor, refused to be educated. The food may have been nourishing, but it was also unappetizing, bland New England staples such as pea soup, corn mush, and Indian pudding dominating the menu. Working class families bred on heartier ethnic fare were likely to agree with the woman who protested, "I don't want to eat what's good for me; I'd ruther eat what I'd ruther." "Scientific nutrition" nevertheless made its way to the masses eventually. The guiding spirit of the New England Kitchen, Ellen Swallow Richards, took her message to higher class women when the poor proved resistant, and it was primarily because of her labors for "euthenics"—whole-

---

[11] Atwater, "Foods: Nutritive Value and Cost," *Sanitarian, 36,* 193–210 (1896) is a concise presentation of his dietary philosophy.

some living through scientific regulation of diet and environment—that the modern home economics movement was born. By the 1920s, home economics teachers were spreading an appreciation of sound nutrition (by now including vitamins) through American colleges, and effecting a significant change for the better in American eating habits.[12]

Unorthodox hygienists of the Progressive years were equally enthused by the recent progress of nutrition, of course, and exploited it for their own ends, but their utilization of science hardly stopped with dietetics. Medical bacteriology was another area of remarkable discovery, bacteriologists having provided, in the short space of the last quarter of the nineteenth century, an understanding, at long last, of the nature of infection. This new science's implications for hygienic ideology were profound—when Holbrook locked horns with female fashion, for example, he did not attack the bulky, ground-length skirts still in style with the crude Grahamite objection that the skirt was too heavy. Rather he forced a gasp from his readers with an account of watching a smartly dressed lady unwittingly drag her skirt "over some virulent, revolting looking sputum, which some unfortunate consumptive had expectorated."[13]

The public's germ consciousness was an appealing target for the new hygiene. Holbrook not only felt a responsibility to transform people's vague fears of microbes and filth into an exact understanding of the nature of bacteria and their modes of transmission, but recognized an opportunity to use that knowledge to promote hygienic philosophy. This was

[12] The poor patron of the kitchen is quoted in Caroline Hunt, *The Life of Ellen H. Richards,* Boston, 1912, p. 124; the New England kitchen is discussed on pp. 121-134. Also see Mary Abel, "Practical Experiments for the Promotion of Home Economics," *J. Home Econ., 3,* 362-366 (1911); Harvey Levenstein, "The New England Kitchen and the Origins of Modern American Eating Habits," *Am. Q., 32,* 369-386 (1980); Edward Kirkland, " 'Scientific Eating': New Englanders Prepare and Promote a Reform," *Proc. Mass. Hist. Soc.,* 86, 28-52 (1974); Robert Clarke, *Ellen Swallow. The Woman Who Founded Ecology,* Chicago, 1973.

[13] *J. Hyg. Herald Health, 46,* 135 (1896).

not just a matter of reminding people that long skirts collected germs and regular bathing washed them away. The whole set of hygienic precepts could be forcefully recommended by the argument that infection was no simple act of contamination, but a dynamic process involving microbe and host. For disease to result, the latter had to provide a suitable culture medium, had to be susceptible. As yet, most physicians were still so excited at having discovered the causative agents of infection that they were paying less than adequate notice to the host. Radical hygienists, however, were bent just as far in the other direction. They were inclined to see bacteria as nearly impotent organisms that throve only in individuals whose hygienic carelessness had made their bodies compost heaps. Tuberculosis is contagious, Holbrook acknowledged, but "the degree of vital resistance is the real element of protection. When there is no preparation of the soil by hereditary predisposition or lowered health standard, the individual is amply guarded against attack." A theory favored by many others was that germs were the effect of disease rather than its cause; tissues corrupted by poor hygiene offered microbes, all harmless, an environment in which they could thrive.[14]

In either case, hygienic extremists were supportive of environmental sanitation. At least for the time being, while the majority of the public lacked full resistance to infection, subjects such as garbage collection and plumbing had to be given space in health journals. But the friendship with sanitation was not merely one of convenience. It grew spontaneously from their genuine mutuality of sentiment that saw health and morality as inseparable. The sanitary reform movement of mid-century had been to a significant degree a project of moral, in addition to medical, rescue. Its leaders had expanded the evangelical equation of ungodliness with uncleanliness to introduce factors of crowding and poverty, and to calculate the moral and physical damage done by

[14] *ibid., 47,* 127 (1897).

miserable living conditions. New York's John Griscom exemplified the sanitationist spirit, introducing his survey of the sanitary condition of his city's laboring population by asking what was the effect of "this degraded and filthy manner of life" upon not only the health and lifespan of slum residents, but also "their morals, their self-respect, and appreciation of virtue." His summation for the implementation of thorough-going public sanitation had as a critical link the argument that a clean population in a decent environment would not be guilty of nearly so much lawlessness, and therefore be less difficult and expensive to govern.[15]

The economic ploy was vital for winning legislative backing of sanitary programs, of course, but for most sanitarians there was a far deeper concern for human lives than dollars. Benjamin Ward Richardson, captain of the second generation of English sanitary reformers, believed that "sanitary science" must continue its campaign against physical disease, but should take as its ultimate goal nothing less than the advancement of "human felicity" by every means possible. In 1875 he even presented blueprints for a city of health—Hygeia—whose citizenry would be as moral as they were healthy. And when twelve years later the American physician Frances White offered her improved plan for the ideal city that could be built by sanitarians, she named it Ethica! The appropriateness of that name was suggested by the title of her address: "Hygiene as a Basis for Morals." Richardson, finally, even planned to write a book elaborating *The Physiology of Sin*.[16]

The book was never written, unfortunately, but the title

[15] John Griscom, *The Sanitary Condition of the Laboring Population of New York*, New York, 1845, p. 11.

[16] Benjamin Ward Richardson, "Felicity as a Sanitary Research," *Asclepiad, 1*, 62–90 (1884); Richardson, *Hygeia, A City of Health*, London, 1876; Frances White, "Hygiene as a Basis of Morals," *Pop. Sci. M., 31*, 67–79 (1887); Lloyd Stevenson, "Science Down the Drain," *Bull. Hist. Med., 29*, 1–26 (1955), p. 13.

alone speaks volumes for the affinity between environmental and personal hygienists in the later 1800s. Their ideological consanguinity was shown in other ways, too. Stevenson has done a masterful study of the motives behind Richardson's and other English sanitarians' opposition to bacteriology and other aspects of the new medical science that rose to dominance toward the end of the century. It was not just an expression of scientific conservatism and resentment at seeing the miasmatic theory (the basis of sanitary reform) supplanted. There was, rather, a religious factor in the "sanitarian syndrome" involving a hatred of any kind of contamination, any impurity, and of any infliction of pain on sentient creatures. Old school sanitarians were thus prominent in the English antivaccination and antivivisection agitations. As those movements spread to America at the end of the century, they won the sympathies of many hygienists. Holbrook's vegetarian beliefs were activated by a more pronounced strain of humane feeling for animals than had been the case with Alcott, and this sentiment spilled over into antivivisectionism. He was convinced, like Shaw in England, that any knowledge gained by mutilating higher animals was not worth the price. Vaccination, on the other hand, he opposed as unnecessary risk taking, when smallpox could be controlled (he supposed) by sanitation and quarantine.[17]

Vivisection and vaccination were but two of the practices of medicine criticized in the late nineteenth century. Therapy also continued to be an object of protest. Although the heroism of standard treatment had declined markedly since mid-century, a prescription was still the reward of any visit to the doctor, and drugless alternatives to healing were appearing in protest. Holbrook published frequent favorable commentaries on the revised water cure system of Germany's Father Kneipp. A combination of baths, herbal teas, and hardening exercises, the system had some vogue in the

[17] Stevenson (n. 14); *J. Hyg. Herald Health*, 45, 276–277 (1895).

1890s before flowing into naturopathy. Holbrook's journal also gave positive notices to osteopathy and "chiropathy" (chiropractic), commending them for not going "to the drug store or ransack[ing] creation for remedies nor load[ing] the blood with poison." But though bathing and musculo-skeletal manipulation were natural and nonpoisonous, Holbrook preferred to give the body complete responsibility for healing itself. Rest and proper diet were the medicines of this doctor who billed himself as a "Hygienic Physician" and censured ordinary physicians for being engrossed with disease rather than health.[18]

Popular discontent with medicine was not so extreme as it had been in Alcott's time, but Holbrook and his comrades did reap some benefit from public suspicion of the effectiveness of therapy, as well as of the motives of physicians. Holbrook's opinion notwithstanding, many physicians of the time were quite interested in preventive medicine, and were even boastful about their newly acquired ability to thwart bacterial invasions with environmental regulation. One manifestation of the ambitiousness of "the new public health" was the campaign waged through the first two decades of the twentieth century to establish a cabinet level National Health Department to conserve the country's human resources. The proposed department's failure to win Congressional approval was due partly to distaste for federal paternalism, partly to lack of organization among its proponents, and not least to a militant opposition that reintroduced the spectre of "medical monopoly." The National League for Medical Freedom drew together worried osteopaths, chiropractors, Christian Scientists, antivaccinationists, antivivisectionists, patent medicine manufacturers, and others fearful of an American Medical Association plot to win total power for the orthodox system of medicine. Progressive health reformers were, as a rule, far less worried about medical designs, and many were outspoken supporters

[18] *J. Hyg. Herald Health, 48,* 54, 232–236, 252 (1898).

of the Health Department plan, but the success of their own ideologies was nevertheless aided by the antimedical mood represented in the League for Medical Freedom.[19]

Another preoccupation of the medical profession that found its way into hygienic ideology was the question of how to deal with the physical effects of stress. Stress management has been made a cardinal feature of contemporary wellness programs. We are constantly being reminded that the pressure-cooker living of the 1980s builds up tensions that have to be regularly released if health is to be preserved. Like most hygienic maxims, the message is not new. Regulation of "the passions of the mind" was Galen's sixth non-natural, and one given heavy emphasis by subsequent hygienic writers down through the Enlightenment. But coping came to take on new dimensions in the nineteenth century, especially in the United States. From the achievement of independence onward, in fact, Americans found themselves wrestling with ambivalent feelings about their country's open political-social system. The precious freedom to get ahead, to capitalize on the main chance, was also responsible for a competitiveness and uncertainty in life that scraped away unceasingly at the individual's mental and emotional reserves. That civilization begets nervousness became a cliché, and it was perhaps unavoidable that as the pace of life quickened, public uneasiness would mount and be translated into medical dogma. Physicians, after all, not only shared the feeling that modern life was nerve-wracking; they also repeatedly encountered patients whose symptoms had no definite pathology but could plausibly be related to the nervous system. Nervousness was a self-fulfilling medical prophecy, and if there was a prophet, it has to have been New York practitioner George Beard. "Neurasthenia," or nerve weakness, was the term Beard applied to what he regarded as the epidemic of advanced civilization. Its manifes-

---

[19] Manfred Wasserman, "The Quest for a National Health Department in the Progressive Era," *Bull. Hist. Med., 49,* 353–380 (1975).

tations were many and protean; his partial list included anxiety, indecisiveness, insomnia, peripheral numbness, "flying neuralgias," variable pulse, sweating hands, involuntary seminal emissions, and every other imaginable imperfection without obvious cause (including ticklishness). By Beard's analysis, neurasthenia was a state of exhaustion brought about by too heavy taxation of the body's nerve force; it was "nervous bankruptcy." To extend his metaphor, civilization always exacted nerve payments, but the rates had gone up spectacularly since the mid-1800s. The telegraph, steamship, telephone, growth of business, and other advances in speed and pressure had added so much to the burden as to make it nearly unbearable. And Americans, as the pacesetters in technological progress, were suffering the most. Beard took the same perverse pride in his country's plight that modern New Yorkers do in the nerve-grating rush and noise of their city. *American Nervousness* (1881), his *chef d'oeuvre*, blared through its title his conviction that no nation on earth approached this one in the degree of its population's nervous exhaustion (and unfortunate as that was, there was considerable satisfaction to be had in knowing that America's nervousness was the proof of its cultural preeminence).[20]

By the 1890s, neurasthenia had been accepted by the American medical community (it did make sense of otherwise baffling clinical experiences), and was being frequently diagnosed. And since, according to Beard, "Nervousness is a physical not a mental state," it could be treated with physical methods. The therapies tested were as numerous as the symptoms they were prescribed for, and could ofttimes be more unpleasant. Beard's later work on the treatment of sexual neurasthenia, for instance, advised bromides (depressants with severe side effects) and, "the most important and efficient remedy," electricity. Both static and galvanic

[20] George Beard, *American Nervousness. Its Causes and Consequences,* New York, 1881, pp. 7–9.

electricity were then popular prescriptions in cases where tonic therapy seemed indicated. Among the forms used by Beard to treat sexual neurasthenia were the static discharging of sparks from the genitals ("franklinization"), and the passage of "mild" currents through electrodes inserted into the urethra and rectum.[21]

The hygiene-minded, naturally, wished for some gentler method of curing or, far better, of preventing neurasthenia in the first place, and the answer was obvious. Alcohol and tobacco were already known to affect the nerves; probably other hygienic abuses depleted the nervous force. Obedience to the laws of health, therefore, would save one's full endowment of nerve energy for parrying the blows of industrial civilization. To be safe, however, it was advisable to take periodic refuge from urban bustle, and to adopt the optimistic outlook advocated by all the theorists of positive thinking who were just then overwhelming the culture. Old hygiene plus New Thought made a perfect remedy for neurasthenia. Holbrook sprinkled discussions of nervous exhaustion and mental suffering liberally over his journal's pages, and early in his career even wrote an entire book on mental hygiene to explain how physical purity and control of the passions would cure nervousness.[22]

What America was to the rest of the world in the neurasthenia hierarchy, woman was to man. Beard accepted his period's assumption that woman has an "impressible, susceptible organization" that makes her show the effects of any physical or nervous irritation sooner than man. "In civilized lands," he conjectured, "women are more nervous, immeasurably, than men, and suffer more from general and special nervous disease." Another remark hit even closer to hygienists' convictions: "The weakness of woman is all modern, and

[21] ibid., p. 17; Beard, Sexual Neurasthenia, New York, 1898, pp. 218, 224, 249–250.

[22] Martin Luther Holbrook, Hygiene of the Brain and Nerves and the Cure of Nervousness, New York, 1873.

it is pre-eminently American." Here hygienists and physicians still agreed; the American woman, a pathetic enough specimen early in the 1800s, had continued to fall until by the last third of the century she had been reduced to "a haggard creature, dull-eyed and sallow, pinched in form, an unfit mother, not a helpmeet, but a drag on the energy, spirits and resolution of her partner in life." The respected New York physician Augustus Gardner attached to this dreary portrait an analysis of causes that dripped vitriol. From the day she was taken from swaddling clothes, he gibed, the American woman was handled like a doll, kept from the sun and breeze, fettered by laces and petticoats, bred for late suppers and dances. And if she managed to escape to boarding school, it would only be to soon tumble into the deadliest trap of all, the "moral epidemic" of self-pollution that ravaged "pubescent, hot-bed brought-up girls."[23]

But if a renovation of her personal hygiene was to be declining woman's salvation, her social role had to be kept unchanged. Doctors and hygienists differed sharply with feminists on the meaning of "the new woman." The aggressive, competitive women who had deserted the home for the marketplace and lecture room and other male preserves were, despite their still small numbers, a bothersome lot by the late 1800s. Health theorists were as upset as other men by these emancipated females, and had no desire to restore the remaining weaker women to health if they intended to exercise that health outside their proper sphere. Fortunately for hygienic strategy, the attempt of women to use their health in masculine ways would eventually result in its loss. A final cause of female neurasthenia, Beard claimed (and most agreed), was the greater cerebral activity of American women and their determination to compete against men (who had innately superior nervous stores). If the "new

---

[23] Beard, *American Nervousness* (n. 18), pp. 185, 207, 336; Augustus Gardner, *Conjugal Sins Against the Laws of Life and Health*, New York, 1870, pp. 199–237.

woman" were to be a healthy woman, therefore, she would have to be a woman in the old role: it was the possession of health that would make her new. Alcott had already cast female hygiene in that mold, but the issue had been far less pressing in the 1840s than half a century later. Holbrook and his contemporaries were much more likely to accompany commentaries on woman's health with comforting pledges that heightened vitality would not be expended in agitating for suffrage. "When the new woman comes," an apologist for outdoor exercise for females promised, "we may be assured that she will be the same sweet, pure, lovable creature on whose shrine we have through endless ages respectfully laid our laurels."[24]

Women hygienists were among those lovable and respectable creatures. Holbrook employed a Jennie Chandler to write the monthly "Hygiene for Women" column in his journal, and she spared no effort to impart to her readers an understanding of all aspects of female health. But she was careful to see the proper end of that health was understood as well. It was not, Chandler protested, to make women like men. Doctors were eagerly seconding that motion. "No woman should forsake an infant for a quadratic equation," a typically overwrought physician warned. Women's pursuit of the same higher education as men, at a period of life when their reproductive systems were maturing toward their grand biological destiny, had to be a major source of female debility. Harvard Medical School's Edward Clarke had given the most influential statement of that position in his 1873 *Sex in Education*. And there was still much respect in the 1890s for his charge that female scholars were vulnerable to seismic disruptions of their "periodic phenomena," including hemorrhaging "that would make the stroke oar of the University crew falter." Chandler was less graphic on

[24] Beard, *American Nervousness* (n. 18), p. 137; Francis Nash, "A Plea for the New Woman and the Bicycle," *Am. J. Obstet., 33*, 556–560 (1896), p. 560.

that point, offering only that "the effort does harm to both health and character." But she was adamant about the uniqueness of women and the necessity of directing hygiene toward the enhancement of feminine characteristics: "The true conception of woman's rights is the right to that which is the best for her as a woman, the right to the very best education and training which her nature requires."[25]

The highest element of her nature, of course, was the maternal, and here Progressive health reformers repeated earlier doctrine, but with redoubled effort. Like their Jacksonian predecessors, they placed special value on female health because of its implications for future generations. To Progressives, however, the stakes seemed higher. Not only had half a century passed with no discernible improvement. There was the new discovery that the modern woman was likely to give birth to fewer children. Contraception and abortion were believed to have risen sharply in recent years, and the 1890 census provided alarming corroboration. The birthrate among the better, Anglo-Saxon, segment of society was revealed to be declining, setting off the cries of "race suicide" that sounded with ever rising volume through the Progressive years. And all the blame could not be stacked upon condoms and abortifacients; surely infertility, miscarriages, and stillbirths could result from corsets, alcohol, and masturbation.

While emergency was the message of the census, hope and power were the bywords generated by the spread of Darwinian biology. Darwin and his popularizer Herbert Spencer did more to reshape the American mind in the late nineteenth century than any other thinkers. Evolutionary theory worked remarkable change in all fields, in science, philosophy, psychology, sociology, political science, history,

[25] Hamilton Osgood, "The Need of a Radical Change in the Education and Training of the American Girl and the Physician's Duty Therein," *Boston Med. Surg. J.*, *104*, 289–292 (1881); Edward Clarke, *Sex in Education*, Boston, 1873, p. 67; Jennie Chandler, "A New Education for Women," *J. Hyg. Herald Health*, *44*, 139–140 (1894).

anthropology—and in hygienic ideology. Spencer made a particularly deep impression on the last area, and not surprisingly, for his writings on education and evolution stamped him as a man kindred in spirit, if not practice. No matter that he had rejected vegetarian diet after a six months trial, believing it lowered his "energy of both body and mind." That error of detail was insignificant within the grand structure of his total philosophy. Spencer valued physical vitality as the source of all happiness and accomplishment in life; his apothegm that "the first requirement to success in life, is to be a good animal" became one of the two most adored shibboleths of Progressive hygienists (the other was *mens sana in corpore sano*). Spencer stressed the necessity of man conforming to nature, recognized the preservation of health as a "duty," and denounced "all breaches of the laws of health" as "physical sins." He scoffed at the notion of illness "as a visitation of Providence," and called on the individual to make his own health and virtue through energetic action. And he modernized these long-cherished principles by setting them within an evolutionary framework. Little wonder that Holbrook (and fellow reformers) believed that, "without doubt," Spencer's philosophy "is the grandest intellectual attainment of this and perhaps any century."[26]

A special attraction of Spencerian thought was its maintenance of the assumption of the inheritance of acquired characteristics, the hypothesis so vital to Jacksonian health ideology. Its employment in that pre-Darwinian period had already, in fact, given a quasi-evolutionary bent to hygiene. The transmission of acquired parental health to offspring had been trusted to accomplish the steady perfecting of the human race over the course of generations, until the ultimate man would, in terms of appearance and health, be al-

[26] Herbert Spencer, *Education: Intellectual, Moral and Physical*, New York, 1881, pp. 57, 103, 282–283; Martin Holbrook, *J. Hyg. Herald Health*, 47, 22 (1897).

most a different species. But *The Origin of Species,* appearing in 1859, introduced a new factor, the mechanism of natural selection, the drama of survival of the fittest. Attainment of the Grahamite world of perfection had required, in theory, the conversion of every last individual to hygiene. It was hoped even the most degenerate might eventually be educated and exhorted into righteousness, but that could take ages, and there really was nothing to keep the unreconstructed from perpetuating themselves indefinitely and conceivably holding back the millennium forever. With the addition of natural selection, though, hygienists acquired a competitive advantage for their kind. Health was fitness to survive; it was strength and endurance and alertness for the struggle. Yet while physical wrecks were individually at a competitive disadvantage, they could still reproduce, and their far greater numbers kept them in the contest and held progress to a crawl. What was needed was the reformation of a critical percentage of the weaklings. Then their ranks would be so thinned as to allow natural selection to operate much more rapidly. Nature would soon weed out completely those who resisted hygienic teaching; "Nature does not forever perpetuate her 'nubbins.' " Conversion of every single person would not be necessary, and the process of human perfection would be accelerated. Holbrook quoted with evident glee Alfred Russell Wallace's aphorism that, "The survival of the fittest is really the extinction of the unfit."[27]

But Progressive hygienists spent much less time pondering the automatic workings of nature than they did speculating about the possible effects of voluntary human action on evolution. For them, the most thrilling prospect opened by the Darwinian revolution was what Wallace denominated "human selection." By that he meant sexual selection in which attractiveness was measured in terms of health, intelligence, and purity. In a society educated to

[27] J. Hyg. Herald Health, *43,* 202 (1893); *ibid., 44,* 240 (1894); *ibid., 45,* 264 (1895).

prize those qualities, Wallace hypothesized, "the man of degraded taste or of feeble intellect, will have little chance of finding a wife, and his bad qualities will die out with himself. On the other hand, the most perfect and beautiful, in body and mind, the men of spotless character and reputation, will secure wives first, the less commendable later, and the least commendable latest of all. As a natural consequence, the best men and women will marry the earliest, and probably have the largest families."[28]

Wallace was described by an interviewer as "leaning forward in his chair with a flushed and eager face" while relating all this, but his excitement was restrained next to that of hygiene reformers who saw "human selection" as the culmination of their dream of hereditary perfectibility. "Take a part in your own evolution," pleaded Holbrook. Select a mate of sound inherited constitution and impeccable hygienic habits, pass your superior health on to your children, and natural selection will do the rest: this was the millennial health message as revised by Darwinism. It presupposed, of course, that acquired characteristics—the pure blood and bounding energy won by meatless, wine-free living—were indeed inherited. Even the determination to tie physical inheritance to the conditions of parents down to the very minute of conception persisted. Trall, for example, reported the sad histories of several families in which parents were normally in good health, and had produced fine children—except for their first born, who were all idiots. "Why? Because of the feastings and dissipations of the wedding occasion" (followed the same evening, according to romantic mythology, by conception of the couple's first child).[29]

Inheritance of acquired characteristics retained its position in biological theory to the end of the century. Darwin

[28] Alfred Russell Wallace, "Human Progress: Past and Future," *Arena*, 5, 157 (1892).

[29] *J. Hyg. Herald Health, 43*, 202 (1893); Russell Trall, *Sexual Physiology*, New York, 1881, p. 257.

himself devised a theory, "pangenesis," to integrate that hypothesis with evolution, and Spencer made acquired characteristics an essential part of his philosophy. The idea was not to be seriously challenged until the 1890s, when the German zoologist August Weismann began receiving a hearing for his studies on chromosomes and his assertions of the independence of hereditary matter from any somatic alterations. Changes imposed upon the body by habit or accident, Weismann realized, did not affect germ cells; acquired characteristics were not inherited, the germ plasm had its own separate, continuous existence. The lesson was only slowly learned, though. As Rosenberg has pointed out, "The absolute distinction between the innate and the acquired was a concept so novel, so contrary to traditional common sense, that it was not generally assimilated until the second decade of the [twentieth] century."[30]

The hold of the inheritance of acquired characteristics was further strengthened by its agreement with Victorian ideals of social progress. Unlike Weismann's deterministic genetics, which made the individual a product of chromosomes beyond his parents' influence, the transmission of acquired traits allowed the benefits of individual actions and environmental changes to be passed to the next generation and carry society on an ever upward path. The force of that attraction was to be tragically demonstrated in the 1930s and 1940s by the Soviet Union's official sanctioning of Lysenko's genetic theories because they agreed with socialist environmentalism. But nineteenth-century hygienists were just as aware of the implications of acquired characteristics. Holbrook voiced an uneasiness many felt when he commented on Weismann's work: "In our opinion if acquired characters were not in some degree inherited there would be little progress." Hygienists wanted human progress, and they

---

[30] Charles Rosenberg, "The Bitter Fruit: Heredity, Disease and Social Thought in Nineteenth-Century America," *Perspect. Amer. Hist.*, 8, 189–235 (1974), p. 225.

wanted people to feel that mistreatment of their bodies amounted to mistreatment of their children and their children's children. Abandonment of the inheritance of acquired characteristics was ideologically difficult, and health reformers clung to it as long as they possibly could.[31]

That loyalty required either stubbornness or ingenuity. Holbrook made a transition from the one to the other. He at first doubted the validity of Weismann's work, suggesting that his experiments in which amputation of the tails of mice through several generations had failed to bring about any inherited shortening of the tail had not been conducted for a long enough period of time. As late as 1894 he congratulated Spencer for having "completely refuted Weismann's theory and . . . [I think] we shall not soon hear any more of it." Just over a year later, however, Holbrook found himself publicly approving Weismann's basic points. More careful consideration of the new theory persuaded him that "education and training do not seem to affect the germ cells in any marked degree." That admission was part of his address to the 1895 Greenacre [Maine] Conference of Evolutionists, a summer symposium adorned with some of the brightest names in evolutionary science. John Fiske, the philosopher who did so much to reconcile religion and evolution, was a participant. So was Edward Cope, an evolutionist who differed with Darwin on major elements of theory, but whose fossil collections were used to support Darwinian ideas. Spencer was unable to attend, but submitted a paper through a colleague. That Holbrook was invited to join such a company indicates that he had some standing as an authority on the interrelations of evolution and hygiene.[32]

His Greenacre remarks on "Evolution's Hopeful Promise for a Healthier Race" present his own mind in evolution from a reliance on the direct inheritability of acquired

---

[31] *J. Hyg. Herald Health, 43,* 23 (1893).

[32] *J. Hyg. Herald Health, 43,* 22 (1893); *ibid., 44,* 112 (1894); *ibid., 45,* 192 (1895); Martin Luther Holbrook, *Stirpiculture; or, the Improvement of Offspring Through Wiser Generation,* New York, 1897, p. 151.

health characteristics to a more subtle accommodation of that hope with Weismannian reality. Much of the talk was a bland reserving of Darwin and Wallace and sexual selection as applied to personal hygiene. It acknowledged that no longer could it be expected that an individual's tighter muscles and expanded lungs and happier stomach would be automatically stamped upon his germ plasm. Specific physical qualities acquired through careful hygiene were no more hereditary than the shortened tails imposed by experiment. That did not, however, mean the door had been completely closed to the genetic transmission of acquired health. "That any gain to the vigor of the constitution can be transmitted to the offspring," Holbrook stated without elaboration, "is very probable"; the germ cells may be immune to the acquisitions of education and training, but "nutrition does affect them."[33]

Precisely what was meant by those generalizations was left unstated at the Greenacre Conference, but Holbrook returned to these themes and developed them in later writings. The key to salvaging hygiene as a hereditary force was to generalize, he saw. Pro-Weismann arguments had concentrated on distinct injuries and malformations: mice did not acquire shorter tails because ancestors had had their tails clipped; the Flathead Indians of the Northwest were not born with elongated foreheads even though their progenitors for centuries had had their heads flatened. Similarly, Holbrook was ready to admit, a bicep enlarged by exercise would not be passed from father to son. But though there was no connection between the bicep and the germ cells, those cells were both a product and a component of the body, and had to be affected by their blood supply. The quality of blood, in turn, was determined by nutrition, by the molecules derived from food. As the germ plasm was high in nitrogen-containing compounds, Holbrook postulated, there must be an adequate supply of nitrogen, or protein, in the diet. Protein de-

[33] Holbrook, *Stirpiculture* (n. 30), p. 151.

ficiency would not produce any specific injury, such as a scrawny bicep, but it had to lower the general strength of constitution of any children, because "the highest form of germ plasm" could not be formed. Malnutrition of germ plasm could as readily result from lack of fresh air and deep breathing. Metabolism, affecting all body cells, including the reproductive ones, required larger amounts of oxygen that could be inhaled by sedentary people spending their lives indoors. Alcohol, also, "in its circulation in the blood, penetrates every part; not even the germ plasm escapes." As a "nervine stimulant," alcohol was responsible as well for "defective nutrition of the nervous centres of the cerebral and spinal substance, during the entire uterine career." And finally, Holbrook had a special concern for chastity. He dedicated an entire book to the subject of the *Physical, Intellectual and Moral Advantages* of sexual purity, presenting it as a necessity for the upward evolution of the race, and maintaining that unchastity damaged reproductive cells. Studies of "the number of spermatozoa in those persons who have lost their virility by excess," he announced, "showed a very great reduction, and the quality also was inferior."[34]

Thus in general, nonspecific sense, "the health of the germ plasm" did depend "on the health of the parents"; not acquired characteristics, but acquired constitution was hereditary. With this nice bit of theoretical juggling, Holbrook was able to maintain his allegiance to Spencer after all, and agree with the English philosopher that parents transmitted "surplus vitality" to children. This inheritance of acquired constitution strategy also provided a solution to the Darwinian dilemma of the conflict of natural selection with humanitarianism. Civilization had developed social and medical measures to save the lives of many who, in a state of nature, would have been quickly eliminated. But by aiding

[34] *ibid.*, pp. 172–174; Holbrook, *Marriage and Parentage and the Sanitary and Physiological Laws for the Production of Children*, New York, 1882, p. 136; Holbrook, *Physical, Intellectual and Moral Advantages of Chastity*, New York, 1894, pp. 59–60.

the survival of the inherently weak, man was lowering the overall fitness of his species. Human moral efforts to benefit the race seemed antagonistic to nature's method, and one had to wonder if the health and improvement of the species necessitated a heartless abandonment of the feeble to the inexorably harsh workings of natural selection. Holbrook's answer of no, explained at length in his Greenacre address, was a simple deduction from the premise that general vitality is hereditary. If weaklings now kept alive by social and medical assistance will heed the rules of health, their descendants will become progressively less weak and the need for survival assistance will eventually disappear. Unfitness can be bred out humanely by hygiene, instead of ruthlessly extirpated by natural selection.[35]

It was nevertheless desirable to encourage a higher reproductive rate among the more fit, and in *Marriage and Parentage* Holbrook advanced a meticulously planned program of accelerated evolution through "sanitary marriage" or "physiological marriage." Proper breeding of humans, he held, required couples to accept the generation of healthy offspring as a social obligation, and to refrain conscientiously from producing children unless they could meet the criteria for sanitary parentage: "For the most physiological marriage we must insist that the father have a good frame, well-developed muscles, a strong heart, energy, ambition, and thoughtfulness; and the mother good digestion, pure, rich blood, good sense, strong love for home and children, and a highly moral nature." The ideal ages for the physiological paragons were thirty to forty for the father, and twenty-five to thirty-five for the mother, and their height differential should be about three inches, in favor of the male. The taller spouse must also be broader across the shoulders, but his mate should have wider hips. Yet Holbrook was sufficient realist to recognize "it would be Utopian to insist that none should marry" unless able to satisfy those exacting and

[35] Holbrook, *Stirpiculture* (n. 30), pp. 146–147, 169.

precise standards. For the while, at least, indifferently endowed individuals might be permitted to reproduce, provided they did all in their power to preserve the middling health they had and educate their children to rise higher. But even for the short run, parenthood was out of the question for invalids or for two people with constitutional tendencies to the same disease or physical deficiencies of the same kind.[36]

Late nineteenth-century advances in biology thus forced alterations in the internal structure of hygienic ideology, yet did not divert it from its millennial orientation. Hygienic evolution must eventuate, Holbrook was confident, in a race of "children of nature, joyous, happy" to whom pain and disease would be unknown; hospitals and jails would survive only as monuments to "an age of ignorance and sin." Perfected agriculture would eliminate any need for animal food, women would dress for health instead of fashion, and "ONE OF ITS GREATEST JOYS WILL BE THE FACT THAT UNCHASTITY WILL BE UNKNOWN." Moreover, "The art of living will then be the greatest of all studies" and "death will not be dreaded."[37]

That higher stage to be reached was also somewhat revised, though, from the millennium of Jacksonian health reformers. The perfect future of hygienists of the Progressive years was still Christian, but, as in schemes of Progressive reformers generally, religious purposes were not so dominant. It was theologically a more sophisticated age, less given to fundamentalist and enthusiastic expectations. Its millennium was more of a utopia, more a secularized kingdom of man than the kingdom of God. Progressive hygienic ideology reflected this changed intellectual environment, so that while it did not reject the moral and religious concerns of an earlier day, it subordinated them to more worldly considerations. One of the more pressing of these was the matter

---

[36] Holbrook, *Marriage and Parentage* (n. 32), pp. 40–43, 63–66.
[37] Holbrook, *Physical . . . Advantages* (n. 32), p. 112.

of racial degeneration. Darwinism had created a consciousness of species, an awareness of well-being at the level of race. It was generally accepted, in Europe as well as America, that the human race was deteriorating, becoming ever weaker in body and mind. Therefore to the old injunction to be healthy as a duty to God, there was now added the obligation to be healthy for the sake of the race, to turn around the decline of the species and cooperate with evolution to achieve genuine progress. The "racial betterment" and like slogans that became so familiar during the Progressive decades ostensibly applied to the human race, but were actually understood by most to have special reference to the Anglo-Saxon strain of the race. Hygienists rarely expressed their belief in Anglo-Saxon superiority with the blatancy of a Grant or Stoddard, but they nevertheless shared the eugenicists' dismay with the declining birthrate of that group and their fear of the apparently feeble-minded and degenerate races of southern and eastern Europe that were pouring through the immigration gates. The yellow and black perils made them nervous as well, but at the same time they held, with other Progressives, to Christian and democratic traditions of helping the disadvantaged. For most health reformers, it would have been out of character to elect the coercive and punitive tactics of sterilization of the unfit and immigration restriction favored by eugenicists. Elevation and assimilation of alien elements was their preference, and not just because it was more civilized, but because it seemed more likely to work. Sanitary marriage and physical perfection might take longer than sterilization, but in the end the race would be standing on a higher plane.

Race retained its double meaning throughout this analysis, though. Human selection and sanitary marriage were to be furthered by education, so only the literate and conscientious class of society would participate in the first stage of advance. Once renovated, they would, by teaching and personal example, carry the message of health down through the remaining layers of society. That this trail-blazing class was

Aryan went without saying. When Holbrook appealed to health educators to make a special effort to teach hygiene to blacks, he justified it with the reminder that evolution had not carried that race "so far from the animal as it has the white." Within the immediate context of American society at the turn of this century, the concept of health as duty to the race was therefore double-faceted: it meant first that the Anglo-Saxon element should regenerate itself, and secondly, that that purified remnant should then rescue the less blessed (and potentially race destroying) portions of humankind.[38]

The new society awaiting the perfected race was not (any more than it had been for Grahamites) an uncivilized Eden. Progressives had an anit-urban bias born of the dirt and crime and foreign population of the slums, and an advanced case of nostalgia for the solid, unchanging virtues of the countryside. But as Schmitt has shown, the Arcadian myth enthralling the Progressive mind was given expression in forms that meshed nature with industrial civilization. Country clubs and landscaped cemeteries were not expeditions into the wilderness, or even a return to the farm: "few seemed frustrated in the suburbs because they could not raise chickens." Arcadianism was tempered by a fascination with technology as a new frontier. Applied science had already demonstrated a power to remove inconveniences and to simplify life which gave Progressive hope that technology could be used to cut through the injustices and jumble of modern civilization and restore a simple natural harmony to life. Thus, as civic reformer William Allen phrased it, the good life was to be found not by returning to nature, but by pursuing "Nature Fore":

> Gifts as well as problems are seen to come with complexity, and civilization flatly refuses to relinquish these gifts. Sound maturity is better than youth or age. . . . Problems of health and of civics can never be solved by appealing to

[38] *J. Hyg. Herald Health, 47,* 192–193 (1897).

Nature Back, when only the few could be healthy, when one baby in three died in infancy, when old age was toothless and childish, when infection ravished nations, when the average life was twenty years shorter than now, and when unspeakable filth was tolerated in air, street, and house. They can all be solved by appeals to Nature Fore, which holds up an ideal of mankind physically able to enjoy all the benefits and to conquer all the dangers of civilization. It is not looking back, but looking in and forward that reveals what natural law promises to those who obey it.[39]

That the present industrial world was so unsatisfactory was not the fault of industry and technology, but of the rapacity of previous human directors of those forces. The ruthless and selfish robber baron had to be replaced by a moral businessman who succeeded through honest work and self-discipline, who truly earned his wealth and used it responsibly. Progressives believed there could be such a thing as ethical acquisition, a "Christian capitalism" that through economic expansion created new opportunities and prosperity for the rest of society. Business success could be hailed as a contribution toward the elevation, rather than subjugation, of one's fellows, and selfishness made respectable since it furthered the interests of the race as a whole. The Progressive devotion to a cult of material (but moral) success was inevitably mirrored by hygienic ideology, and a chair in the boardroom became a regularly promised reward of healthful living.[40]

The connections between hygiene and success in business (and other fields) were clear enough. The climb to the top demanded strength, determination, and mental acuteness, all qualities long associated with correct physiology. But

[39] Peter Schmitt, *Back to Nature. The Arcadian Myth in Urban America*, New York, 1969, p. xvi; William Allen, *Civics and Health*, Boston, 1909, pp. 399–400.

[40] J. G. Cawelti, *Apostles of the Self-Made Man*, Chicago, 1965.

more than anything else, to the Progressive mind, it required the new power of efficiency. Originally a technical-mechanical concept, and a commonplace and unassuming one, efficiency expanded into a social gospel at the end of the nineteenth century. The appeal of efficiency grew apace with social critics' awareness of the corruption and waste in industry and government, and then with the bureaucratic and managerial ethic fostered by Progressive reform. By the early 1900s, reverence for efficiency had pervaded every cranny of society; it had become a word to conjure with. Efficiency in business, government, or any other endeavor was accepted as a moral responsibility, the *sine qua non* of effective labor. And conversely, inefficiency, wastefulness, any squandering of resources, signified an immoral self-indulgence that would lead to corruption. A college dean was merely echoing well-established popular philosophy when he advised that, "efficiency and morality may not be synonymous, but they are mighty good chums."[41]

Efficiency had always been chummy with physiology, too. Although they did not use the term, Jacksonian health reformers aimed at improving physical efficiency by eliminating the stimulants that placed a wasteful drain on vitality. As efficiency advanced as a distinct attribute at the end of the century, though, hygienists became almost absurdly self-conscious about saving the body from any unnecessary activity. Holbrook's women's editor, Jennie Chandler, warned that "economy of strength" would be lost by such unthinking acts as scratching the head, tapping the foot, frowning, gritting the teeth, and other useless motions. "The body is a bank and the currency is the various kinds of energy," she explained. "You cannot spend the nickels and dimes of energy too freely without finding the total large enough to cramp your activities in the large things of life." Her physical-fiscal analogy was well adapted to Progressive

---

[41] Thomas Hunt, quoted by Charles Rosenberg, *No Other Gods, On Science and American Social Thought,* Baltimore, 1976, p. 141.

hygienic ideology. Hygienists could approach the body as health accountants, evaluating function in terms of deposits of food and rest, and withdrawals of exertion and self-neglect. The quantity, and quality, of the deposits and withdrawals would determine the degree of physiological wealth, and wise management would yield efficiency of operation— maximum production with minimum waste. And since increased capacity for work improved one's chances for success, physical efficiency actually did translate into fiscal efficiency. Even stripped of its economic meaning, the "efficient life" was more valued by hygienists than the "strenuous life" so commonly associated with the Rooseveltian age. As YMCA leader Luther Gulick saw it, "To be strenuous is no end in itself. It is only when being strenuous is an aid to efficiency that it is worth while."[42]

The anticipated product of physiological efficiency was, aside from his financial success, much the same as his Jacksonian predecessor: strong and energetic, intellectually agile, morally upright, and dedicated to lifting all fellow creatures to his level. He was expected to be a good Christian as well, but his religious characteristics were muted, and he was in fact frequently placed on a pagan pedestal. Progressive society was captivated by the Greek ideal of harmonious physical and mental development. "A healthy mind in a healthy body" was a generally popular formula with which hygienists differed only in the degree of health they imagined the body and mind could achieve. Thus overall, despite the significant differences in their individual programs of physical salvation, Progressive health reformers spoke a *lingua franca* in which the crucial adjectives were natural, harmonious, evolutionary, successful, and efficient.

[42] *J. Hyg. Herald Health, 44,* 75 (1894); Luther Gulick, *The Efficient Life,* New York, 1909, p. 50.

☆☆☆☆☆☆☆☆☆☆☆☆☆☆☆☆☆☆☆☆☆☆☆☆☆☆☆☆☆☆☆

CHAPTER SIX
PHYSIOLOGIC OPTIMISM

☆☆☆☆☆☆☆☆☆☆☆☆☆☆☆☆☆☆☆☆☆☆☆☆☆☆☆☆☆☆☆

NO ONE SPOKE THE LANGUAGE OF PROGRESSIVE HYGIENIC ideology with more fluency and charm than Horace Fletcher. That alone would qualify him to serve as the main representative of the style of radical hygiene that had evolved by the beginning of this century. But Fletcher deserves the spotlight as much for his impact on the public, fellow hygienists, and health scientists as for his typification of a new mode of thought. And certainly not least among his credentials for special consideration is the fact that his was no ordinary health reformer's life, soured by chronic illness and impoverished by asceticism. Fletcher, in fact, lived one of the few hygienic lives that might excite general envy.[1]

Born in Lawrence, Massachusetts in 1849, he submitted to a conventional childhood until age fifteen. Then shipping out on a whaler, he visited feudal Japan (establishing a lifelong love for the country) and China at the close of the Tai-Ping rebellion (somehow wandering into brief membership in a crew of Chinese pirates). Some schooling at Dartmouth followed, then more travel in the Orient, and finally marriage and temporary settlement in San Francisco. There

---

[1] This chapter is a condensed version of an article, "'Physiologic Optimism': Horace Fletcher and Hygienic Ideology in Progressive America," *Bull. Hist. Med.,* in press. For details of Fletcher's life, see Horace Fletcher, *Happiness as Found in Forethought Minus Fearthought,* New York, 1898, pp. 8–15; Arthur Goodrich, "The Philosophy of an Adventurous American," *American Mercury, 62,* 198–203 (1906); *The National Cyclopedia of American Biography,* vol. 14, supp. 11, New York, 1910, pp. 39–40; *Dictionary of American Biography,* vol. 6, New York, 1931, pp. 464–465.

Fletcher amassed his fortune by manufacturing ink and importing Japanese art and other merchandise. He also became well-known in San Francisco society as a talented painter, all-around athlete, and exceptional marksman. In the early 1890s, the restless Fletcher moved on to manage a New Orleans opera company, to serve as art correspondent for the Paris edition of the New York Herald, and try his hand at other tasks. By 1898, he had circled the world four times and could recall thirty-eight distinct occupations; and he had yet to embark on his career as a hygienist. He was living by then in a thirteenth-century palace on Venice's Grand Canal, but he issued forth regularly for lecture tours and global adventuring such as hacking through Phillipine jungles and hiking through Himalayan blizzards. His grand tour of life continued until 1919, when he died in Copenhagen following exhausting welfare work in Belgium.

As his love of variety suggests, Fletcher had a considerably less rigid personality than most hygienic evangelists. Contemporaries almost invariably bowed to him as "Mister Horace Fletcher," described him as robust and cheerful, and characterized him with such friendly images as "Santa Clause without the whiskers." Thus while Fletcher shouldered the light man's burden, he carried it with an uncommon ease, with little of the deliberate earnestness that stiffened his counterparts. In their juvenile ebullience, his hygienic expositions often sound like those of *Arrowsmith*'s Almus Pickerbaugh, but they are generally free of the stern pietism with which Pickerbaugh restrained his. And Fletcher was as congenial in practice as in preachment. He warned of the dangers of alcohol and tobacco, but he also admitted to an occasional cigar, or glass of wine, or even cocktail, and did not consider himself damned for the indulgence.[2]

[2] Frances Bjorkman, "Horace Fletcher and Fletcherism," *Independent, 64*, 623–626 (1908), p. 624; Horace Fletcher, *Fletcherism, What It Is*, New York, 1913, pp. 32–35; Isaac Marcosson, "Perfect Feeding of the Human Body," *World's Work, 7*, 4457–4460 (1904), p. 4458.

He nevertheless had courted damnation, in a physical sense, by the excesses of his early life. By age forty gourmandism had bloated his once athletic five-foot seven-inch frame to an unwieldy 217 pounds. Overweight, dyspeptic, constantly plagued by "that tired feeling," and subject to frequent attacks of influenza, he came to feel like "a thing fit but to be thrown upon the scrap-heap."[3] When his application for a life insurance policy was denied, Fletcher resolved to regain his health, and his transformation from *bon vivant* to health reformer began. The discovery of his specific reform, however, was to take some time, and to be arrived at circuitously. At the same time his body was being rejected by the insurance company, Fletcher's mind was being swamped by the wave of positive thinking that rolled over America at century's end. By nature a man of action and an optimist, Fletcher was attracted by the supposition that obstacles are imaginary and a person can do whatever he believes he can. The offspring of his analysis of mind power was *Menticulture* (1895). This first book was pedestrian psychology, even by New Thought standards, but in his unabashed offering of banalities disguised as profundities Fletcher completed the first rough draft of his design for health. At this stage, mental and emotional health was his preoccupation. He cheerfully assured readers that clearness of thought, peace of mind, calmness of behavior and other rewards unlimited awaited those who would take the simple step of immediately purging their minds of the two roots of all evil passions: anger and worry. Most of the book was given to repetitious exhortations to be happy and to descriptions of the glorious state that would follow "Mental Emancipation." It is in these descriptions that Fletcher reveals the already Progressive frame of mind that would endure through his transition from mental to physical hygiene.

Menticulture was regarded by its formulator as the

[3] Quoted in Michael Williams, "Horace Fletcher's Philosophy," *Sunset, 24,* 284–290 (1910), p. 286.

surest method of building a "Twentieth Century Hope," of restoring to purity an America whose "Democracy has become an Oligarchy of Greed." (Fletcher had a Germanic strain in his soul compelling him to capitalize important words). He several times expressed admiration for Edward Bellamy's *Looking Backward* (1887), the remarkably popular account of the socialist utopia of the year 2000. With Bellamy he deplored the waste and brutality of *laissez-faire* capitalism, and longed for a society in which all citizens were assured employment and a fair share of the fruits of their labors. Where Fletcher broke with Bellamy was on the question of the means to these ends. Bellamy's mechanism of "the reaction of a changed environment upon human nature" was the reverse of Fletcher's conviction that human nature could be easily changed, by Menticulture, and the new nature would react upon environment. For Bellamy's socialism, Fletcher substituted "altruism." "We will catch up with Mr. Bellamy's prophecy," Fletcher prophesied, "long before the time specified in *Looking Backward,* by the simple unravelling of a silken skein of endless possibilities from the free end within ourselves."[4]

The assertion that industrial abuses were not inevitable products of the capitalist system but only temporary expressions of perverted human nature, was characteristic of Progressive hygienic ideology, and allowed hygienists to reconcile the two goals of social justice and individual success. In the manner of "welfare capitalism" economists, Fletcher argued that modern industry could produce such an abundance of goods "that a moderately sensible distribution of them would render every inhabitant comfortable and happy." And menticultured minds, freed of anger and worry, would gladly assent to a sensible distribution of goods. But the assurance of a generous minimum standard

[4] Horace Fletcher, *Menticulture, or the A-B-C of True Living,* Chicago, 1898, pp. 135, 154–158; Edward Bellamy, *Looking Backward, 2000–1887,* New York, n.d. (Random House), p. 225.

of living for all should not prevent individuals from striving to become more comfortable and happy. "Greedy ambition" was despised by Fletcher as the most base of passions and the source of social degeneracy, but when cleansed of greed, ambition became noble: "Neither must friendly rivalry, nor ambition to excel, be classed as aggressions; as they are phases of growth." Rather than a vice, the desire for success was a natural trait intended to spur each person to the realization of his potential. Capitalism could be a game of courteous competition in which there were no losers, but some could deservedly win more than others. And the transition to the new order seemed so easy. It required only the denial of one's evil passions (greedy ambition) and then joyous pursuit of the natural instinct to succeed. "Human nature is good nature," Fletcher allowed, "if freed from fear and restraint, and if it seem profitable to be good there is a double incentive." Elsewhere he wrote, "The practical benefit of the emancipated mind to the individual, and of the emancipated individual to the community, can not be overestimated. In every walk in life Emancipation is invaluable to the worker, and the most potent aid to success. The emancipated peanut vendor will have more customers than his worm-eaten neighbor. The emancipated merchant will find that trade will pass the door of his calamity-howling rival and come to him."[5] The worm-eaten neighbor and calamity-howling rival suffered, it is clear, not because of any unfairness in the competitive system, but because they had not yet emancipated themselves so they could be winners too.

The link between emancipation and success was efficiency. Likening the body to a power plant, Fletcher proposed eliminating the circuits of worry and anger and hooking the Divine Spark (vital energy) to lines running to good thought and acts. One did not have to be an electrical engineer to appreciate the switchover would allow the plant to "perform every duty better, and with less fatigue."[6]

[5] Fletcher, *Menticulture* (n. 4), pp. 19, 37, 39, 65.
[6] *ibid.*, pp. 19–20, 49.

Beyond such hints about the mechanisms of success, Fletcher gave little attention in this first work to the matter of physical health. His nearest approach was a passing observation that his digestion had improved since emancipation, and perhaps the perfect health hoped for by Christian Scientists was a possibility.[7]

The sequel to *Menticulture* appeared three years later under the name *Happiness as Found in Forethought Minus Fearthought.* True to its effervescent title, *Happiness* was an optimistic rehash of his first book. Its only advance beyond the earlier work was the identification of fear as the "taproot" of anger and worry, and the assurance that it was the evil emotion which had to be eliminated before full happiness could be attained. But aside from promising that "a healthy mind insured a healthy body," Fletcher moved no closer to the subject of physical hygiene.[8]

Now addicted to writing primers on life, and to exercising his gift for cryptic titles, Fletcher soon presented *That Last Waif or Social Quarantine* (1898) to the public. This was an attack on the complacent assumption that a sizeable segment of the population must always be poor, and a plea to begin the eradication of poverty and the evils it engenders by rescuing and nurturing neglected and abused children. Only when the last waif has been saved, Fletcher preached, can society rest satisfied that justice has been done and a higher plane of living achieved. The institutional and procedural details of the system of social quarantine were left hazy, though Fletcher did identify the kindergarten as a central agency. One who read only *That Last Waif* must have supposed the author fancied himself a sociologist rather than a physiologist. Yet his leap to physiology had already been taken during the preparation of that book, and with time Fletcher came to see social quarantine as an outgrowth of nutrition. The preface to the 1903 edition of *That Last Waif* included several provocative suggestions, such as that

---

[7] *ibid.,* p. 36.
[8] Fletcher, *Happiness* (n. 1), pp. 29, 90.

"many of the *worries* of existence take their everlasting flight from the atmosphere of the rightly nourished," and that "health, morals, temperament, physical efficiency, and all the requirements of virtue and good citizenship could be mended or modified by mere attention to the ingestion of food and more careful eating."[9]

This preface was as obscure about the precise relation of nutrition to good citizenship as the text was about the particulars of waif rescue. But other works published in the interim had subjected the connection of eating with ethics to careful scrutiny—and made Fletcher, if not a physiologist, at least a physiological *cause célèbre*.

The physical Fletcher has been left in search of a remedy for obesity and related ills. In 1898, various "cures" having failed him, he turned to reading books on hygiene, particularly with an eye toward the relation of eating and health. One aspect of that relation which he surely discovered before reading very far was the necessity of careful mastication of food. Americans' haste in eating had been a subject for reproachful humor since the Revolution at least. "We *do not* bolt our food," Alcott protested in the 1850s, "but *throw* it down our throats. . . . We seem to be in a perpetual strife with each other to see who can throw nearest the walls of the aesophagus without hitting!" Holbrook, following four decades after, complained of the frequency of "buccal indigestion" caused by infrequent chewing, and saw "slow eating" as "one of the most necessary hygienic reforms of the time."[10]

Fletcher nevertheless seems to have become committed to mastication only after determining its value through personal reasoning and experience. He was unable, he claimed, to find a consensus regimen in the writings of the supposed

[9] Fletcher, *That Last Waif or Social Quarantine*, New York, 1903, pp. xii, xxvi.

[10] William Alcott, *Lectures on Life and Health*, Boston, 1853, p. 57; Martin Holbrook, *J. Hyg. Herald Health*, 45, 8 (1895); *ibid.*, 46, 152 (1896).

experts on hygiene, and so "determined to consult Mother Nature herself."[11] This consultation was primarily an exercise in "Mother Logic" (common-sense reasoning about the designs of Mother Nature), and allowed Fletcher to display his simple and complete faith in the wisdom and goodness of nature. The discoveries to which he was led by his logic were to be described and redescribed in a series of books of such titles as *The New Glutton or Epicure* (1903), *The A. B.—Z. of Our Own Nutrition* (1903), and *Optimism. A Real Remedy* (1908). Together with the previously mentioned works, these comprised what Fletcher dubbed the "A. B. C. Life Series," a set of encyclopedias of self-help sufficiently popular to require several printings for most volumes.

Pared to its fundamentals, Fletcher's philosophy of perfect living was indeed nearly as simple as A B C. It was woven from two premises: nature does not err, so that any condition lower than the highest health is due to human transgressions of natural law; and the physical basis of full health is proper nutrition. Therefore, employing Mother Logic, nutritional sins are committed while food is in the mouth, since once swallowed, it passes into the control of unsinning nature. In the upper end of the alimentary tract, "the three inches of personal responsibility," there are several natural powers subject to abuse: appetite, taste, saliva, and mastication. Appetite is nature's announcement of fuel and repair requirements, and has qualitative as well as quantitative instructions. One should eat only when appetite urges, select the food or few foods which seem especially appetizing at that moment, and eat only so long as appetite remains a strong impulse. The second power, taste, is nature's gift of pleasure in nutrition, and one should keep every food item in the mouth until the last trace of taste is extracted. Foods and beverages naturally try to linger on the tongues of even the most wolfish, and can almost be heard supplicating: "I am tasty; don't you want to taste me:

[11] Fletcher, *Fletcherism* (n. 2), p. 5.

When I am swallowed my gustatory charm is dead and gone forever; please let me leave my taste with you, good Mr. Taste."[12]

Saliva is the first agent of digestion, and would not have been provided unless nature wanted it mixed thoroughly with food before swallowing. Salivation is also a signal that natural appetite is aroused. The final agent, mastication, is nature's mechanism for mixing saliva and extracting taste.

As convincing as this exposition of nature's genius was on paper, it still had to be given the practical test. In mid-June 1898, Fletcher weighed about 205 pounds and carried a waistline of 44 inches; by mid-October, as a result of systematically masticating his one daily meal until every bit of taste was withdrawn, he had dropped to 163 pounds and a waist measurement of 37 inches. His nagging ailments had also fallen along the way and he had gained in their stead an energy and eagerness for activity that had been lost for twenty years. The experiment also uncovered still more of nature's provisions for full nutrition. Careful mastication, for example, withdrew delightful new taste sensations from foods. Taste was more intense and prolonged, and built to a climax unknown to careless chewers, an "indescribably sweet flash of taste, which Taste offers as a *pousse café* to those who serve it with respect." Of more physiological import, as thoroughly chewed food was reduced to a creamy pulp, it naturally flowed toward the back of the mouth where, as the last bit of taste was released, it was suddenly and involuntarily swallowed, naturally sucked into the body. The swallowing impulse, Fletcher decided, was nature's means of assuming responsibility for food once mouth preparation was complete. As experience demonstrated that the reduced food was not always swallowed completely, but that sometimes a nonliquefied sediment was left behind and had to be expelled into the napkin, Fletcher was led to discover nature's "Food Filter," the body's power to discrimi-

[12] *ibid.*, p. 121.

nate between nutritious and innutritious matter and reject the latter.[13]

The cooperation of these various digestive agencies largely comprised what Fletcher termed "head digestion." But it was also clear that digestion was affected by one's mental-emotional state, so the practice of forethought was needed to complete proper head digestion. The final proof of correct head digestion, though, was derived from the other end of the alimentary tract, in the form of "tell-tale excreta." Ideally, it would seem, there should be no excreta to tell tales. Nature's food filter effectively prevented any innutritious material from being swallowed, and complete chewing assured total digestion of swallowed material. Experience, however, even Fletcher's, proved otherwise, and it was necessary to admit defecation as a normal function. One could nevertheless distinguish the usual from truly physiological feces, and the distinction held such fascination for Fletcher as to almost make him a coprophiliac. Some of his most eloquent, nearly rhapsodic, passages are in his discussions of the properties of "Economic Digestion Ash," a phrase adopted not as a euphemism (Fletcher prided himself on being free of prudery), but as a concise summary of the virtues of proper digestion. Perfect excreta resembled ash by being small in proportion to the quantity of food consumed. Fletcher even maintained that most fecal material was not waste from food, but was composed of detached particles of intestinal mucosa and condensed solids of used digestive juice, what he imaginatively called "dandruff of the alimentary canal." So slowly would such ash accumulate, further, that a healthy individual would feel nature's urge to evacuate only every six to ten days, and even then the quantity expelled should not exceed two to four ounces.[14]

Ash was an appropriate term also because healthy excreta were almost dry and, apparently most important in

[13] Fletcher, *The New Glutton*, New York, 1903, pp. 182, 188–190.

[14] *ibid.*, pp. 73–83, 142–150; Fletcher, *The A. B.-Z. of Our Own Nutrition*, New York, 1903, pp. 10–12; Fletcher, *Fletcherism* (n. 2), pp. 93–94.

Fletcher's view, odorless. Bacterial decomposition was presumed to occur only in intestines fouled with hastily chewed and swallowed food. "Offensive excreta," he pronounced, "are quite certain evidence of neglect of the self-controllable parts of our own nutrition.... HEALTHY HUMAN EXCRETA ARE NO MORE OFFENSIVE THAN MOIST CLAY AND HAVE NO MORE ODOR THAN A HOT BISCUIT." Fletcher attached extraordinary value to cleanliness, and seems to have regarded hygiene as a kind of internal sanitary reform. As early as his New Thought period, he had compared people who insist on discussing disagreeable topics to sewers, and averred that, "Every time I think of anything mean I fancy I can smell it." Hence odor, and taste, became for him a measure of naturalness. Good taste in food was ecstatically hailed as one of nature's highest gifts, and the disappearance of taste regarded as the sign of completed mastication. An unusually resistant green onion once parried more than seven hundred chews before surrendering to Fletcher's swallowing impulse, and his first observation about the "tussle" was that no onion odor was left upon his breath. Those, on the other hand, who stopped short of the requisite number of mastications, were repeatedly chastised for letting "dirt" into their bodies and warned of the "sewer gas" that would be generated by indigestion. By this esthetic rule, natural feces could not be malodorous. But for final persuasion of any who lacked his conviction of nature's daintiness, Fletcher presented experimental proof. He unblushingly published an objective scientist's eye-witness account of two of his evacuations, with the witness's testimony that all criteria of perfect digestion ash were met.[15]

---

[15] Fletcher, *The A. B.-Z.* (n. 14), p. 11; Fletcher, *Happiness* (n. 1), pp. 187–189; Fletcher, *The New Glutton* (n. 13), pp. 127, 147–150, 203. Fletcher's habits of eating relatively small amounts, selecting foods of low fiber content (milk and potatoes were favorites), and rejecting any food constituents he could not chew to pulp all encouraged small, dry, infrequent stools. He claimed not, however, to experience the difficulty of evacuation one would expect of constipation.

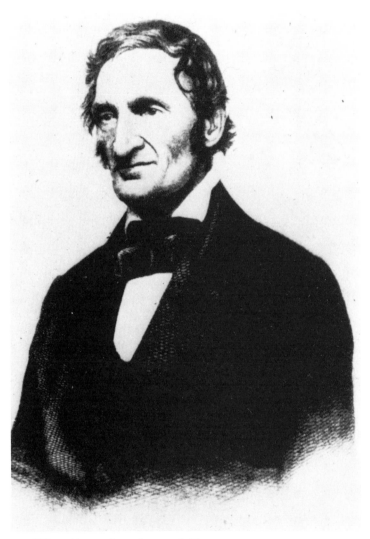

1. William Alcott, about the age of fifty.

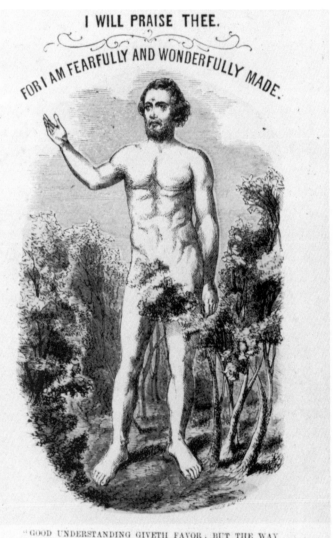

2. Frontispiece from Larkin Coles, *Philosophy of Health*, Boston, 1857, exemplifying the health reform philosophy of Christian physiology.

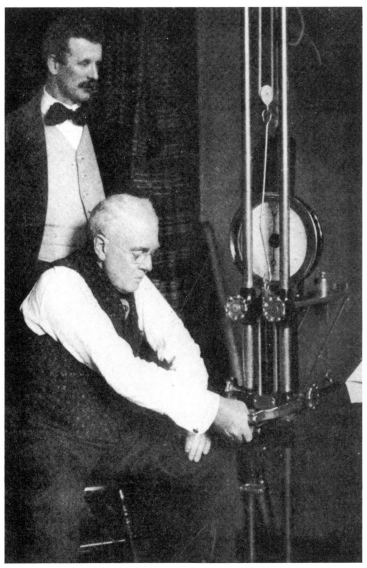

3. Horace Fletcher taking one of the endurance tests supervised by
   Yale gymnasium director William Anderson (background).

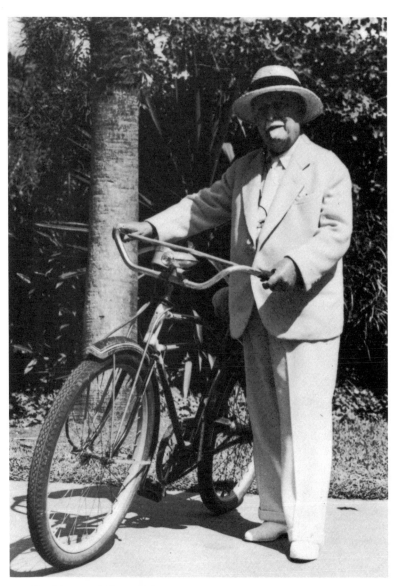

4. John Harvey Kellogg, M.D.

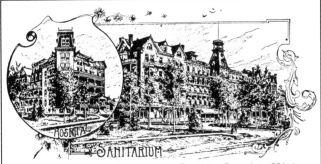
5. Ad for Kellogg's Battle Creek Sanitarium.

6. Ad for Protose, one of Kellogg's meat substitutes manufactured for the vegetarian market.

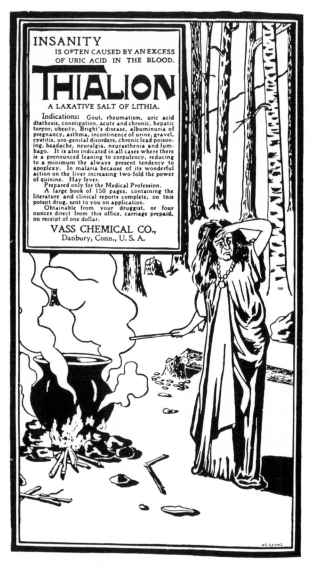

7. Ad for Thialion, the most aggressively promoted of the many uric acid solvents.

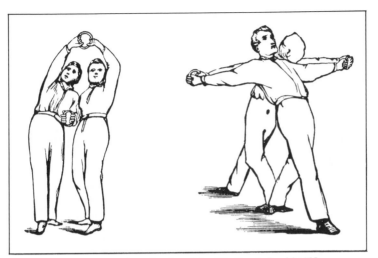

8. Two of the ring exercises developed by Dio Lewis for his "New Gymnastics."

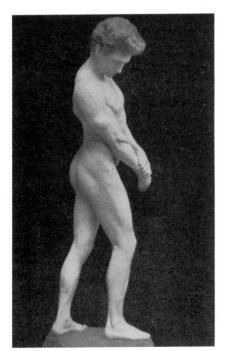

9. Bernarr Macfadden displaying the fruits of physical culture.

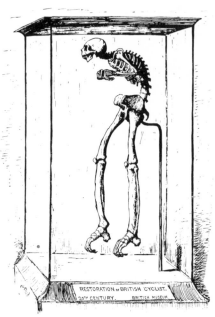

10. Anticycling commentary from *Punch*.

A WARNING TO ENTHUSIASTS.

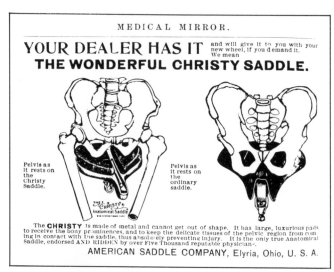

11. Ad for one of the most popular makes of "anatomical" bicycle saddles to relieve perineal pressure and consequent injury.

That ash was also described, it will be recalled, as "economic," an apt term certainly for any digestive system that produced so little waste, but one with far broader implications for Fletcher. "Economic" suggested "efficient," and total efficiency was the ideal he had held in view from his first formulation of menticulture. Indeed, efficiency assumed a religious significance for him. He warned that food should never be "carelessly and dirtily served," but "treated as if it were incense on the sacred altar of Highest Efficiency." On another occasion, when a member of the New York Academy of Medicine questioned the propriety of his phrase "Dietetic Righteousness," Fletcher responded in "righteous indignation": "By George! . . . Is there anything more sacred than serving at the altar of our Holy Efficiency?" Experimental study of his own physical health, however, had led to an awareness of the inefficiency of unnatural digestion and the conviction that menticulture itself rested on a physical basis of proper digestion. By 1903, Fletcher was defining menticulture as "the discovery that the best mental results could not be accomplished in a body weakened by any indigestion, any mal-assimilation of nutriment, any excess of the waste of indigestion." Contemplation of the beauties of economic digestion ash could move him to beg readers to ask themselves: "With All Eternity ahead of me, cannot I afford at least 1/48 of my time [the estimated time needed for thorough mastication] for careful feeding of my body in a manner known to favor physical health; mental keenness; firmness of character; enjoyable temperance; sexual vigor without morbidity. In fact, general respectability and efficiency?"[16] It is not pure facetiousness to credit Fletcher with a revived and unprecedentedly ambitious *Dreckapotheke.* How else might one describe a complete prescription for successful living derived from human excreta?

Discussions of the individual and social effects of the pre-

[16] Fletcher, "Appetite and Hunger," in Olympian Society, *The Olympian System of Physical and Mental Development,* 4 vols., Chicago, 1919, 2:195–203, 199; Fletcher, *Fletcherism* (n. 2), p. 128; Fletcher, *The A. B.-Z.* (n. 14), pp. xxi, 5.

scription are scattered through Fletcher's writings. The most concise presentation is to be found in *Optimism. A Real Remedy*, the 1908 work where his penchant for grandiloquent terminology was given its freest rein. His optimism, Fletcher explained, was fundamentally the same as William James' "Meliorism," and might be more accurately denominated "Physiologic Optimism." It surpassed the "Halfblind Optimism" of Christian Science by admitting the existence of evil (but offering a means to escape evil) and by fixing attention on health instead of disease. Though its blending of "Forethought" and "Physiologic Mastication" was now familiar, physiologic optimism promised some startling individual and social transformations. As individuals achieved perfection of physical efficiency, they would become immune to disease and longer-lived by at least twenty years. And when death came, it would be a peaceful crossing. With a healthy, pain-free body and a mind rid of fear, one might even welcome death as a "promotion" along "the road of evolution." Over the course of generations, furthermore, that evolution would carry masticators "towards higher and higher supermanhood."[17]

As supermanhood was approached, physicians would no longer be required, at least not as therapists, and doctors would perforce become "directors of health and consultants in hygiene." Efficient health would be its own reward, and the means to still higher ends. Not only would the consumption of less food save one at least one dollar a day, but the resultant health would be something that one might "use in his business and profit by," and which might end "if not in money itself, in the power to earn money." Again the apology for this apparent selfishness was that it gave one the power to help others, though now Fletcher called it "Altruistic Opportunism." Already its power had been demonstrated by converts such as the young woman whose initial

[17] Fletcher, *Optimism. A Real Remedy*, Chicago, 1908, pp. 43–44, 77; Fletcher, *Fletcherism* (n. 2), pp. 134, 173.

failures as an authoress had pressed her into the darkest pessimism, down even to the consideration of suicide. At virtually the last moment, she discovered physiologic mastication: "Rest, recuperation, health, renewed energy, successively developing bright ideas, progressively marching popularity, remunerative authorship, congenial matrimony. This was the sequence. The seemingly helpless girl became queen of a happy household, and she is the envied of Fame."[18]

Suppose, Fletcher concluded, that "all the world should reverse the lever of its thought-automobile, should stop its backward motion in thinking, and should use its collective power to go ahead instead of astern.... What would happen?" For once, his imagination was stymied; the possibilities were too brilliant to be clearly seen, but would undoubtedly exceed, he crowed, anything yet dreamed even by Jules Verne. And the road to that glorious future was already being cleared, according to his closing embellishment, by the swelling army of appreciators of "physiologic enlightenment," seekers after "the millennium of nutrition normality."[19]

At the head of these enlightened comrades was Hubert Higgins, a surgeon and demonstrator of anatomy at Cambridge University. Higgins met Fletcher in 1901, at a time when he had been suffering for years with "goutiness" and excessive weight. Ripe for conversion, he became a Fletcherite and watched his weight plummet from 282 to 178 pounds while his health rose as dramatically. Higgins' gratitude and acquired insight were expressed in *Humaniculture* (1906), a wok whose text fulfilled all the optimistic implications of its title, but that nevertheless had a more reasoned and controlled tone than Fletcher's treatises on the sociology of swallowing. His more sophisticated style, his deep exploration of buccal anatomy for the purpose of demonstrat-

---

[18] Fletcher, *Optimism* (n. 17), pp. 15–16, 28, 53, 57, 64.
[19] *ibid.*, pp. 76–79; Fletcher, *Fletcherism* (n. 2), 79.

ing the operation of a swallowing impulse, and his relative indifference toward the economic implications of correct chewing imparted an air of respectability to the book. Yet the work was also unsettling for its intimations of the racial consequences of neglecting proper nutrition. Fletcher often dropped ominous hints about degenerate slum children and diluted stock and growing pauper and criminal classes, but never fastened on racial decline as the overriding evil to be conquered by hygiene. Higgins, however, began and ended his book with warnings of the urgency of arresting racial decay, and haunted the interim pages with spectres of lunatics and "inefficients." To be sure, it was tame beside many degeneracy scare sheets, but the work still confronted the reader with an emotionally charged threat, then cooly directed him to see natural nutrition as his escape. At one point humaniculture was defined as "the all-inclusive science of Human Physiology"; at a later one, it was "the golden science of perfect man." Guided by this science, America could realize its destiny of greater-than-Athenian glory, and to facilitate that rise a "Department of Humaniculture" should be established in the federal government. Higgins even outlined the work of the department's officers (most of them to be physicians educated to prevent rather than cure), and declared that "the discovery of the principles and practice [of humaniculture] will lead on to the millennium."[20]

Higgins' passion was hardly the characteristic response of biological scientists to Fletcher, but a surprising number did yield him respectful attention and even some measure of tribute. Indeed, rarely, if ever, has a lay health reformer been given so positive a reception by scientific luminaries, and had such impact on scientific opinion. Physiologists and biochemists, after all, were occupied with questions of efficiency too, and their curiosity was naturally aroused when

[20] Fletcher, The New Glutton (n. 13), pp. 226–235; Hubert Higgins, Humaniculture, New York, 1906, pp. 170, 215, 217, 231–235, 242, 247. Also see Higgins, "Is Man Poltophagic or Psomophagic?," Lancet, 1905 (i), 1334–1337, 1417–1419.

Fletcher suddenly appeared announcing himself as a virtuoso of efficiency—and bearing documentation to prove it. Fletcher himself was unaware at first of the extent of the powers mastication had given him. Logic might have suggested that natural digestion should allow his body to do more with less food, but just how much more had to be revealed by experience. In 1897, a year before the launching of his dietary experiments, Fletcher had succumbed to the bicycling craze that had been the rage throughout the decade. He even took up daily riding, but found that a run of as much as fifty miles (a relatively easy jaunt for serious wheelmen) left him exhausted. His cycling was apparently soon abandoned, until the summer of 1899, a year after his discovery of economic digestion. Then, finding himself in Paris on the Fourth of July, Fletcher decided to observe his homeland's birthday by bicycling to an artist friend's studio near Fontainebleau. The going was so easy that he cycled some miles with his friend, then returned awheel to Paris the same day. To his amazement, he realized he had accomplished more than one hundred miles (the century run so prized by cyclists) without fatigue, and without muscular soreness the following day. This revelation of the physiological efficiency of his nutritional practice moved Fletcher to issue himself a greater challenge. In August, with no special training in the interim, he celebrated his own birthday (his fiftieth!) by pedalling one hundred and ninety miles, and was so free of fatigue and stiffness as to ride another fifty miles the next morning. In subsequent trials, he demonstrated an astonishing power to move easily from long periods of inactivity to the performance of demanding feats of endurance. A certain amount of this physical improvement can be accounted for by the loss of excess weight following his adoption of careful mastication, but his ability to forego training and still outperform trained athletes half his age must transcend simple weight loss. Fletcher apparently had an exceptional natural athletic prowess, freely exercised in his youth, then submerged by middle-aged obesity. As the fat receded, however, his genius for endurance returned to the surface and, coupled with zeal for demonstrating the benefits of mastication, enabled him to shatter the conventions of physical conditioning.[21]

Fletcher's climb to scientific attention began in November 1900, when he made the acquaintance of Dr. Ernest Van Someren, a self-described "young and obscure general practitioner" of Venice. Being already engaged in dietary experimentation in an effort to relieve his own illness, Van Someren was intrigued by Fletcher's claims. He tried Fletcherizing, quickly benefited, joined Fletcher in experiments on others, and in less than a year was standing before the British Medical Association offering a detailed physiological rationale for the importance of mastication, the action of the swallowing reflex, and the inoffensiveness of his evacuations. While his address met with the predictable skepticism, it also roused the interest of Sir Michael Foster, the renowned professor of physiology at Cambridge University. Consequently, Fletcher and Van Someren travelled to Cambridge late in 1901 in order to have their claims tested by Foster and Frederick Gowland Hopkins, professor of physiological chemistry (and eventual Nobel Prize winner). Their findings, derived from the study of a number of volunteers (including physicians), were that the Fletcher system created an appetite for simple foods in small amounts; allowed healthy functioning on a caloric intake less than half the value commonly taken; brought about improvement in the "sense of well-being" and in "working powers"; and produced smaller, less objectionable stools. Foster felt compelled to stress, however, that the experiments had lasted only a few weeks, and should be extended and made more thorough before the findings could be regarded as anything more than preliminary. The Cambridge laboratories, he regretted, lacked the equipment and funds for a conclusive study.[22]

---

[21] Fletcher, The New Glutton (n. 13), pp. 84–100.

[22] Ernest Van Someren, "Was Luigi Cornaro Right?," Brit. Med. J., 1901 (ii), 1082–1084, p. 1082; Michael Foster, "Experiments Upon Human Nutrition," in Fletcher, The A. B.-Z. (n. 14), pp. 48–52.

Among the laboratories that were suited for an adequate investigation was that of Russell Henry Chittenden, the director of the Sheffield Scientific School of Yale University and the pioneer in physiological chemistry in the United States. Chittenden learned of Fletcher through correspondence with Foster in 1902, invited Fletcher to New Haven, and actually entertained him in his home for several months, all the while subjecting the cooperative Fletcher to close physiological study. Part of Chittenden's investigation was a measure of his subject's physical fitness, supervised by William G. Anderson, M.D., director of the Yale Gymnasium and a commanding figure in the period's physical education-physical culture revival (Figure 3). Just two years earlier, Anderson had published in a popular magazine his views on "the making of a perfect man." There he presented his belief that the ideal of physical and intellectual vigor could be reached only from a foundation of rigorous physical training and proper nutrition, both to be observed through the entire life span. He was particularly insistent on the possibility of maintaining strength and endurance in advanced years, and so must have felt fully vindicated as a prophet by the time Fletcher left his gymnasium. Putting the fifty-four year old hygienist through four days of the Yale University Crew exercises (he regarded rowing and football as the most demanding and effective programs of physical training), he was, as he modestly phrased it, "surprised." Fletcher, Anderson continued, had performed the exercises "with an ease that is unlooked for. He gives evidence of no soreness or lameness and the large groups of muscles respond the second day without evidence of being poisoned by carbon dioxide. . . . Mr. Fletcher performs this work with greater ease and with fewer noticeable bad results than any man of his age and condition I have ever worked with."[23]

[23] Hubert Vickery, "Biographical Memoir of Russell Henry Chittenden, 1856–1943," *Nat. Acad. Sci., Biographical Memoirs, 24,* 59–104 (1947), pp. 80–81; Russell Chittenden, "Physiological Economy in Nutrition," *Pop. Sci. M., 63,* 123–131 (1903), p. 130; William Anderson, "The Making of a Perfect Man," *Munsey's M., 25,* 94–104 (1901). For ad-

Anderson's surprise turned to amazement four years later, when Fletcher returned to New Haven for a second battery of tests. Now approaching his fifty-ninth birthday, and for some reason twenty pounds heavier than he had been in 1903, Fletcher could hardly have been expected to equal his previous performance. Instead, he surpassed it, and in one test, a measure of the endurance of the soleus and gastrocnemius muscles, he actually doubled a Yale student record! The student record, moreover, had been established by an athlete in training, but Fletcher insisted he ignored physical training (a claim confirmed by his statistics of five-feet seven and one-half inches height, one hundred seventy-seven pounds weight, and seventy-five resting pulse rate). Anderson marveled that never in his thirty-five years as a physical educator had he "tested a man who equalled this record. . . . What seems to me the most remarkable feature of Mr. Fletcher's tests is that a man nearing sixty years of age should show progressive improvement of muscular quality merely as the result of dietetic care and with no systematic physical training."[24]

Anderson was not alone in his puzzlement. As the result of Fletcher's exploits, in fact, the relation of dietary practice to muscular endurance had already become a question of excited debate among physiologists. Anderson supposed the phenomenon might be explained easily, as "due to moderation in living." Fletcher agreed, though he would have substituted "efficiency" for "moderation" and claimed his unusual endurance was but the normal expression of nature

---

ditional biographical information on Chittenden, see George Cowgill, "Russell Henry Chittenden," *Science*, *99*, 116–118 (1944); Howard Lewis, "Russell Henry Chittenden (1856–1943)," *J. Biol. Chem.*, *153*, 339–342 (1944); and E. Neige Todhunter, "Russell Henry Chittenden," *Alabama J. Med. Sci.*, *2*, 337–341 (1965).

[24] William Anderson, "Observations on the Results of Tests for Physical Endurance at the Yale Gymnasium," *N.Y. Med. J.*, *86*, 1009–1013 (1907); Russell Chittenden, "The Influence of Diet on Endurance and General Efficiency," *Pop. Sci. M.*, *71*, 536–541 (1907), p. 541.

freed from excess indigestible food. He went even further, unfortunately, offering a quaint refinement of theory that blamed too much protein in the diet for a "putrid decomposition" which released carbon dioxide which caused muscular fatigue. One might "throw off or burn up the mephitic products" by regular strenuous exercise, or one might prevent their formation in the first place by giving "careful buccal treatment" to a diet low in protein. Then the body "is always in training," naturally, and has no need for artificial regimens of exercise.[25]

Fletcher's scientific innocence is patent, even without his citation of alcohol as an example of "superabundant proteid." But his concern for the amount of protein eaten was the reflection of a sophisticated scientific discussion that he had kindled, and which was being led by Chittenden. The professor of physiological chemistry had been amused by the layman's faith in "some hypothetical deglutition center," and had realized that the significant feature of Fletcher's chewing and swallowing was not the mechanism but the quantity of food. "To me the chewing business became unimportant," Chittenden recalled in later years, "except in so far as it tends to diminish the craving for food and thus results in the appetite being satisfied by a small amount. Hence to me the center of interest shifted at once to the question, how much do we really know as to the amount of food the human body requires to meet daily needs under the different conditions of life, especially of protein food? ... These were the thoughts that led to my planning the investigation."[26]

These investigations, still hailed by nutritionists as a "revolution" in their science, ended in a drastic reduction of

[25] Anderson, "Observations" (n. 24), p. 1013; Fletcher, "Possible Progressive Growth in Muscular Efficiency After Fifty Years of Life Without Systematic Physical Exercise," N.Y. Med. J., 86, 1005–1009 (1907), p. 1008.

[26] Fletcher, "Possible Progressive Growth" (n. 25), p. 1008; Chittenden quoted by Vickery, "Biographical Memoir" (n. 23), p. 81.

188 ★ PHYSIOLOGIC OPTIMISM

the estimated protein requirement. Prior to meeting Chittenden, Fletcher had never worried himself about the quantity of protein, or calories, in his diet. Trusting nature to request all that was needed, he had cheerfully chewed his way through a diet that averaged only about forty-five grams of protein and, he claimed, 1600 calories per day. His ability to maintain vigor on such Spartan fare, however, defied nutritional canons. Authoritative standards ranged from 118 to 165 grams of protein per day, depending on the authority. The most respected was that of Carl von Voit of the University of Munich, who suggested 118 grams a day for men of moderate activity, and 145 grams for hard workers (including, presumably, men undergoing varsity crew exercises). The belief that a high protein intake is essential for health was so firmly embedded in scientists', and the public's, minds that "the words nutritious and nitrogenous are almost synonymous." But the Voit and other standards had been arrived at simply by the analysis of the food actually consumed by people who could afford to eat as much as they wanted. That method was open to objection on logical grounds—it is invalid, indeed naive, to assume people's appetites will constrain them to eat only as much as their bodies require—and on empirical grounds. Even before Fletcher burst upon the scene, several studies had reported cases of seemingly healthy people maintaining nitrogen equilibrium on as little as 25 to 50 grams of protein daily. The Swedish physiologist V. O. Sivén drew particular attention, and denunciation, with his claim of health on 25 to 30 grams, and the Copenhagen physiologist Mikkel Hindhede had also begun his experiments of maintaining himself on a largely potato diet containing only 15 to 20 grams of protein per day. But it was Fletcher who finally brought about sober reconsideration of the protein standard, by the impression he made upon Chittenden. So forceful was that impression, that Chittenden launched his reevaluation of protein needs by adopting a Fletcher-like diet himself, in spite of warnings from physician friends. And far from experiencing the predicted deterioration, he found himself suffering less from a rheumatic ailment of his knee, indigestion, and "sick headaches," and actually growing in strength and endurance (while losing about sixteen pounds weight). In the meantime, Chittenden had also procured funds from a number of sources (both the National Academy of Sciences and Horace Fletcher were among the contributors) to finance an elaborate study of the effects of low protein diet on sedentary workers (Yale professors), moderate workers (U.S. Army volunteers), and heavy workers (Yale athletes). Between autumn 1903 and summer 1904, each group lived, for periods ranging from five to eight months, on a diet containing less than half the Voit protein allotment. There was no medical evidence of decline in health among the participants, and gymnasium tests revealed a significant rise in strength over the course of the experiment. One of the athlete volunteers, Gymnasium Director Anderson's son, even won two national gymnastic championships while on the diet.[27]

The study convinced Chittenden that most people consumed much more protein that was required, and that the excess was an unnecessary tax that lowered body efficiency. The mechanism by which superfluous protein inhibited strength and endurance could not yet be explained with certainty, but Chittenden was clearly quite comfortable in his own mind with the theory that the products of protein catabolism inhibit muscular function. He also feared these metabolites might injure the nervous system, and was sure they must overburden the liver and kidneys. Chittenden's

[27] Vickery, "Biographical Memoir" (n. 23), pp. 80–82; Elmer McCollum, *A History of Nutrition*, Boston, 1957, pp. 191–196; Chittenden, "Physiological Economy" (n. 23), p. 129; W.D.H., "Physiological Economy in Nutrition," *Nature, 73*, 328–330 (1906), p. 328; Chittenden, *Physiological Economy in Nutrition*, New York, 1904, pp. 4–17, 440; V. O. Sivén, "Zur Kenntnis des Stoffwechsels beim erwachsenen Menschen, mit besonderer Berücksichtigung des Eiweissbedarfs," *Skan. Arch. für Physiol., 11*, 308–332 (1901); Mikkel Hindhede, *Eine Reform Unserer Ernährung*, Leipzig, 1908.

rationale for lowered efficiency was considerably more elegant physiologically than was Fletcher's, but his underlying premise was the same: nature rebels at extravagance. The title selected for his book reporting the study—*Physiological Economy in Nutrition*—might just as well have been used by Fletcher for any of his works.[28]

One man's economy, it soon became apparent, is another man's parsimony. Chittenden's conclusions fueled a lively controversy in which his observed results of improved health were attributed to general dietary temperance and a regular schedule, or were scorned as unlikely to continue over a longer period of time. The debate was too involved to be explored here except to note that while the question was argued on a scientific plane beyond Fletcher's reach, discussion nevertheless frequently echoed his concerns for efficiency, productivity, and racial vigor. Chittenden repeatedly warned that, "there is no more important question before the medical profession today than how to increase the efficiency of the individual and of the race," and felt that overnutrition was a massive obstacle blocking "that high degree of efficiency which every enlightened man desires to attain." Therefore it was a "menace to the health and welfare of the human race as [serious as] many other evils more striking in character," even "alcoholic drink." Impropriety with protein was responsible for financial, as well as physical, inefficiency, and Chittenden could envision a marvellous train of social benefits that might follow a 50 percent reduction in purchases of that most expensive class of foods.

The saving to the community, to the family, might well amount to enough to constitute the difference between pauperism and affluence. . . . Further, there is ground for

---

[28] Chittenden, *Physiological Economy* (n. 27), pp. 455–470; Chittenden, *The Nutrition of Man*, New York, 1907, pp. 208–209; Chittenden, "Economy in Food," *Century M., 70*, 859–871 (1905); Chittenden, "The Importance of a Study of Nutrition," *Am. Med., 10*, 816–818 (1905), p. 817.

thought in the possible economy of time which an improved condition of health would result in for the working members of the family. If greater economy in diet will diminish the number of sick days in the year, thereby increasing the working power of the wage earner, . . . the economic value of the proposition is at once apparent. Finally, happiness and contentment, which usually appear in direct proportion to the health and prosperity of the individual, may be counted upon as becoming more conspicuous in the life of the community.

Elsewhere he predicted mental and moral progress for the race as well.[29]

But although Chittenden's promise of a happier world had limited effect on the actual level of protein consumption by Americans, his experiments did force reconsideration of the daily protein recommendation, and a lowering of its value until finally he was vindicated. The present official protein allowance is essentially the same as the figure established by Chittenden in his investigations—investigations that had been inspired by Fletcher.[30]

Fletcher's influence on Chittenden was paralleled by the impact he had on other individuals and groups concerned for Americans' health. Foremost among these was Chittenden's Yale colleague Irving Fisher, the respected professor of political economy. Fisher's involvement with Fletcher might eventually have developed from purely professional

[29] Chittenden, "Discussion on the Merits of a Relatively Low Protein Diet," *Brit. Med. J.*, 1911 (ii), 656–662, p. 657; Chittenden, "Economy" (n. 28), p. 864, 871; Chittenden, "Over-nutrition and Undernutrition, with Special Reference to Proteid Metabolism," *Brit. Med. J.*, 1906 (ii), 1100–1102, p. 1102; Chittenden, *Physiological Economy* (n. 27), pp. viii, 473.

[30] Ruth Leverton, "Building Blocks and Stepping Stones in Protein Nutrition," *J. Nutr., 91*, supp. 1, 39–43 (1967); National Academy of Sciences, *Recommended Dietary Allowances*, Washington, 1980, p. 46: current recommendations for daily protein consumption are 56 grams for a 70 kilogram man and 44 grams for a 55 kilogram woman.

considerations, as there were both direct and metaphoric connections between Fletcherism and economics. As it happened, however, Fisher, like Chittenden, was led to the dietary scheme by personal health experience. In the early years of his career, he admitted, he had been "blind to what health conservation means." But a three-year battle with tuberculosis, beginning in 1898, cured that blindness, and in fact made Fisher into something of a zealot. He read James' *Varieties of Religious Experience,* for example, as soon as it was published in 1902, and professed to seeing a great deal of himself in the religion of healthy-mindedness. Within a decade he was having to apologize to his wife for being such "a health prude" and making her irritated with his constant hygiene lectures to their children. His colleagues as well found him tiresome, and brilliant though his work in economics was, his professional standing finally suffered from his reputation as a health fanatic. Yet Fisher felt that he did "want before I die to leave behind something more than a book on Index Numbers," and was unembarrassed to list his crusade against the waste of health alongside the careers of Jesus, Socrates, and Buddha.[31]

It was through Chittenden that Fisher became aware of Fletcherism and the advantages of a low protein diet, and was persuaded to direct an experiment involving nine of his own students. As a political economist, Fisher was concerned with long-term productivity of the labor force. Thus the physiological quality that captured his attention was endurance, rather than strength (he frequently stressed the difference, pointing out that a muscle's strength "is measured by the utmost force it can exert once; its endurance, by the number of times it can repeat a given exertion within its strength."). Chittenden, he felt, had demonstrated that a low protein diet increased strength, but had not adequately

---

[31] Irving Fisher, *Life Extension,* Poughkeepsie, N.Y., 1917, p. 8; Irving Fisher [Jr.], *My Father, Irving Fisher,* New York, 1956, pp. 83–85, 152, 214.

determined its effects on endurance. Nor had the relationship between Fletcherizing and endurance been fully tested. In January 1906, Fisher's students organized an "eating club" for the purpose of evaluating Fletcher's system. For nineteen weeks they devoted their table time to "thorough mastication and implicit obedience to appetite." During the second half of the experiment they were also actively encouraged to eat less protein ("when the appetite was *entirely* willing."). As might by now be predicted, the subjects soon found themselves wanting less food and voiding less offensive feces. And, of course, they all the while grew in endurance. Tests requiring repetitive exercises, such as calf-raises, knee-bends, and dumbbell lifts, were administered at the beginning, middle, and end of the test. All but one of the volunteers improved dramatically (from fifty to more than two hundred percent) between January and June, and it seemed more than coincidence that the exception was the student who had failed to reduce his protein consumption until near the experiment's end, and whose fecal improvement rating was one of the lowest. Fisher carefully analyzed the experiment to be certain the improvement could only have come from diet, and he concluded by giving roughly equal credit to Fletcher and Chittenden—thorough mastication and low protein together built endurance.[32]

Fisher had apparently already begun to practice what he preached, and it was perhaps the resulting endurance that allowed him to leave tuberculosis behind and work so tirelessly to do for his discipline what Fletcher had done for

[32] Fisher, "The Influence of Flesh Eating on Endurance," *Yale Med. J., 13*, 205-221 (1906-7), p. 205; Fisher, "The Effect of Diet on Endurance, Based on an Experiment with Nine Healthy Students at Yale University, January–June, 1906," *Trans. Conn. Acad., 13*, 1-46 (1907), pp. 3, 4, 16-33, 45. In June 1907, Fisher had the honor of meeting Fletcher and using him to test a machine he had invented to measure endurance. According to Fletcher, "I made such a good showing" that Chittenden and Anderson insisted on the second set of gymnasium exercises discussed on p. 186 Fletcher, "Possible Progressive Growth" (n. 25), p. 1007.

physiology, to in fact use physiology to make political economy, the "dismal science," optimistic. He saw as clearly as anyone the significance of health for labor and productivity, and more clearly than most the importance for health of personal (as opposed to environmental) hygiene. The dietetic precepts he had confirmed could thus be given an influential place in the renovation of society. It would be but one place among many, however, for Fisher appreciated the complexity of both public health and sociology. His complete design for the healthful society was first given as a report for the National Conservation Commission that had been established by Theodore Roosevelt in 1908 to study the mineral, water, soil, and forest resources of the nation. An investigation of human resources and their waste was also included among the commission's duties, and Fisher was appointed to direct that survey. His report, issued the following year, began with a proclamation that perfectly captured the ethos of Progressive physiologic optimism. "The problem of conserving natural resources," Fisher explained, "is only one part of the larger problem of conserving national efficiency. The other part relates to the vitality of our population. . . . The prevention of disease . . . increases economic productivity." His elaboration of that theme embraced a host of environmental and personal factors: quarantine, urban sanitation, food and drug legislation, regulation of working conditions, etc. In the realm of personal hygiene, special emphasis was given to the waste caused by "undue fatigue," a waste, he felt, "probably much greater than the waste from serious illness." Most of the causes of fatigue identified by Fisher were commonplace (alcohol, tobacco, too long working days), but "excessive amounts of the protein element" was not so predictable, even in the midst of the Chittenden controversy, nor was the suggestion that "thorough mastication leads instinctively to a reduction in protein." And in expansive general remarks on the possibilities of "conservation through personal hygiene," Fisher presented Horace Fletcher as a prime example of what can be achieved when the individual assumes personal responsibility for his health.[33]

That same year, Fisher cooperated with Fletcher in founding the Health and Efficiency League of America, an organization devoted to building an understanding of health and an awareness that "the goal of 'efficiency' covers nothing less than the entire field of human life and activity, and includes the mind and the will as well as the body." The first lesson taught by the league was "learning how to chew and 'properly taste food.' " The league proved a short-lived enterprise, but Fisher found other organizations for the promotion of his health ideas. He was already president of the Committee of One Hundred on National Health, a collection of prominent physicians, health officials, educators, economists, and others prodding the federal government to establish a national department of health (the committee included among its members such medical celebrities as William Henry Welch, Herman Biggs, and Prince Morrow, as well as Chittenden—and Horace Fletcher). One of his projects as committee president was the persuasion of life insurance companies to underwrite the work of the committee. National implementation of his health program, he promised, would prolong the lives of policy holders and increase insurance company profits. His success in converting company presidents was limited, but he stayed by his plan. When the prospects for a national department of health dimmed, he organized the Life Extension Institute, a nonprofit foundation dedicated to making periodic low cost health examinations available to the public. He hoped, in fact, to convince insurance companies to provide for free examinations for policy holders, and at least one company that adopted the proposal did realize a considerable savings. Fisher's lectures on behalf of the institute included lessons learned from Fletcher, such as that Americans' "hurry

[33] Fisher, "The Influence" (n. 32), p. 206; Fisher, *Report on National Vitality*, Washington, 1909, pp. 1, 4–5, 83.

habit" at the table was responsible for an unnecessarily high incidence of high blood pressure and kidney disease.[34]

With the passing of time, Fisher became much more worried about another American disease: race suicide. Alarmed by the "rising tide of color," afraid that Americans were about to "quietly lie down and let some other race run over us," he threw himself into the eugenics movement. But even there Fisher retained his hygienic orientation. His 1921 presidential address to the Eugenics Research Association, for example, was largely an appeal to his comrades to recognize the eugenic usefulness of hygiene. He clearly suspected that denials of the inheritance of acquired characters did not preclude the possibility of germ plasm being injured by defective nutrition, and he called for a major investment of research into the dysgenic effects of poor hygiene. Fisher summarized his point by suggesting that "hygiene and eugenics should go hand in hand. They are really both hygiene—one individual hygiene and the other race hygiene—and both, eugenics—one indirectly through safeguarding the quality of the germ plasm and the other directly through breeding." He moved on to consider other challenges to eugenics, but returned in his concluding remarks to another evocation of Fletcher. Fisher was still advocating a national department of health, and in describing the hygienic and eugenic education such a department could provide the American public he selected a curious word to denote it—"humaniculture."[35]

Examples of Fletcher's wide-ranging influence might be

---

[34] "The Health and Efficiency League of America," *Hyg. Phys. Ed.*, *1*, 980–982 (1909–10), p. 982; William Schieffelin, "Work of the Committee of One Hundred on National Health," *Ann. Amer. Acad. Pol. Soc. Sci.*, *37*, 321–330 (1911); Fisher, *My Father* (n. 31), pp. 116, 163; Fisher, *Life Extension* (n. 31), pp. 18–19.

[35] Fisher, "Impending Problems of Eugenics," *Sci. M.*, *13*, 214–231 (1921), pp. 219–220, 228, 230. Several of Fisher's articles included footnote references to Higgins' *Humaniculture*. Also see [Life Extension Institute], *The Review of Reviews Course in Physical Training, Health and Life Extension*, New York, 1920, lesson two, pp. 6–10, 17–19.

multiplied, and would have to include Upton Sinclair, the socialist novelist whom Mencken characterized as a "wholesale believer in the obviously not so." Sooner or later, Sinclair sampled just about every hygienic prescription on the market—and publicly espoused a number of them—but he began with Fletcherism. Sinclair's health problems started while he was in college, in the late 1890s. He suffered increasing distress for several years until, in 1902 or 1903, he chanced upon a magazine piece on Fletcher. The article was "one of the great discoveries of my life" (this was exactly the same period, 1902–1903, that he was discovering socialism). To condense his story, he began Fletcherizing, converted a young writer friend, Michael Williams, and they recovered health together. In the process, their appreciation of "the virtue of good eating" insinuated itself into their grand "dream of the new humanity." The result was still another book extolling Fletcherism as a major step toward the salvation of a declining America. The work also gave much space to Chittenden and Fisher, and to advice on breathing, bathing, toothcare, etc., but its thrust was toward Fletcher and the vigor and endurance his example promised a weak nation. Sinclair was to pass on to a number of other dietary programs, yet through all his hygienic hopscotching, he remained true to Fletcher. At least into the 1920s, he was still stressing the importance of cooperation with one's food filter.[36]

Among the other figures who felt Fletcher's impact were the leaders of physical education, who were forced by Fletcher's feats to reconsider their ideas about athletic training; temperance crusaders who were excited by Fletcher's discovery that proper mastication caused the thirst for strong drink to wither—a Fletcherized martini, one rejoiced, tastes like kerosene—while a group of Seventh

[36] Mencken quoted by Leon Harris, *Upton Sinclair: American Rebel*, New York, 1975, p. 180; Upton Sinclair and Michael Williams, *Good Health and How We Won It*, New York, 1909, pp. 4, 7, 41–50; Sinclair, *The Book of Life*, 2 vols., New York, 1921, 1:145.

Day Adventist students in Tennessee claimed to have rescued hundreds of mountaineers from their enslavement to
moonshine by teaching them to Fletcherize; and Irving
James Eales, an osteopathic physician whose system of
"Healthology" drew heavily from Fletcher.[37]
The list could be made so long as to become indigestible.
And for every Fletcherite who made it into print, there were
apparently many more who chewed quietly beyond public
notice. Fletcher believed two hundred thousand American
families were abiding by his precepts by the 1910s, and his
publishers estimated he had helped millions to discover
healthy living. Popular journalists could quip that only the
"African hunter" received more attention than Fletcher
from the press, or make reference to the "Chew-Chew Club"
without feeling any need for further explanation. Fletcher's
ideas were so pervasive that the noted authority on American Indian culture, George Wharton James, argued that Indians had been natural Fletcherizers for centuries, and attributed much of their physical endurance to the habit. That
habit even spread to England, where some London elite
amused themselves with "munching parties." Novelist
Henry James (William's brother) also adopted Fletcherism,
entertained Fletcher in his home, and distributed copies of
The New Glutton to his English neighbors. After six years
of the system, however, he developed stomach troubles that
the great clinician William Osler blamed on improper eating habits (and there were rumors that many more Americans suffered from "Bradyfagy, a disease arising from the
habit of eating too slowly.").[38]

---

[37] Walter Chapin, "Diet—the Proteids," *Am. Phys. Ed. Rev.*, *12*,
121–125 (1907); Elmer Berry, "The Effects of a High and Low Proteid
Diet on Physical Efficiency," *Am. Phys. Ed. Rev.*, *14;* Eugene House,
"Diet and Endurance," *Am. Phys. Ed. Rev.*, *21*, 490–502 (1916); Elbert
Hubbard, "The Gentle Art of Fletcherizing," *Cosmopolitan*, *46*, 48–53
(Dec., 1908), p. 51; Fletcher, *Fletcherism* (n. 2), pp. 151–157; Irving
Eales, *Healthology*, London, 1913, pp. 126–132.

[38] Fletcher, *Fletcherism* (n. 2), pp. x, 43; Williams, "Horace Fletcher's
Philosophy" (n. 3), p. 284; "The Lounger," *Putnam's*, *5*, 762 (1909);

Gastric distress had, of course, long been predicted by Fletcher's critics, who from the beginning had found his writings a rich lode for jests about insufficient food, jaw fatigue, and long, boring meals. One jeered at Fletcher for believing that by chewing "our one mouthful of food long enough we shall delude the stomach into magnifying it into ten, and can dine sumptuously on a menu card and a wafer biscuit." Another reported that a popular New York restaurant had placed instructions for Fletcherizing on each table, but discontinued the experiment after three weeks because slow-chewing customers "gave the cash drawer indigestion and heart failure."[39]

Fletcherism was no easier on its would-be practitioners. As Van Someren warned the British Medical Association, "the habit of a lifetime cannot be changed in a few days or weeks." The shortest period in which the swallowing reflex had been reestablished, he reported, had been four weeks, and that early triumph had required avoidance of meal-time conversation so that concentration could be directed entirely toward chewing. Many who tested Fletcherism must have lacked the necessary perseverance, and even those who finally mastered mastication could not be certain how much of any improvement in health should be credited to chewing and how much to reduced food consumption. That none were able to equal Fletcher's vitality and endurance is testimony that the founder was exceptional, that he was, as a colleague called him, a "physiological puzzle."[40] That his method was

---

George Wharton James, *What the White Race May Learn from the Indian*, Chicago, 1908, p. 124; Fletcher, *The New Glutton* (n. 13), p. 272; H. M. Hyde, *Henry James. At Home*, London, 1969, p. 138; Gay Allen, *William James, a Biography*, New York, 1967, p. 474; Élie Metchnikoff, *The Prolongation of Life*, New York, 1908, p. 159.

[39] Woods Hutchinson, "Some Diet Delusions," *McClure's, 26,* 611–623 (1906), p. 611; "Shall We Fletcherize," *Lit. Dig., 47,* 130 (1913).

[40] Van Someren, "Was Luigi Cornaro Right" (n. 22), p. 1084; Fletcher, *The New Glutton,* (n. 13), p. 58. Fletcher's critics were inclined to place him in the category of "physiological freaks": James Crichton-Browne, *Parcimony in Nutrition*, London, 1909, p. 73.

laborious and less than satisfying for most people is evidenced by its rapid disappearance after death removed Fletcher's inspiring presence.

Yet if few conversions to Fletcherism were permanent, the system undoubtedly expanded public awareness of the need to eat more slowly and chew more attentively, and thus helped wean Americans from the "gobble, gulp and go" table manners of the nineteenth century. The standard hygiene text for high school and college use during the first half of this century, Irving Fisher and Eugene Fisk's *How to Live*, continued to cite Fletcher as the discoverer of the importance of thorough mastication through the twenty-first (and last) edition of the book in 1946. As one of his obituaries proclaimed, "Horace Fletcher taught the world to chew."[41]

---

[41] "Horace Fletcher Taught the World to Chew," *Lit. Dig., 60,* 92–93 (Feb. 8, 1919). A recent study of the effects of thorough mastication on fat absorption has suggested Fletcherism may have had some distinct nutritional value: Allen Levine and Stephen Silvis, "Absorption of Whole Peanuts, Peanut Oil, and Peanut Butter," *New Eng. J. Med., 303,* 917–918 (1980). I am indebted to Dr. Steven Helgersen of Seattle for calling my attention to this article.

CHAPTER SEVEN
MUSCULAR VEGETARIANISM

☆☆☆☆☆☆☆☆☆☆☆☆☆☆☆☆☆☆☆☆☆☆☆☆☆☆☆☆☆☆☆☆☆☆☆☆☆

ANOTHER WHO TAUGHT THE WORLD TO CHEW WAS THE ONLY
health reformer to outshine Fletcher during the Progressive
years. John Harvey Kellogg, in fact, even cast a shadow over
Graham, for the assorted precooked breakfast cereals, peanut butter, nut-based meat substitutes, and other delicacies
concocted by this culinary inventor comprised a health food
smorgasbord beside which the Graham cracker shrank to
pauper's fare.

Kellogg's head table was set at his Battle Creek Michigan
Sanitarium, originally a Seventh Day Adventist institution
designed to perpetuate Grahamite philosophy. Such, at
least, was the sanitariums design in effect. In theory,
though, Adventist health doctrine was free of any ties to the
Jacksonian health reform movement. It was an indepen-
dently acquired body of knowledge, not discovered by
clumsy human probing, but revealed by the Creator of the
laws of hygiene Himself. The Adventist "prophetess of
health" was the nascent church's spiritual director, Ellen
White, a woman who through most of her life experienced
visions (occurring unpredictably five to ten times a year) in
which she was instructed by angels, Christ, and often God.
Her early visions, beginning in 1844, dealt with theological
issues, but from 1848 onward, healthful living was increasingly the subject. Tobacco, tea, and coffee, she was told, had
to be forsworn by those awaiting the Second Coming. Subsequent communications, which ran into the 1870s, lengthened
the list by adding meat, gluttony and grease, drugs and doctors, corsets, unnatural sex, even artificial hair. If that
seems a rather uninspired list to have come from divine revelation, it must be remembered that the word of God should

be the same whether heard indirectly through science or immediately in vision. But though White's catalogue of hygienic evils was necessarily identical to Alcott's and Graham's, it was not necessarily derived purely by direct illumination, uninfluenced by earlier mortal opinions. It was difficult for a literate person of the mid-1800s to grow to adulthood totally unaware of health reform teachings. Numbers has recently argued that White was not just familiar with standard health reform works by the time of her most important visions, but that some of her writings actually borrowed prodigally, but without acknowledgement, from an early philosopher of health, Larken Coles.[1]

Although Numbers' case is convincing, White perhaps did receive genuine revelations, and conceivably outraged Adventists are correct in seeing his book as a Satanic "deception." Those are questions for theologians rather than historians. What is historically certain is that whether divinely informed or terrestrially tutored, Ellen White accepted hygiene as a religious duty, and also came to see healing and health education as a responsibility of the church to its members. In a vision experienced Christmas day 1865, she was told that sick Adventists, who hitherto had sought treatment at hydropathic institutions "where there is not sympathy for our faith" and where sometimes "the sophistry of the devil" ruled, should have their own establishment for recovery of health. Within a year there opened in Battle Creek, Adventist headquarters, the Western Health Reform Institute, a hospital employing water and other natural therapies (air, light, diet) and staffed by a "Faculty" dedicated to discharging no patient until he had been "instructed as to the right mode of living."[2]

But nobility of purpose was not enough to save the insti-

[1] Ronald Numbers, *Prophetess of Health: a Study of Ellen G. White*, New York, 1976.

[2] *ibid.*, pp. 100, 105. The Adventist charge that Numbers' book is part of "the very last deception of Satan" is discussed in *Time*, *108*, 43 (Aug. 2, 1976).

tute from a troubled first decade, and it was on the verge of being closed when it was rescued (in 1876) by the appointment of a new, more dynamic physician-in-chief, John Harvey Kellogg (Figure 4). Son of the institute's treasurer and largest stockholder, Kellogg had nevertheless won his new position mostly on merit. Born in 1852, he had been a sickly child, "threatened with an early death from tuberculosis." This satisfying of the first requirement for becoming a health reformer had been followed, at age fourteen, by the reading of a work by Graham and conversion to vegetarianism. Six years later, Kellogg journeyed to New Jersey for a term at Trall's now struggling Hygeio-Therapeutic College, then moved on to earn his medical degree at New York's Bellevue, one of the better medical schools at the time. Kellogg maintained his affiliation with the regular profession throughout his life, and included surgery in his practice. His biographer even identifies him as "one of America's foremost surgeons," though that assessment would appear to be somewhat inflated in light of a marginal note made by the previous owner (a midwestern Adventist) of my copy of the biography: "Why then was Mother's scar such a horrible thing?" Kellogg was nevertheless a competent surgeon, but his distrust of drugs and advocacy of "natural" methods relegated him to fringe status in the eyes of most orthodox practitioners.[3]

His professional standing was made shakier still by his energetic espousal of "biologic living," the term he coined for what was essentially the same hygienic system as health reform. Kellogg's inkwell fed a flood of hygienic counsel that swirled unabating through the late nineteenth and early twentieth centuries. His volumes were the most elaborate defenses of vegetarianism, the most scathing denunciations of alcohol, the most merciless attacks on sexual misconduct

[3] John Harvey Kellogg, *The Natural Diet of Man*, Battle Creek, Mich., 1923, pp. 188–189; Richard Schwarz, *John Harvey Kellogg, M.D.*, Nashville, 1970, is overly reverential, but the only full biography of Kellogg. Also see Gerald Carson, *Cornflake Crusade*, New York, 1957.

(parents were encouraged to make unannounced nighttime raids on their children's rooms to catch youthful masturbators in the act, and to cure their prey with cauterization of the clitoris or circumcision without benefit of anesthesia). *The Evils of Fashionable Dress, Harmony of Science and the Bible, The Itinerary of a Breakfast,* and his nearly fifty other books were accompanied by uncounted public lectures, and a popular periodical, *Good Health,* which commanded an audience of more than twenty thousand subscribers at times, and continued in existence until 1955. Articles were contributed to a number of independent journals as well, and even his wife Ella added several books to the cause. A buoyant liver to the age of ninety-one, Kellogg seems truly to have been, as Irving Fisher described him, "a tireless steam engine" and "a wonderful advertisement for his own theories."[4]

Kellogg's biologic living was most effectively taught at the Battle Creek Sanitarium, as he had renamed the Western Health Reform Institute soon after his takeover (Figure 5). The "San," the name by which it came to be known to all Americans, was also opened to other denominations (and eventually, under Kellogg's direction, it was separated from the Adventist Church). Revitalization accompanied all this reorganization. Finding himself with only twelve patients when his tenure began, Kellogg developed programs and a reputation that were soon attracting several thousand patients a year. By the time he died in 1943, he had hosted more than three hundred thousand patients at the San, including such celebrities as President Taft, John D. Rockefeller, Jr., Alfred DuPont, J. C. Penney, Montgomery Ward, and grape-juice magnate Edgar Welch.[5]

All were students as well as patients, for Kellogg was determined that his establishment be a "University of Health,"

[4] Kellogg, *Plain Facts for Young and Old,* Burlington, Iowa, 1886, pp. 292, 326–326; Schwarz, *John Harvey Kellogg* (n. 3), p. 92; Irving Fisher [Jr.], *My Father, Irving Fisher,* New York, 1956, p. 109.

[5] Schwarz, *John Harvey Kellogg* (n. 3), pp. 75–76.

a "place where people learn to stay well." One rule taught to patients from early in the San's history was the importance of complete mastication to aid digestion and prevent overeating. Kellogg also required his dyspeptic patients to begin each meal with hard toast or a similar hard-to-manage item so as to force attention to careful chewing at the outset of the meal. But after Fletcher visited the San in 1902, Kellogg began stressing mastication even more. In a subsequent letter to Fletcher he assured him: "We are all in training to find our [swallowing] reflexes, and are expecting to make a great deal of this." Another envelope brought a copy of a "Chewing Song" that Kellogg had written to entertain and instruct sanitarium patients (but sadly no vestige of the tune can be found in Kellogg's papers today). In another letter Kellogg announced that he had told his patients that Fletcher "had done more to help suffering humanity than any other man of the present generation." In published articles, Kellogg offered such provocative suggestions as that an effective means of combatting race degeneracy would be to substitute grade school instruction in "the fine art of . . . Fletcherizing" for such sterile exercises as memorizing the *Aeneid*. The verb "to fletcherize" was in fact minted by Kellogg, who also erected a large "Fletcherize" sign at the head of the San dining room. Kellogg was also involved in the founding of the Health and Efficiency League of America (as well as a member of the Committee of One Hundred on National Health), and though he became frustrated with Fletcher's concentration on chewing at the expense of other elements of biologic living, he continued to praise the masticator at least into the 1920s.[6]

The probably gleeful "Chewing Song" notwithstanding,

[6] *ibid.*, pp. 46–47, 62; Horace Fletcher, *The New Glutton*, New York, 1903, pp. 50–67; Kellogg, "Suggestions Toward Checking Race Degeneracy Due to the Conditions of School Life," *Hyg. Phys. Ed.*, 1, 245–51, 312–314, 402–405 (1909–1910), p. 402; Kellogg, *The Natural Diet of Man*, Battle Creek, Mich., 1923, pp. 336–337; Carson, *Cornflake Crusade* (n. 3), p. 236.

Kellogg esteemed Fletcher less for his masticatory reformation than for his triggering of Chittenden's reevaluation of the daily protein requirement. The foundation of biologic living, as with Grahamism, was vegetable diet, and the lowering of the protein recommendation was a grand cause for celebration for Progressive vegetarians. They had already endured half a century of charges that their protein intake was too low. The objection had lost some weight in recent years, as increasing numbers of Pythagoreans had permitted themselves the luxury of milk and eggs (there was considerable diversity within vegetarian ranks by the end of the 1800s, from highly conservative fruitarians, who also ate nuts, to the comparatively profligate lacto-ovo vegetarians who comprised a new majority). Even those who were not "VEM" (Vegetables, Eggs, and Milk) practitioners were probably consuming more protein because of the popularity of nut-based imitations of meat dishes. Kellogg's products—peanut butter, Protose, Nuttose, Battle Creek Steaks, and Battle Creek Skallops—dominated the health food market (Figure 6). But there were numerous competitors—Plasmon, Tropon, Emprote, etc.—vying for the favor of vegetarian converts of wavering willpower.

Vegetarian strictures on gluttony still checked liberal eating, however, and kept average protein consumption well below the levels recommended prior to Chittenden. Vegetarians were a source of concern to orthodox nutritionists also because of the recent realization of the body's less efficient utilization of vegetable protein. Several experiments performed during the last quarter of the nineteenth century had established that the cellulose of vegetable foods interferes with the digestion of protein and results in a lower rate of absorption than for flesh protein.[7]

Even as these objections lost much of their force in the aftermath of Chittenden, scientific opinion remained solidly

---

[7] For a good review of these studies, see Elbert Rockwood, "The Utilization of Vegetable Proteids by the Animal Organism," *Am. J. Physiol., 11,* 355–369 (1904).

antivegetarian. It was admitted that lacto-ovo vegetarians, at least, had an adequate diet, and even occasionally acknowledged that it was probably more healthful than a diet rich in meat and short on vegetables. But most nutritionists bristled at the assertions that vegetarianism was the only natural diet for man and was far superior to any regimen containing meat. The most indignant of all, vegetarianism's chief nemesis during the Progressive years, was Woods Hutchinson, a New York physician with a special interest in interpreting medical and biological matters for the public. Evolution was one of his favorite subjects (the title of an early work, *The Gospel According to Darwin*, reveals his allegiance), and when turned against the scientific pretensions of vegetarians it yielded two weighty arguments. First, Hutchinson reiterated the long-standing judgment that the human teeth and intestinal tract had structures intermediate between those of carnivores and herbivores, and submitted that the race must therefore have evolved on a mixed diet. Secondly, he noted that through most of his evolutionary history, man had been a pure animal, governed wholly by instinct. Reason, with its power to decide wrongly and mislead, had emerged relatively late. The natural food of man, then, the diet for which he was fitted by evolution, was the food that appealed to his instinct, not that which satisfied his reason: "To 'taste good' is nature's stamp of approval upon a food." The vast majority thought meat tasted not just good, but best; the one thing that primitive, barbarous, and civilized man shared, he observed, was a longing for the "fleshpots of Egypt," for (he taunted) "Meat! R-r-red meat, dr-r-r-ripping with b-l-lood, r-r-reeking of the shambles." Vegetarians defied that instinct, suppressing it with a reasoned moral decision, and thus punished themselves with an unnatural diet. "The man in the street follows his God-given instincts and plods peacefully along to his three square meals a day. . . . Here, as everywhere, instinct is far superior to reason, and a breakfast diet of sausage and buckwheat cakes with maple syrup and strong coffee has carried the white man half round the world; while one of salads and cereals, washed down with post-mortem subterfuge, would leave him stranded, gasping, in the first ditch he came to."

The sounds of imperialism were not always muffled. Civilizations evolved according to their compliance with instincts too, Hutchinson stressed, and "it may be stated that vegetarianism is the diet of the enslaved, stagnant and conquered races, and a diet rich in meat is that of the progressive, the dominant and the conquering strains."[8]

There were two types of debilitating vegetarian foods that Hutchinson particularly despised. Graham bread, or any other bread heavy with bran, he believed, was less nourishing than white bread, and too irritating to the bowels. Human instinct had always shown a preference for white over black, brown, "or other mulatto tint" of bread. "White flour, red meat, and blue blood," Hutchinson proclaimed, "make the tricolor flag of conquest." But even more contemptible than bran bread was the recent fad of breakfast cereals. Hutchinson's instincts were for bacon and eggs, and cereal he counted as no breakfast at all. The oatmeal-eating Scottish race may have distinguished themselves, but then "any nation trained to survive a diet of oatmeal and the shorter catechism could survive anything and flourish anywhere." Such adaptability was less likely for people brought up on the nutritionless precooked cereals that were issuing in profusion from Battle Creek. Kellogg's success had attracted imitators, and the market was awash with a "whole brood of 'Fierce,' 'Foodle,' 'Gripe Nits,' 'Fush,' 'Grapogripo-grits,' 'Shredded Doormats,' 'Eata-heapa-hay,' 'Uneeda-paira-blinkers,' etc.," which Hutchinson insisted "will not support life; easily upset digestion, destroy the appetite, and calorie for calorie are exceedingly expensive."[9]

---

[8] *Dictionary of American Biography,* vol. 9, New York, 1932, p. 443; Woods Hutchinson, *Instinct and Health,* New York, 1909, pp. 18, 34, 46–47; "The Dangers of Undereating," *Cosmopolitan, 47,* 385–393 (1909), p. 388.

[9] Hutchinson, *Instinct and Health* (n. 8), pp. 37–51; Hutchinson, "Some Diet Delusions," *McClure's, 26,* 611–623 (1906), pp. 619–620.

Kellogg was too busy to be long distracted by such slights to his dietary creations and his doctrine, and shrugged off Hutchinson's criticism as "pernicious piffle." Piffle or not, the public at large continued to laugh at the vegetarian message, and to propose prizes for vegetarians capable of "the quickest demolition of the largest quantity of turnips," or the disposition of "one hundred heads of celery with the utmost celerity." Nor did vegetarians aid their cause by advertising the wonders of their cookery. Some of the most frightful sins ever committed in a kitchen were on the head of Ella Kellogg, whose cookbook of vegetarian recipes instructed newcomers to the fold to perpetrate such crimes as boiling pasta an hour; "toothsome and tempting viands" indeed![10]

But the world's mocking was nothing new, and was hardly capable of extinguishing vegetarian spirit. Progressive vegetarians, in fact, were in a positively victorious mood, even before the low protein diet became respectable. Experience and scientific theory had combined in the late nineteenth century to produce new evidence for the superiority of vegetable diet, and that in turn had spurred Pythagoreans to uncharacteristic aggressiveness in the presentation of their message. Possessed of new confidence, formerly defensive vegetarians were flexing their muscles, and no one more proudly than Kellogg.

In truth, the vegetarians of earlier days had not always been the retiring sort: "What is John Bull, with his beef and beer," Alcott had challenged, "but a mass of incipient putrefaction." Yet in that same address, he had chastised his listeners for being so timid, and called them "to change their mode of conducting the controversy, and boldly wage eternal war against customs fraught with evil." But even as he spoke, his forces (the members of the American Vegetarian Society) were dwindling and before two decades had passed

[10] Kellogg, *The Natural Diet* (n. 6), p. 368; Charles Forward, *Fifty Years of Food Reform*, London, 1898, p. 31; Ella Kellogg, *Science in the Kitchen*, Battle Creek, Mich., 1892, pp. 3, 106.

George Beard could write of "the history of the rise and fall of vegetarianism" as if the movement had gone the way of the Roman empire. And after another two decades, Holbrook, considerably more sympathetic to the fleshless diet than Beard, was still forced to upbraid vegetarians for not making use of science to win more followers.[11]

Holbrook's prodding was more symptom than cause of the end of vegetarian quietism. A reconditioning of doctrine to keep it in pace with science had already begun, and was building toward a turn-of-the-century rush of books, periodicals, and pamphlets bulging with modernized critiques of flesh food. Yet as updated as vegetarian theory was, it might be observed, many positions from older times were retained. One of Kellogg's treatises on dietary reform, for instance, opened its analysis of the natural diet of humanity with the same comparisons of teeth, intestinal tracts, and extremities (hooves and claws) that the writers of the early 1800s had relied upon to answer the question. Coverage of those points did not exhaust the discussion for him, though. Kellogg (and his contemporaries) pursued the argument from comparative anatomy much further, calling for consideration of the salivary and mammary glands, tongue, skin, tail, posture, and singing habits (songbirds live on grains and fruits, while carnivorous birds can only croak and caw, according to his generalization): in all cases, human structure was closest to that of the frugivorous primates.[12]

The resemblance of man to ape had already been emphasized by health reform vegetarians without any hints from Darwin, but in the wake of *The Origin of Species* the human-primate relation took on profound new significance. Biblical man, as an independent creature designed similarly to, but still separately from, the ape, was not necessarily in-

---

[11] Alcott, *Am. Veg.*, 4, 174 (1854); George Beard, *Eating and Drinking; a Popular Manual of Food and Diet in Health and Disease*, New York, 1871, p. 91; Holbrook, *J. Hyg. Herald Health*, 44, 137–139 (1894).

[12] Kellogg, *Shall We Slay to Eat*, Battle Creek, Mich., 1905, pp. 22–32, 139. Also see Francis Newman, *Essays on Diet*, London, 1883, p. 90.

tended to subsist on the ape's diet. But evolutionary man, a descendant of apes (a creature who once was an ape!), could not so easily distance himself from meatless diet. If his fruit- and nut-eating ancestors had been favorably selected by nature over untold millennia, his recent experimentation with flesh food could hardly be accepted as natural or desirable.

Carnivores, incorrigible to the end, resisted that conclusion with evolutionary musings of their own. Their stock responses were either the one offered by Hutchinson, or a revived version of the thesis of Bell's 1835 essay, the one which had set off the first fleshpot tempest. While man had descended from the ape through time, this argument ran, he had risen far above the animal in culture. His superior intelligence allowed him to select a variety of foods and alter them to meet his needs by the application of the cooking art. And since omnivorousness had been accompanied by a steady climb to civilization, the diet must have been evolutionarily advantageous. Indeed, the process had gone so far that human nutrition no longer bore any relation to simian diet, or even to primitive man's: "the gulf that separates Shakespeare and Newton from the Papuan is wider than that which separates the Papuan from the gorilla and the chimpanzee; and therefore it is easier for the lowest order of human beings to live after the manner of the apes than for the highest orders of humanity to live after the manner of the savages."[13]

If a meat-eating Shakespeare found it impossible to follow the diet of a savage (let alone an ape), vegetarians returned, the difficulty was not in nature, but in the strength of depraved habit. Original man had lived happily on fruits and nuts, they maintained, until in the course of geological evolution harsh environmental changes caused shortages of vegetable food in some regions of the globe and forced inhabitants to turn to flesh. During the same epoch, the discovery of fire, needed for survival in the new, colder ennvironment,

[13] Beard, *Eating and Drinking* (n. 11), pp. 106–107.

also enabled man to make meat palatable. As consumption of the stimulating food increased, addiction developed, "habit became so strong as to enslave." Kellogg actually went so far as to maintain that all animals were originally nut eaters. His own success making nut-based meat substitutes apparently convinced him that nuts were very close to meat in composition, so it was easy to suppose that some catastrophic failure of nut supplies in remote ages had forced many species to turn to the most similar food—the flesh of other animals. Hence the appearance of carnivorousness in the evolutionary scheme. Kellogg even proposed that canine teeth, so efficient at rending flesh, had evolved originally for tearing the husks of coconuts and similar noncarnivorous tasks.[14]

That wolves had once been tranquil nibblers of acorns was of far less moment, though, than that human beings had degenerated into voraciousness. Vegetarians had to admit that meat-eating man had far outstripped his herbivorous ancestors in intellectual evolution, but, after all, once hunting had become the norm, natural selection had favored ingenuity as well as bloodthirstiness. And much of what was called civilization and advanced culture had been won by conquest, by the rapine and slaughter that were the ultimate consequences of an appetite for flesh food. The evolutionary attainments of carnivores were thus tarnished and incomplete, and were now even being reversed. The advance of civilization had always been precarious while associated with the flesh diet, and it was merely a question of time before a species "altogether perverted," as Kellogg saw man, would begin "stumbling down the steep declivity of race degeneracy." The stumbling had in fact begun, and the only way it could be checked was to return the race to its proper place

[14] Gustav Schlickeysen, *Fruit and Bread. A Scientific Diet,* New York, 1877, p. 95; Kellogg, *Shall We Slay* (n. 12), p. 32; Kellogg, *The Itinerary of a Breakfast,* Battle Creek, Mich., 1919, p. 184. Also see Newman, *Essays* (n. 12), p. 91, and Otto Carqué, *The Foundation of all Reform,* Evanston, Ill., 1904, pp. 12–16.

within the evolutionary dynamic. The rejection of flesh food would reverse the downward slide, moreover, not just by improving the fitness of individuals, but also by changing overall social health. Vegetarians had long associated temperament with diet, blaming selfishness and quarrelsomeness on meat, and attributing generosity and cooperativeness to vegetable diet. Intuition and comparative zoology provided the evidence: "The habits of flesh-eating animals are not pleasant," the Honorable Rollo Russell explained with disgust. "In hiding during the day, and skulking in the twilight, or sneaking on silent feet during the night hours, . . . they are enemies of all peaceable beings." How different from these stealthy and ferocious beasts were "the grain-eating tribe": "The social creatures are the happiest, the best fitted to survive and replenish the earth." And when humankind was included among the "social creatures," their fitness to survive was not only moral, but physical. Human vegetarians resented nature's violent redness, and resisted the intrusion of "survival of the fittest" into the social sphere. They were, as a group, highly receptive to the reaction against social Darwinism and its substitution of mutual aid for struggle in the evolutionary process. Believing that cooperation accomplished more (and peaceably) than competition, and assuming a cooperative spirit to be the natural product of vegetable diet, they could not help but expect vegetarianism to lift the race to a higher and climactic stage of evolutionary advance: "In ignorance and want man left his early paradise: through knowledge and industry he will regain it, but with all the achievements of art and science he will make it 'far happier than that of Eden,' and with a conscientious life according to the laws of nature there will be no danger of a return to the misery and savagery of previous ages."[15]

Evolution could even be used to reinforce the humane argument for vegetarianism. By abolishing the separateness of

---

[15] Kellogg, *Natural Diet* (n. 6) pp. 14–15; Rollo Russell, *Strength and Diet*, London, 1905, pp. 110–111; Carqué, *Foundation* (n. 14), p. 16.

man and making him one with the rest of nature, evolutionary theory had taught man his kinship with the animals,
and encouraged him to attempt mutual aid with his fellow
creatures rather than slaughter them.[16]

The objection to slaughter did not derive entirely from
humane feeling and moralistic interpretations of science,
however. Equally distressing to most vegetarians was the association of disease with the slaughterhouse. That diseased
animals were often butchered and sold for food had been
known to vegetarians of the Jacksonian period; Graham had
suggested the meat eater's stomach might be regarded as "a
kind of 'potter's field' to receive the unknown dead of every
disease."[17] But in the 1830s, the possibility of many diseases
spreading by contagion was not so widely feared, and the
actual agents of infection were unknown. By the end of the
century, though, the germ theory had not only provided an
understanding of the nature of infectious pathogens and
their communicability from one animal to another, it had
excited a general public dread of microorganisms and filth of
any sort. That queasiness about germs and dirt was at the
seat of the national wave of nausea and anger following
Upton Sinclair's *The Jungle*. That sensational exposé of
conditions in Chicago's meat-packing plants, written to gain
sympathy for the stockyard workers and generate support
for socialism, instead so sickened Americans that they demanded protection from tainted meat and forced through
passage of the 1906 Food and Drugs Act. As Sinclair soon
realized, he had set his sights too high; aiming at the public's
heart, he had hit its stomach.

The year before *The Jungle*, one of Kellogg's works had
described the abbatoir in comparable retch-inducing detail,
but with a shotgun attack that intentionally aimed at heart
and stomach, and head, at once. The heart was hit first, the

[16] Henry Salt, *The Logic of Vegetarianism*, London, 1906, pp. 25–30.
[17] Sylvester Graham, *Lectures on the Science of Human Life*, 2 vols.,
Boston, 1839, 2:375.

very title of the volume—*Shall We Slay to Eat?*—forcing readers to confront the moral implications of their eating habits. Reminders of the gentleness of unoffending livestock, creatures with whom man was bound by evolution, were followed by stark descriptions of the butchering process and the squealing and bleating of the dying animals. Kellogg provided pictures as well, photographs of cattle jammed into holding pens, paraded unsuspectingly before sledgehammer-wielding "assassins," piled lifeless at the feet of their smirking killers. Those pictures attacked the stomach too, giving horrifying witness to his blood-drenched prose, to the "tide of gore," the "quivering flesh," the "writhing entrails." It was classic slaughterhouse style, but added to it was sober comment on the frequency of trichinosis and other diseases among the butchered animals, and the dirtiness and carelessness of the butchers. In the final analysis, it was the intellectual reaction that was expected to win the reader to vegetarianism. Love for fellow creatures and hatred of animal suffering had been appealed to for centuries, with very limited results. Mass conversion, as always, had to come from selfish motives, from fear for personal well-being, and the threat of infection from germ-infested meat was as frightening a hazard as vegetarians could convincingly pose. "Each juicy morsel" of meat, Kellogg disclosed, "is fairly alive and swarming with the identical micro-organisms found in a dead rat in a closet or the putrefying carcass of a cow and in barnyard filth." Methusaleh would never have become a byword for longevity had he eaten such stuff:

> No fish was he fed,
> No blood did he shed.
> And he knew when he had eaten enough.
> And so it is plain
> He'd no cause to complain
> Of steaks that were measly or tough.
> Or bearded beef grimy,

Green, moldy, and slimy,
Of cold-storage turkeys and putrid beefsteaks,
With millions of colon germs,
Hams full of trichina worms,
And sausages writhing with rheumatiz-aches.
Old Methuselah dined
On ambrosia and wined
On crystal pure water from heaven-filled springs.
Flesh foods he eschewed,
Because, being shrewd,
He chose Paradise fare and not packing-house things.[18]

Scientific experts quoted to the same effect lacked Kellogg's touch for imagery, but were disturbing nonetheless.

But the danger of specific infections such as trichinosis or tuberculosis was still less upsetting to Kellogg than the threat of a general, more difficult to define meat-induced condition. The most villainous of all germs, in his opinion, were the various species responsible for putrefaction, the decomposition of protein into a host of compounds, of which many are extremely malodorous (e.g., indole, skatole) or toxic (e.g., neurine, putrescine, cadaverine). These putrefaction products are generally present in human feces as a result of the bacterial decomposition of residual dietary protein in the intestines. Many of them, particularly from the latter (toxic) group mentioned above, were isolated by the German scientist Brieger in the 1880s, and classed together under the heading of *ptomaines* (from the Greek for corpse). The unfounded fear of "ptomaine poisoning" that Brieger's work excited (and that has lingered to the present in the public mind) renewed the primitive human suspicion of bowel contents as pathological, a suspicion that quickly grew into its most sophisticated form yet in the theory of "autointoxication." This idea that the body could poison itself by absorption of ptomaines and/or other putrefaction

[18] Kellogg, *Shall We Slay* (n. 12), pp. 145–167; Kellogg, *Natural Diet* (n. 6), p. 107; Schwarz, *John Harvey Kellogg* (n. 3), p. 40.

products from the colon, had a definite superficial allure. There was no doubt that those products were toxic. There was equal certainty that constipation (the retention of ptomaine-producing feces) was accompanied by an array of symptoms, including mental and physical lethargy, poor appetite, headache, and coated tongue. Constipation was also a frequent complaint of patients presenting no definite pathology, those exasperating unfortunates who in earlier times would have been diagnosed as hypochondriacs or neurasthenics. Now they became sufferers of gastrointestinal autointoxication (or else, as will be seen in the next chapter, of uricacidemia). The plausibility and usefulness of autointoxication outweighed, for many physicians, its lack of experimental or clinical documentation. The leaders of the profession during the 1910s and 1920s had to repeatedly admonish their colleagues for using autointoxication "as a convenient cloak for ignorance." "Time and again," a San Francisco practitioner complained, "I have been put to the embarrassment of having to point out to some brother physician that his beautiful case of 'autointoxication' was really an aortic regurgitation, a chronic nephritis, a myxedema, a high blood pressure, tuberculosis, or some other well-known disease." The renowned Logan Clendening was less diplomatic, dismissing the medical literature on autointoxication as "mad, maudlin, jumbled, mystic, undigested" and "sophomoric."[19]

The theory's proponents had acted with sophomoric haste. They had jumped to their conclusions on the basis of the evidence mentioned above, and experiments in which intestinal contents and fecal extracts had poisoned animals when injected directly into the bloodstream. But they had not shown that the putrefaction products were absorbed from the

[19] Walter Alvarez, "Intestinal Autointoxication," *Physiological Rev.,* *4,* 352–393 (1924), p. 353; Alvarez, "Origins of the So-called Autointoxication Symptoms," *JAMA, 72,* 8–13 (1919), p. 8; Logan Clendening, "A Review of the Subject of Chronic Intestinal Stasis," *Interstate Med. J., 22,* 1191–1200 (1915), pp. 1192–1193.

human intestine in sufficient amounts to cause injury, or escaped detoxification by the body's defenses. In fact, it was demonstrated by opponents, little of the poison could be absorbed through the colon, and any that was would be neutralized in the intestinal wall and liver. And the fact that purgation gave immediate relief from the symptoms associated with constipation was final evidence against autointoxication. If poisons absorbed from impacted feces were the cause of the headache and malaise, the discomfort should continue for some time after the purging, while the toxins continued to circulate. Immediate improvement indicated the symptoms had a physical, not chemical, origin related to the mechanical distention of the rectum. Duplication of symptoms in volunteers who allowed cotton to be packed into their rectums closed the case against autointoxication as a common disease entity.[20]

Or at least it should have. By the time it encountered strong opposition, though, the autointoxication theory had gathered sufficient momentum to carry it into the 1920s. It received its early impetus in the 1880s, from the work of Charles Bouchard, a Paris physician whose *Lectures on Autointoxication in Disease* became the authoritative text on the subject. A major boost was given by Sir Arbuthnot Lane, a giant of surgery who unfortunately ended his career being accused of an obsession with autointoxication. Convinced that the colon was a "cesspool," Lane made it his mission to transform "human derelicts ... into useful and happy people" by removing their colons or otherwise remodelling intestinal tracts reeking with poisons. His "short-circuiting" procedure set off "an epidemic of operative surgery" which had reached the point by the mid-1910s that "now surgeons (some surgeons) are everywhere seeking to remedy almost any condition by removing ceca, colons, and sigmoids, or all three, or by making unnatural intestinal

---

[20] Alvarez, "Intestinal Autointoxication" (n. 19); J. George Adami, "An Address on Chronic Intestinal Stasis," *Brit. Med. J.*, 1914 (i), 177–183.

anastomoses." Bad results were apparently common: Clendening remarked of his fellow physicians who performed the Lane operations that "to find some of their patients you must ask the sexton."[21]

Less risky, and for a season more popular, was the remedy offered by the most prominent of the autointoxication theorists. Élie Metchnikoff, director of the prestigious Pasteur Institute and winner of the 1908 Nobel Prize for his contributions to immunology, was in fact a true philosopher of autointoxication. His "Optimistic Philosophy," or orthobiosis, is too complicated a creation to be explored closely, though its ultimately Faustian reaching was bound, however intricately, to the same old hatred of intestinal putrefaction. Driven to grapple with the big questions of life and mortality by his own "precocious and unhappy old age." Metchnikoff discovered that senility was due in large measure to the poisons generated by the intestinal flora. Of pivotal importance to this conclusion were the two observations that lactic acid (the product of the fermentative bacteria that sour milk) inhibits the activity of putrefactive organisms, and that exceptional longevity was most common in societies making heavy use of soured milk preparations. Bulgaria was particularly rich in centenarians, Bulgarians consumed much yogurt, yogurt was produced by an especially active lactic acid generating microbe: in condensed form, those were the steps by which Metchnikoff arrived at his conviction that seeding the gastrointestinal tract with the "Bulgarian bacillus" would displace putrefactive bacteria and retard the aging process.[22]

His full argument was persuasive enough to make yogurt,

[21] Arbuthnot Lane, "An Address on Chronic Intestinal Stasis," *Brit. Med. J.*, 1913 (ii), 1125–1128; Lane, *The Operative Treatment of Chronic Intestinal Stasis*, London, 1915; Adami, "Address" (n. 20), p. 179; Paul Woolley, "Intestinal Stasis and Intestinal Intoxication: a Critical Review," *J. Lab. Clin. Med.*, 1, 45–54 (1915–1916), p. 45; Clendening, "Review" (n. 19), p. 1192.

[22] Élie Metchnikoff, *The Prolongation of Life*, New York, 1908, pp. 82, 171–182, 327. Also see R. B. Vaughan, "The Romantic Rationalist. A Study of Élie Metchnikoff," *Med. Hist.*, 9 201–215, (1965).

buttermilk, special new milk products like "Vitalait," and even dried tablets of "Lacto-bacilline" all the rage among the health conscious. "For several months," at least, "one heard of nothing but the Bulgarian bacillus. The bacillus shared with Mr. Lloyd George's budget the honor of monopolizing the conversation at the dinner tables of the great. He [Metchnikoff] dominated Belgravia, frolicked in Fulham, and bestrode Birmingham and the whole of the British Isles. [But] whether he did any good to any one except the chemists and the purveyors of milk there is some reason to doubt." Most judges felt no hesitancy at all about expressing doubt; to them Metchnikoff cut a ridiculous figure as "the modern Ponce de Leon searchng for the Fountain of Immortal Youth and finding it in the Milky Whey."[23]

As devoted a worrier about autointoxication as Kellogg was, he nevertheless agreed with that evaluation of Metchnikoff, as well as the still more disparaging assessments of Lane's approach. Kellogg represented the vegetarian position on intestinal self-poisoning, which was quite distinct from those competing views. Lane he found the more offensive, for though Kellogg was an avid practitioner of surgery himself, extirpation of the colon seemed an unnecessarily heroic operation. His hygienist's faith in nature's wisdom made it impossible to accept "that Nature has made so great a blunder as to provide the human race with a useless and even mischievous organ." The organ clearly was designed as a temporary reservoir for the indigestible—and nonputrefying—cellulose constituents of fruits and vegetables. "The fault with the modern colon is not that it is superfluous," therefore, but that it was so regularly abused by erroneous diet.[24]

Metchnikoff's dietetic alternative was to be preferred, but while Kellogg gave ready second to the idea that autointoxi-

---

[23] "Metchnikoff and Buttermilk," *JAMA*, *67*, 939 (1916); Edwin Slosson, *Major Prophets of Today*, Boston, 1916, p. 175.
[24] Kellogg, *Itinerary* (n. 14), p. 163.

cation was "the cause of old age," he could only scowl at Metchnikoff's method of combatting it. A whole chapter of his *Autointoxication,* in fact, was entitled "Metchnikoff's Mistake," and all but delighted in the Parisian's early demise at age seventy-one. Metchnikoff's mistake had been to only add yogurt and buttermilk to his diet, and not eliminate flesh. One of Kellogg's treasured anecdotes was the response he solicited from one of Metchnikoff's assistants: "Metchnikoff eats a pound of meat and lets it rot in his colon and then drinks a pint of sour milk to disinfect it," the man had reported. "I am not such a fool. I don't eat the meat."[25]

Meat was the critical item in the vegetarian analysis of autointoxication. As developed by Kellogg, that analysis started from the position that the ordinary meat-containing diet was so high in protein as to greatly encourage the growth and activity of proteolytic (or putrefactive) bacteria in the colon. As the microbes operated on undigested flesh food, the body would be "flooded with the most horrible and loathsome poisons," and brought to suffer headache, depression, skin problems, chronic fatigue, damage to the liver, kidneys, and blood vessels, and other injuries totalling up to "enormous mischief." Anyone who read to the end of Kellogg's baleful list must have been ready to agree that "the marvel is not that human life is so short and so full of miseries, mental, moral, and physical, but that civilized human beings are able to live at all."[26]

The adjective "civilized" was a crucial distinction, of course, but while Kellogg's hygienic reform predecessors and contemporaries all strove to help whole people return to nature, his attention was concentrated on their colons: if that organ could be restored to its natural condition, he felt, the rest of the body would quickly follow. "Civilized colon" was the worst of all the degenerations consequent to man's

[25] Kellogg, *Autointoxication or Intestinal Toxemia,* Battle Creek, Mich., 1919, p. 311.

[26] Kellogg, *Itinerary* (n. 14), pp. 25, 36, 82; Kellogg, *Autointoxication* (n. 25), p. 131.

desertion of nature, but the affliction went generally unnoticed because it was so tied to cultural habits as to appear normal. Actually, the typical colon was much more sluggish than nature intended, having been devitalized by a combination of civilization's errors. Sedentary living, first of all, had weakened the abdominal muscles and decreased their power to push forward the colon's contents. A second mistake was the civilized custom of sitting instead of squatting to evacuate (toilet seats, in Kellogg's opinion, should be much lower and sloped backwards, to imitate natural defecatory posture). Thirdly, there was the habit of ignoring nature's call to evacuate because to answer would be inconvenient or impolite. Civilization's concern for manners had made man as house-broken as the dog, Kellogg scoffed, forcing him onto an artificial schedule that gradually paralyzed the colon's natural movements.[27]

But the worst offense of all was civilized diet. Modern man ate too concentrated a diet, with insufficient bulk and roughage to stimulate the bowels to action. Fletcher's mistake, Kellogg never wearied of explaining, had been to reject all foods that he could not reduce to liquid by mastication. He had entirely eliminated fiber from his diet, and thereby made himself a victim of constipation and, ultimately, autointoxication. A vegetarian diet, he added for the unaware, was high in roughage. Its other advantage was that it was low in protein. The high protein diet common to flesh eaters was ideal fodder for the putrefactive microorganisms of the colon, while its low fiber content reduced its rate of movement to a crawl that gave the microbes time to convert all unabsorbed protein to ptomaines. In the meat eater's sluggish bowels, Kellogg believed, lay "the secret of nine-tenths of all the chronic ills from which civilized human beings suffer," including "national inefficiency and physical unpreparedness," as well as "not a small part of our moral and social maladies."[28]

[27] Kellogg, *Itinerary* (n. 14), pp. 71–95.
[28] *ibid.*, pp. 87, 93.

That moral and social purity required physical purity was a premise of too long standing in hygienic ideology not to be enlarged upon as an aspect of autointoxication. Vegetarian polemicist W.R.C. Latson, editor of *Health Culture* magazine, perhaps carried the question to its limits: "This condition of food intoxication may lead to acts of violence or immorality, at the memory of which the perpetrator looks in horror and amazement. The diner leaves the table intoxicated with a dozen poisons. A heated argument, a word too much, a moment of frenzy, a sudden blow; and the next morning he awakens to find himself a criminal. Or a hand is laid on his arm, a voice whispers in his ear; and he turns aside to follow the scarlet woman—the scarlet woman whose steps lead down to hell." Warnings of the multifaceted dangers of autointoxication, which seemed the required content for Progressive vegetarian publications, contributed to the creation of what Kellogg called the "sensitive colon conscience" needed to rescue civilization from the "race-destroying effects of universal constipation and world-wide autointoxication."[29]

That "universal constipation" was, in Kellogg's estimation, "the most destructive blockade that has ever opposed human progress." It was thus not enough to reject meat and reduce protein intake, for there were natural internal secretions containing proteins, as well as dietary protein, which could putrefy in even the vegetarian's colon. All waste had to be passed through the intestines quickly if autointoxication were to be prevented. By Kellogg's analysis, that meant that even the popular ideal of one daily movement was inadequate: "one bowel movement means constipation of a pronounced degree." For instruction in natural evacuation, man had to turn again to his evolutionary forbears, the primates. Kellogg supposed apes to possess as much authority for the exit of the human alimentary tract as for its en-

---

[29] W. R. C. Latson, *Food Value of Meat*, New York, 1900, p. 68; Kellogg, *Itinerary* (n. 14), p. 99.

trance, and personally inquired of the directors of the London and Bronx zoos how often their primates moved their bowels. The answer of three to four (and more) times a day was gladly accepted as the human norm. A colon returned to nature by low protein, vegetable diet, abdomen-strengthening exercise, and proper defecation posture would freely move after every meal, as well as first thing each morning. To promote that regularity, Kellogg recommended the inclusion of bran or other roughage with each meal, as well as a dose of paraffin oil to lubricate the intestines. Bulky feces and slippery bowel walls also assured such a speedy passage that any putrefactive bacteria chancing to enter the body would be swept through the colon before they had time to establish a footing (vegetable diet would have already substituted fermentative bacteria for the putrefactive microbes resident during the colon's "civilized" days). A final blessing was the disappearance of foul odors from the bowel discharges.[30]

If Kellogg repeated Fletcher in that respect, his stool-frequency measure of bodily efficiency was antipodal to the masticator's. Yet he expected multiple daily movements to build that same physical endurance which had distinguished Fletcher. Endurance was a cherished goal of other vegetarians too; indeed, the most distinctive feature of the Progressive period's muscular vegetarianism was its apotheosis of muscle. Chest-thumping advertisement of the athletic accomplishments of vegetarians became the obligatory climax to any Pythagorean presentation. That was a significant change of tactics. The older strategy had preferred the selection of examples of strength and endurance from the animal kingdom (and in keeping with tradition, Kellogg also offered a defense of Graham's selection of the rhinoceros as ruler of the jungle). Human cases had been

---

[30] Kellogg, *Itinerary* (n. 14), pp. 33–35, 93; Kellogg, *Autointoxication* (n. 25), pp. 97–99, 139; Kellogg, *Natural Diet* (n. 6), p. 114. Also see Schlickeysen, *Fruit and Bread* (n. 14), p. 137.

offered all along as well, but they had been less plentiful and forwarded with less confidence. Usually they were simply reports of ordinary people managing to maintain health, not of extraordinary athletes. This type of subdued testimonial continued into the new age also. One of the favored subjects was William Penn Alcott, the only son of the Jacksonian health reformer. A life-long Pythagorean, he too suffered from consumptive troubles as a child, but overcame the weakness and went on to become a Congregational minister and to take an active part in the affairs of the American Vegetarian Society. His first wife and their three children were not vegetarian, and all died early; but he was more careful in selecting his second mate, and they enjoyed a long and healthy life together. Early in his second marriage, in fact, he gave up fine flour (the father's curse of becoming a Grahamite was visited upon the son), and soon escaped the slight rheumatic troubles which previously bothered him. He lived until 1919, and the age of eighty-one.[31]

Such lives were admirable, but they lacked the magnitude of physical accomplishment needed to dispel the belief that strength required meat. That idea, already having solid intuitive standing, had been braced during the mid-1800s by the authority of Justus von Liebig, the preeminent developer of physiological chemistry in its emergent period. Liebig's skill at juggling chemical formulae and his arrogant determination to simplify the chemical mechanisms of life had led him to a theory of metabolism maintaining that all body heat is produced by the oxidation of fats and carbohydrates (the respiratory foods), and the energy for all muscular movement by the oxidation of protein (plastic food). An extension of the latter position was that an individual's protein consumption should be proportional to the amount of

---

[31] Kellogg, *Natural Diet* (n. 6), p. 50; *J. Hyg. Herald Health*, 45, 221–224 (1895); Forward, *Fifty Years* (n. 10), p. 49; Donald Winslow, "A Lasell Neighbor a Century Ago," *Lasell Leaves*, 79, 4 (1954).

muscular work he had to do. Heavy laborers and athletes apparently required a high protein diet.[32]

This aspect of Liebig's thought was most unwelcome to vegetarians. Since the typical fleshless diet contained significantly less protein than the standard, vegetarians were theoretically incapable of prolonged exertion. Many ignored the Liebig challenge, but there were others who made embarrassing attempts to rationalize working power on a low protein dietary. The English Pythagorean John Smith, for example, struggled to prove that vegetarians manufactured much of their tissue protein from the nitrogen inhaled from the air—why else, he asked, would nature have put so much of that gas in the atmosphere? He also suspected atmospheric nitrogen might be swallowed with food and get into the blood from the stomach.[33]

Fortunately Liebig's theoretical obstacle was soon dismantled. Experiments performed in the 1850s and 1860s measured protein metabolism by the quantity of urea (protein's chief metabolite) excreted, and found no relation between the amount of muscular work accomplished and the quantity of protein oxidized. Instead it became clear that muscular energy was derived from carbohydrates and fatty acids, which implied vegetarians might enjoy an advantage in working power. Only vegetarians noticed that implication, though, for while it was supplanted as an energy source, protein continued to enjoy undeserved status for its plastic properties. The large quantities of protein consumed by athletes and heavy laborers (who earned hearty appetites and found protein-rich foods to be especially palatable) were rationalized by the assumption that the protein appetite was a physiological craving representing the body's demand for repair of muscle worn down by exercise. The high protein diet of athletes, which was actually only a custom, was thus accepted by nutrition scientists as a physical necessity. The

[32] Justus von Liebig, *Animal Chemistry*, Cambridge, 1842, pp. 204–210.

[33] John Smith, *Fruits and Farinacea. The Proper Food of Man*, New York, 1854, pp. 133–137.

very same dietitians who sniped at Liebig for having recommended superfluous protein for energy, in the next breath recommended superfluous protein for tissue maintenance. Pre-Chittenden protein allowances for athletes were far above the amount of protein taken by the typical vegetarian competitor.[34]

The pressure on vegetarians to prove that their diet could support any degree of vigorous living thus continued into the twentieth century. It was in fact increased by the growth of competitive athletics in the later 1800s, and the popularization of meat as the staple of the training table. Ever since the ancient Greek Olympic hero Milo of Croton won fame on a reputed training diet of twenty pounds of meat and eighteen pints of wine a day (as well as twenty pounds of bread), it had been popularly assumed that athletes required flesh food for victory. In the early 1870s, Beard had been evidently upset by Harvard's loss to Oxford in a London boat race. He vented his distress in snide comments that if the American crew had allowed its enemy to prescribe a dietary for them they could not have done worse than with the high vegetable, relatively low meat diet they had followed on the recommendation of "ignorant writers in our country." "They failed not for lack of strength," he added, "in which they were superior to their rivals; but for lack of staying power." Far better results would have been achieved with a regimen of restrained vegetable consumption and lots of lean and rare beef and mutton.[35]

Beard's advice was being taken to heart by the end of the century. The standard diet for collegiate teams consisted of two kinds of meat at all three meals, supplemented with "a moderate quantity" of fruits and vegetables. No less an au-

[34] Elmer McCollum, *A History of Nutrition*, Boston, 1957, pp. 123–127; Francis Benedict, "The Nutritive Requirements of the Body," *Am. J. Physiol.*, *16*, 409–437 (1906), pp. 411–412; J. C. Dunlop, *et al.*, "On the Influence of Muscular Exercise, Sweating, and Massage, on the Metabolism," *J. Physiol.*, *22*, 68–91 (1897–98).

[35] H. A. Harris, *Greek Athletes and Athletics*, London, 1964, pp. 110–112; Beard, *Eating and Drinking* (n. 11), pp. 135–136.

thority than W. O. Atwater fully approved of this training diet including "especially large amounts of protein." His careful studies of the food taken by the crews of Yale and Harvard (now submissive to Beard) found 150 to 170 grams of protein to be the daily average; generally at least two-thirds of the protein was taken from animal sources. Other inquiries revealed college football teams often consumed more than 200 grams per day, the University of California players ingesting a robustious 270 grams. Sandow, the most celebrated strongman of the day (he was a blockbuster attraction with Ziegfeld) ate nearly 250 grams of protein, and an English prize fighter approached 280 on his regimen of one pound of mutton three times·daily, and a bit of bread and ale. Most training guides made a point of advising that beef be served rare or "underdone," seemingly agreeing with the ancient vegetarian charge tht carnivorous eating habits created an aggressive carnivorous behavior. According to Holbrook, meat was so rare at some training tables the athletes referred to it as "red rags."[36]

That vegetarian "athletes" might stand up to boys trained on red rags was an amusing, absurd proposition. Spencer ridiculed vegetable-built muscles as "soft and flabby"; Beard sadly recalled a vegetarian hiker he had met, a young man of "pale and feminine features, tinged with an unnatural flush," whose attempt to maintain a mere twenty miles a day pace had killed him (with consumption naturally) within a year. And when London's Vegetarian Society announced the formation of an athletic and cycling club, meat-eating sportsmen could scarce contain their merriment:

---

[36] W. O. Atwater and A. P. Bryant, *Dietary Studies of University Boat Crews*, U.S. Department of Agriculture, Office of Experiment Stations, Bulletin No. 25, Washington, 1900, pp. 66–72 especially; Russell Chittenden, *The Nutrition of Man*, New York, 1907, p. 156; Martin Holbrook, *Eating for Strength: or, Food and Diet in Their Relation to Health and Work*, New York, 1888, pp. 149–154. Also see James Slonaker, *The Effect of a Strictly Vegetable Diet on the Spontaneous Activity, the Rate of Growth, and the Longevity of the Albino Rat*, Palo Alto, Cal., 1912.

We shall hear of the vegetable "scorcher" [racing cyclist] and gymnast, of the athlete who is trained on artichokes, and the pacemaker who is built up with asparagus. It is a dangerous competition, into which the vegetarians are urged by overweening ambition. Evidently there are men amongst them who are not content with a spiritual mission, who say, "let us produce a record-breaking cyclist; let us have our own strong man; only by such prodigies can the world be converted." This challenge to the eater of beef must cause some misgiving amongst the orthodox. Suppose the vegetarian athlete should be tempted from the faith by the success of his carnivorous compeers? He may forget that it was vegetarianism he was appointed to vindicate, and not the egotism of his thews and sinews.[37]

But vegetarians did not forget their purpose, and so strong was their desire to vindicate their diet that carnivorous compeers were soon covered in their dust. In 1896, for example, the aptly named James Parsley led the Vegetarian Cycling Club to easy victory over two regular clubs. A week later, he won the most prestigious hill-climbing race in England, breaking the hill record by nearly a minute. Before the summer was out, Parsley had set a new fifty mile record, as well as several records for shorter distances on a tandem, and for London to Brighton and back on a tricycle. Other members of the club (numbering altogether about ninety, including thirteen ladies) also turned in remarkable performances, and none gave any evidence of being "soft and flabby." Their competitors were having to eat crow with their beef.[38]

American vegetarian cyclists were soon in hot pursuit of the English. Will Brown, who in the 1890s switched to vegetable diet to save himself from an early death with consumption, gained so much strength in just three years as to batter

---

[37] Herbert Spencer, *Education: Intellectual, Moral, and Physical,* New York, 1881, p. 236; Beard, *Eating and Drinking* (n. 11), p. 94; "The Vegetarian Creed," *Living Age, 216,* 128 (1898).

[38] Forward, *Fifty Years* (n. 10), pp. 154–157.

all records for the 2000 mile ride. And Margarita Gast established a women's record for 1000 miles on a diet of fruit, zwieback, raw potatoes, and, shockingly, "sometimes a little claret."[39]

Cycling, moreover, was only one sport in which vegetarians were trouncing the opposition. Long distance walking races were also very popular in the 1890s, and were regarded as an ultimate test of endurance. In the 1893 race from Berlin to Vienna, the first two competitors to cover the 372-mile course were vegetarians. They required 155 and 156 hours respectively; the next finisher, a meat eater, arrived 22 hours later. A 100-kilometer race held several years later in Germany also attracted much attention, for of the first fourteen finishers, eleven were vegetarians. A similar outcome attended a 70-mile walking match in which contestants were required to complete the course within fourteen hours. Six of the eight vegetarian entrants met the standard, and the other two failed only for having gotten lost and travelled an extra five miles. Not a single flesh eater could meet the fourteen-hour limit, and only one could even finish the race; according to Kellogg, he "straggled in, very much exhausted."[40]

Runners throve on vegetarian diet too. To consider only one example, Jonathan Barclay, secretary of the Scottish Vegetarian Society, in 1896 competed in some twenty races at distances from the half mile to ten miles, and won eleven while never finishing lower than third (some years later, in 1912, the vegetarian Kolehmainen became one of the first men to complete the marathon under 2:30). Comparable records were compiled by vegetarian swimmers, tennis players, and other athletes, including the West Ham Vegetarian Society's undefeated tug-of-war team. So impressive did the vegetarian athletic record become, that when Berlin's Wil-

[39] Latson, *Food Value* (n. 29), pp. 60–63.

[40] Forward, *Fifty Years* (n. 10), p. 156; Jacques Buttner, *A Fleshless Diet*, New York, 1910, pp. 163, 170–171; *Lancet*, 1893 (i), 1396–1397; Kellogg, *Shall We Slay* (n. 12), p. 106.

helm Caspari published his unprecedentedly thorough studies of vegetarianism and physiology (1905), he devoted a lengthy concluding section to the analysis of vegetarian athletic success. The focus of his discussion was the 1902 walking race from Dresden to Berlin, a contest which drew thirty-two competitors. Prior to the race, Caspari selected the leading vegetarian and flesh-eating contenders, and subjected each to thorough physical evaluation, including measurements of oxygen capacity per kilogram of body weight at rest and work. The vegetarian champion was a twenty-eight year old man who had adopted the vegetable diet eight years before, and for the last two years had made heavy use of Kellogg's health food products, especially peanut butter. He had developed, in Caspari's judgment, a "physique like Sandow," and still more surprising, had the highest oxygen capacity yet measured. The vegetarian subject went on to capture the race handily, in record time (26 hours, 58 minutes), while the meat-eating cofavorite Caspari had tested failed to finish. Places two through five, incidentally, were also won by flesh abstainers.[41]

Caspari nevertheless refused to credit vegetable diet "in itself as decisive" for the humiliation of the carnivorous walkers. Since vegetarians were more self-conscious about health, he reasoned, they were more likely to live regular, hygienic lives year-round, and particularly to refrain from the use of alcohol (the meat eater who had dropped out had refreshed himself during the race with wine). But the physical advantage from healthful living was minor, in Caspari's estimation, to the psychological advantage of vegetarians. Having already called attention to the importance of will power for the completion of feats of endurance, he now presented the vegetarian life as a daily training ground for perseverance and determination. Not only was the diet itself

[41] Forward, *Fifty Years* (n. 10), pp. 158–160; Jules Lefèvre, *A Scientific Investigation into Vegetarianism,* London, 1923, p. 162; Wilhelm Caspari, "Physiologische Studien über Vegetarismus," *Pflüger's Archiv, 109,* 473–595 (1905), pp. 569–572, 580–583.

painful to adhere to, but the frequent social embarrassment accompanying refusal to eat meat demanded psychological firmness of practitioners. When to these considerations was added the regular necessity of defending unusual principles, one could easily see vegetarian strength of will becoming fanaticism. And it was this *Fanatismus,* Caspari insisted, which carried so many vegetarians to victory. Athletes on ordinary diet saw the contest solely as a sporting event, but vegetarians approached it as a struggle to justify their life ideals and demonstrate physical and moral superiority to their adversaries.[42]

The vegetarian's zeal for vindication, it might be argued, was even more important during training than in the competition itself. Any veteran of endurance contests knows that will power may hold one up to the end, but by itself cannot produce respectable, let alone winning, times. Rigorous training is the difference between running well instead of merely finishing, and vegetarians undoubtedly benefitted from the relatively lenient attitudes toward training in the early 1900s. The training programs recommended for young and serious distance runners at that time, for example, were considerably less demanding than the schedules followed by thousands of middle-aged marathoners today. The vegetarian's desire to win for his philosophy was a spur that could goad him beyond the accepted boundaries of training, give him the fortitude to put in the extra miles at extra effort. The high oxygen consumption rate of the Dresden to Berlin winner suggests a rigorous training regimen.

But stiffer training was perhaps not all. Despite Caspari's certainty that there was no dietary advantage to vegetarianism, there probably was. Numerous studies in recent years have documented the value of a high carbohydrate diet for endurance performance. Athletes engaged in competition extended over several days (such as the Dresden walkers) are especially likely to benefit from the ability of a car-

---

[42] Caspari, "Physiologische Studien" (n. 41), p. 585.

bohydrate heavy diet to restore depleted muscle glycogen to high levels after each day's contest. There surely was a significant difference in the carbohydrate content of the vegetarian athlete's training diet and that of the conventional athlete who followed the standard advice to maintain himself on a high protein diet. Vegetarian temperance was an advantage too. Athletes at the turn of the century made free use of alcohol as a stimulant. It was reportedly standard practice for runners to quaff champagne or brandy immediately before a race. Several marathoners at the 1908 Olympics drank cognac during the competition to keep up their strength, and a walker in a 100-kilometer contest in Germany the same year was reported to have consumed twenty-two glasses of beer and half a bottle of wine. These dietary factors combined with more serious training and fanatical will power to resist fatigue to give vegetarians the competitive edge needed to win.[43]

The victors' own explanations were similar, but with the inclusion of autointoxication. Putrefaction poisons depressed muscular function, and also mental power, so that the vegetarians' superior determination was physiological rather than fanatical. The muscular efforts of flesh eaters were further hampered by the action of "fatigue poisons" present in meat, a product of the animal's own struggles before death. Kellogg (and others) also tackled the worship of protein as muscle fuel, patiently outlining the carbohydrate basis of muscular energy and even discoursing on muscle glycogen levels.[44]

Nonvegetarian athletes were not invariably losers, and

[43] Malcolm Ford, "Distance Running," *Outing, 18,* 205–210 (1891); Ford, "Training," *Outing, 19,* 421–424 (1891–92); Randolph Farles, "On Training in General," *Outing, 30,* 177–182 (1897); Adolphe Abrahams, "Athletics and the Medical Man," *Practitioner, 86,* 429–446 (1911), p. 445; Graham Chambers, "Observations on the Urines of Marathon Runners," *Brit. Med. J.,* 1911 (i), 490–491; Ernst Jokl, "Notes on Doping," *Med. and Sport, 1,* 55–57 (1968), p. 56.

[44] Kellogg, *Shall We Slay* (n. 12), pp. 101–103.

apologists for flesh food defended themselves with examples of meat-built stamina such as Johnnie Hayes, the winner of the 1908 Olympic marathon. Hayes' workouts were supported by two flesh meals daily, and he expressed confidence that "plenty of meat such as steaks, chops and roast beef and lamb are beneficial while training." His faith was apparently corroborated by the results of the Pittsburgh marathon the following year, in which 70 percent of the flesh-eating entrants finished, but only 60 percent of the vegetarians could complete the course. But such results were the exception rather than the rule, vegetarians could reply, for not only was the overall Pythagorean athletic record impressive, there were experimental studies to document a genuine physiological superiority for flesh abstainers. The Belgian Schouteden carried out tests in 1904 on twenty-five students separated into vegetarian and meat-eating groups. For each he determined the endurance of the hand muscles by measuring the maximum number of times each subject could lift a weight on a pulley by squeezing a handle. The mean number of contractions for vegetarians was 69, for meat eaters 38, and the vegetarians as a rule recovered the ability to squeeze much more quickly than the flesh eaters.[45]

Contracting the hand was at best a marginally athletic exercise, though, and vegetarian claims to muscularity benefitted much less from Schouteden's work than from the experiments done three years later by Irving Fisher. As a logical extension of his study of the relation of endurance to a low protein dietary (discussed in the last chapter), Fisher examined the influence of meatless low protein diet. His forty-seven subjects were divided into three groups—Yale

---

[45] Hayes quoted by Elmer Berry, "The Effects of a High and Low Proteid Diet on Physical Efficiency," *Am. Phys. Ed. Rev.*, *14*, 288–297 (1909), p. 296; Watson Savage, *et al.*, "Physiological and Pathological Effects of Severe Exertion (The Marathon Race)," *Am. Phys. Ed. Rev.*, *16*, 1–11 (1911), p. 3; McCollum, *History of Nutrition* (n. 34), p. 198. Also see Irving Fisher, "Diet and Endurance at Brussels," *Science*, *26*, 561–563 (1907).

athletes trained on a full flesh regimen, athletes who abstained from meat, and sedentary vegetarians (nurses and physicians from the Battle Creek Sanitarium). Each was tested to determine the maximum length of time he could hold his arms out horizontally, and the maximum number of deep knee bends and leg raises he could perform. The final tally—"much to my surprise," Fisher avowed—was heavily in favor of the flesh abstainers. Only two of the fifteen meat eaters, for example, were able to maintain the arm hold more than fifteen minutes; none achieved half-an-hour. Of the vegetarians, however, twenty-two (of thirty-two) exceeded a quarter-hour, and fifteen broke the thirty-minute barrier. In fact, nine doubled that time, and one surpassed three hours. But the final touch to the carnivores' embarrassment was given by the six-year old son of one of the San volunteers, who, curiously imitating his father, "held his little arms out, and did not drop them until 43 minutes had elapsed."[46]

The meat eaters were similarly humiliated in the other tests, and the results could not, Fisher maintained, be explained by Caspari's hypothesis. While a few of the vegetarians had exhibited some degree of "fanatical desire," it had not been evident in the majority. Most of the subjects were clearly moved by pure competitive drive, by the determination to break the records set by others, whatever their dietary persuasion. Fisher even warned his flesh eaters that their performances would be recorded as evidence of Yale athletic ability, confident that "Yale spirit" would prove "as great a stimulus as any 'vegetarian' spirit could possibly be." In one case, Fisher reported in a letter to his wife, he stood in front of a Yale track man and continually urged him to hold out his arms for the glory of his school; the spiritless lad gave out in less than ten minutes.[47]

Other factors—training, amount of sleep, work load, use

---

[46] Irving Fisher, "The Influence of Flesh-Eating on Endurance," *Yale Med. J.*, *13*, 205–221 (1906–07), p. 214.

[47] Fisher [Jr.], *My Father* (n. 4), p. 111.

of alcohol and tobacco, etc.—were considered, but there was nothing to reasonably account for the vegetarians' performance except diet. Whether the crucial factor was lack of meat, or merely of excessive protein, however, could not be determined, for the vegetarians were all low protein feeders. The experiment thus may have been nothing more than an ornate repetition of Chittenden's investigations. Fisher concluded low protein and vegetable diet both contributed to endurance, but presented no supporting evidence. He eventually changed his mind, deciding low protein by itself, whether of animal or vegetable origin, was responsible for endurance.[48]

Two years later Kellogg reported a similar study, and results, from Battle Creek, but the subject seems to have been pursued no further. Scientists had long before become jaded by vegetarian exaggerations, and neither Fisher nor Kellogg could be regarded as disinterested or accomplished physiologists. Their studies are still occasionally cited in discussions of diet and fitness, but are dismissed as "dated" and not credible. The official position is that there is no basis for advocating either a balanced vegetarian or ordinary mixed diet for athletes.[49]

Muscular vegetarians of the Progressive period had still more ammunition in stock, including an answer to the briefly popular notion that fish is brain food. The phosphorous required for the maintenance of nervous tissue, Pythagoreans advised, could be obtained from cereals too, which, unlike fish, did not readily putrefy. That explained why fishermen had never been celebrated for their intellectual achievements! Vegetarians were already linking a meat diet to cardiovascular disease also, and by the late 1910s were capitalizing on the recent discoveries of vitamins to

[48] Fisher, "The Influence" (n. 46), p. 219; Fisher, *Report on National Vitality*, Washington, 1909, pp. 4, 43.

[49] McCollum, *History of Nutrition* (n. 34), p. 198; Melvin Williams, *Nutritional Aspects of Human Physical and Athletic Performance*, Springfield, Ill., 1976, p. 303.

extol the advantages of their system. There is inadequate space for exhaustive discussion of Progressive vegetarian science, but its integration of traditional argument with modern theories spun from the advancing edges of contemporary science, and aggressive backing of theory with performance, should be already clear. The examination of Progressive vegetarianism cannot be concluded, however, without a reminder that its aim was to make muscle a racial, and not simply an individual, trait. That vegetarians shared their contemporaries' dismay at the physical and moral deterioration of the race, and saw purified diet as the remedy, has been noted in an earlier chapter. It might be added here that Kellogg led this campaign as well. One of the last holdouts for inheritance of acquired characteristics, he expected that not just improved health, but reformed health habits themselves could be transmitted through heredity. These ideas were forwarded through the work of a Race Betterment Foundation he organized and used to sponsor national Race Betterment Conferences in 1914 and 1915. At the second conference, he even proposed that an eugenics registry be organized to record the names of individuals distinguished for vigorous health. This "human pedigree" book might then be used to assist people concerned to practice what Holbrook had called sanitary marriage.[50]

Kellogg's eugenics work was soon halted by the escalation of American involvement in World War I. Even had plans for the registry continued without interruption, however, sanitary marriages could not have been joined quickly enough to save his football team. In 1923, Kellogg opened Battle Creek College, a four-year program in physical education and home economics that soon expanded its curricu-

---

[50] John Coppock, "Hygiene of the Brain," *J. Hyg. Herald Health, 48,* 1–3 (1898); Lady Walb. Paget, "Vegetable Diet," *Pop. Sci. M., 44,* 100 (1893); Kellogg, *Shall We Slay* (n. 12), p. 109; F. X. Gouraud, *What Shall I Eat,* New York, 1911, p. 350; Lefèvre, *Scientific Investigation* (n. 41), pp. 33–37; Josiah Oldfield, "Vegetarian Still," *Nineteenth Cent., 44,* 246–252 (1898); Schwarz, *John Harvey Kellogg* (n. 3), pp. 220–223.

lum—and fielded a football team. It was the director's hope that with a training regimen of "biologic living" the squad would so overwhelm opponents as to win them, and the rest of the public, to vegetable diet. The team was disbanded after its inaugural season, though. The college administration's official reason was that the game was too violent, but the team's poor won-lost record was undoubtedly a consideration. It was not a shining denouement for muscular vegetarianism.[51]

[51] Schwarz, *John Harvey Kellogg*, (n. 3), p. 102.

☆☆☆☆☆☆☆☆☆☆☆☆☆☆☆☆☆☆☆☆☆☆☆☆☆☆☆☆☆☆☆☆☆☆

CHAPTER EIGHT
URIC ACID AND OTHER FETISHES

☆☆☆☆☆☆☆☆☆☆☆☆☆☆☆☆☆☆☆☆☆☆☆☆☆☆☆☆☆☆☆☆☆☆

FEW CHEMICAL COMPOUNDS HAVE SO UNENVIABLE A HIS-
tory as uric acid. White, odorless, and tasteless, it is saved
from being utterly nondescript only by its vulgar origins
and pathological involvements. As a metabolic end-product,
it is normally encountered in animal evacuations, in the
urine of primates, and the excrement of creatures such as
birds, serpents, and slugs. It was discovered, in 1776, in uri-
nary calculi, the kidney and bladder stones that have been
the cause of so much human misery. And before the close of
the eighteenth century, uric acid had also been identified in
tophi, the deposits that torment the joints of gout sufferers.
In 1848, the London physician Alfred Garrod detected the
substance in the blood of gout patients and asserted it to be
the cause of the disease. The final blows against the compound's character, however, were reserved for the turn of
the twentieth century, when the acid came to be accused of
an astonishingly long and varied list of medical crimes: "Of
all words connected with disease," a commentator on *Fads
and Feeding* wrote, "probably uric acid is more universally
known than any other. One hears it continually spoken of as
though it were the most familiar substance on this earth, and
advertisements of some preparation which will seemingly
expel this arch-fiend from the system meet one's gaze some-
where on the pages of every daily paper or periodical." So
devoted were physicians and patients alike to the menace of
the compound that an exbeliever could describe the Progressive period as an age possessed by "the uric acid fetish."[1]

---

[1] William Kelley and Irwin Weiner, eds., *Uric Acid*, Berlin, 1978, pp.
1–11; W. S. C. Copeman, *A Short History of the Gout*, Berkeley, Cal.,

The "High Priest of uric acid," as Clendening dubbed him, was another London physician, Alexander Haig. Born in 1853, he took an unconventional route to his career as health reformer: the affliction of his youth was not consumption, but migraine. Finding no relief in medicine, he finally turned, at age twenty-nine, to dietary treatment. He first eliminated sugar, then tea, coffee, and tobacco, but all sacrifice came to naught until he swept his table clean of animal foods (except cheese and milk). Once the switch to lacto-vegetarian diet was made, he steadily overcame the headaches that had cost him one to two days of lost work each week during his student career at Oxford and St. Bartholomew's Hospital. The triumph generated Haig's first scientific publication, an 1884 paper that displayed already the cavalier handling of biochemistry which was to become his trademark. His migraine, he confidently theorized, had been due to impure blood, the impurity probably being an alkaloid produced by intestinal fermentation of excessive protein in his diet. His educated speculation took a new course, however, as Haig accumulated clinical experience. He discovered that several authorities believed migraine was often a manifestation of a gouty constitution. He also knew that the classic treatment for gout was a low protein diet such as the one which had banished his headaches, and that one of the favored drugs in gout therapy—salicylic acid—was also used against headache. Closer examination revealed several signs of gout in his personal and family history, so that by 1886 there could be little doubt in his mind that the migraine poison was none other than "our old friend uric acid."[2]

1964, pp. 9–10; C. Stanford Reads, *Fads and Feeding*, New York, 1909, p. 94; Eustace Miles and C. H. Collings, *The Uric Acid Fetish*, London, 1915.

[2] Logan Clendening, "A Review of the Subject of Chronic Intestinal Stasis," *Interstate Med. J.*, 22, 1191–1200 (1915), p. 1199. For biographical data on Haig, see "Obituary. Alexander Haig, M.D. OXF., F.R.C.P. LOND.," *Lancet*, 1924 (i), 825–826; Haig, *Uric Acid. An Epitome of the*

That term "friend" was intended to be facetious, but was, in fact, prophetic. Haig was in the process of forming a life-long partnership with the substance, one to which he would apply extraordinary persistence and imagination in order to find a place for uric acid in every pathological situation. Born through personal experience, this devotion was to be nurtured by his scientist's desire to simplify medical theory, and by an inadequate schooling in analytical and physiological chemistry allowing him to invariably discover ways to make uric acid the simplifying factor. Every one of Haig's many papers was to have some connection to uric acid, as would his several books. His *magnum opus, Uric Acid as a Factor in the Causation of Disease*, went through seven editions, each of which offered more than nine hundred pages of praise to the malevolence of the compound.

The friendship was too involved to permit coverage of all intimate details, but a general description of its development is easily given. Haig's suspicion that uric acid was the source of his headaches was soon confirmed by analysis of his own, and other migraine patients', urine. Managing to find a direct correlation between the level of uric acid excreted and the occurrence of headache, Haig supposed that excess uric acid in the blood—uricacidemia—initiated headache, in which case administration of a small dose of an acid to lower blood pH and reduce uric acid solubility should give relief. Almost predictably the therapy worked, but it did bring a surprise. The clearing of uric acid from the blood was followed by new symptoms of shooting pains in the joints, symptoms suspiciously like those of gout. And when these pains were removed by dosing with alkali, Haig had his mo-

---

Subject, London, 1906, pp. 1–13; and Haig, *Uric Acid as a Factor in the Causation of Disease,* 6 ed., Philadelphia, 1903, pp. 1–4. Haig, "The Physics of the Cranial Circulation and the Pathology of Headache, Epilepsy, and Mental Depression," *Brain, 16,* 230–258 (1893), p. 241; Haig, "Influence of Diet on Headache," *Practitioner, 33,* 113–118 (1884); Haig, "Further Notes on the Influence of Diet on Headache," *Practitioner, 36,* 179–186 (1886), pp. 179–180.

ment of revelation, his sudden appreciation of the wondrous simplicity of what he came to call "the human test-tube."[3]

In this test tube, he could see, the poison uric acid could exist in solution or as a precipitate. Its condition depended on pH and temperature, just as in an ordinary test tube, and in either event, whether in the blood or tissues, it caused disease. That deposits in the tissues would produce irritation was obvious enough, but the mechanism by which dissolved uric acid played havoc required some deduction. Since his migraine pain was aggravated by stooping and relieved by applying pressure to the arteries of the neck, Haig concluded the immediate cause of the headache must be elevated blood pressure. And as high uric acid levels were also associated with migraine, there seemed to be a direct relation between acid in the blood and blood pressure. Finally, Haig had already observed that test tube solutions of urates could be chemically manipulated to form gelatinous colloids, and imagined it was "quite possible" a similar phenomenon might occur in the blood. In one of his frequent blithe leaps from *in vitro* to *in vivo,* Haig formulated the condition of collaemia, "the presence of uric acid as a colloid in the blood stream and its action as an obstructor of the tiny capillaries." By impeding the flow of blood, colloidal uric acid forced an increase in blood pressure throughout the body, and also, Haig reasoned, served to depress the metabolic rate (or, to use his homely analogy, acted like "a wet blanket on a fire.").[4]

This combination of deficient combustion and excessive blood pressure was a highly versatile theoretical construct that could be employed to explain a remarkable assortment of clinical problems. Inhibited metabolism, for example, allowed sugar to pass through the body unoxidized, and was thus the cause of diabetes. High blood pressure, on the other

[3] Haig, *Uric Acid as a Factor* (n. 2), p. 176. One of Haig's papers was entitled "The Human Body as an Analytical Laboratory," *Brit. Med. J.,* 1901 (ii), 1078–1082.

[4] Haig, *Uric Acid as a Factor* (n. 2), p. 174; Haig, *Uric Acid. An Epitome* (n. 2), pp. 37, 54.

hand, was responsible for coma (after all, Haig reminded, patients emerging from coma often complained of severe headache, and he had already demonstrated headache to be a product of abnormal blood pressure). Similar reasoning was used to complete the list of collaemia diseases, a catalogue running through insomnia, asthma, menstrual dysfunction, neuritis, atherosclerosis, anemia, Bright's disease, Grave's disease, insanity, and hemorrhoids, to report only a few. Another that should not be left out of the recital was the telltale collaemic face, a woeful visage marked by puffy skin and bulging eyes. Haig boasted he could estimate a patient's blood pressure merely by the severity of his facial collaemia.[5]

Unfortunate as it was, collaemic face represented only the ailments associated with excess uric acid in the blood. There remained the problems caused by deposition of the compound in the tissues, the "local or precipitation group" of uric acid diseases. Gout headed this list, of course, but all bodily tissues were subject to localized uric inflammation, so that conditions ranging from gastritis and jaundice to eczema and flatulence could be credited to uric acid. And the account was still not completed by the addition of these precipitation diseases, for it was clear to Haig that uric acid could be a predisposing factor as well as exciting cause. Microbic infection, the pathological process with which most other physicians were preoccupied, could also be interpreted as a collaemic phenomenon. Germs, Haig argued, flourish only in impure and sluggish blood, "while those falling into the brightly burning fire of a quick combustion with fine circulation and small accumulation of waste products are themselves burnt up and cannot produce disease." Thus, he eventually came to maintain, "uric acid is the factor that controls the results of microbic invasion, and a life free from excess of uric acid is to a large extent a life immune from microbic injury."[6]

[5] Alexander Haig, *Uric Acid. An Epitome* (n. 2), pp. 49–51, 59–60.
[6] *ibid.*, p. 105; Haig, "The Circulation as a Factor Which Determines the Effects of Microbic Invasion," *Med. Rec., 78*, 391–394 (1910), p. 394.

The final element of wickedness in uric acid's nature was its ability to easily move back and forth between blood and tissues, thereby subjecting its victims to alternating bouts with collaemic and precipitation diseases. Blood pH was one determinant of the substance's location: the more alkaline the blood, the more uric acid it would hold, and the more collaemic the sufferer would be. Highly alkaline foods, such as potatoes, he believed, would foster one set of diseases, acidic foods the other. Environmental temperature acted in a similar way, with heat drawing uric acid into the blood, cold driving it out. With this tidy scheme of pathological chemistry in hand, no clinical history and no epidemiological observation could evade Haig's analysis. Other doctors might have been mystified by the case of the Englishman who came down with an acute attack of gout after he returned to India from a vacation in his homeland. But Haig discovered that while in England the patient had eaten heartily of foods productive of uric acid; that he had been bothered by the extreme heat on the Red Sea during his return passage, and then exposed to cool March winds in Bombay. What could be clearer than that the uric acid deposited by his English diet had been all brought into the blood by the Red Sea heat, then violently precipitated in his now gouty joints by the chill of India? Just as obvious was the chemical basis of the bit of folk wisdom that "May is the month of suicides and murderers." Uric acid was largely confined to the tissues during the winter because of cold weather and the English taste for oranges and other acid fruits during those months. But warm weather brought more alkaline diet, and thus a "spring cleaning" of the tissues. And as uric acid rushed into the blood, exerting its collaemic effects on brain and nerves, it brought on sudden melancholy or irritability.[7]

Even love was given a uric acid equation. The reason a

[7] "Some Cases in which Arthritis and Endocarditis were Produced by Drugs which Diminish the Solvent Powers of the Blood for Uric Acid," *Brit. Med. J.*, 1895 (ii), 1602–1605, p. 1605; Haig, "Freedom From Uric Acid and How to Obtain It," *Med. Rec.*, *68*, 332–335 (1905).

young man's fancy turned the way it did in the spring, Haig intimated, was because of his uric-acid-induced blood pressure. Nature's outlet for that spring tension was sexual intercourse, for the exertion of the act lowered the blood pH, thereby precipitating uric acid and lowering blood pressure. Thereby a biochemical basis was provided for the observation of statisticians that April, May, and June were the peak months for conceptions in Europe. The same theory also offered hope for handling the still disturbing problem of masturbation. In Haig's view, the practice was an instinctive effort to relieve collaemic tension, and could not be suppressed "with such feeble weapons as mental and moral suasion"; the wretched onanist, like virtually everyone else, was a captive of his circulation, and could be liberated only by purified diet.[8]

Onanism, melancholy, and gout, however, were but way-stations on the road to final calamity. The uric acid deposits in an individual's tissues would steadily grow in quantity as the years passed and as his constitutional vigor ebbed, until at last, Haig forecast, "the long pent up store of urates breaks its dams and rushes into the circulation with an overwhelming flood." If not destroyed on the rocks of apoplexy, the hapless victim would be swept onward to heart failure, Bright's disease, or a like fate.[9]

One of the worst of those fates was cancer, which Haig supposed was caused by long-term irritation by uric acid deposits, and should therefore be responsive to dietetic therapy. In 1911–1912, he actually attempted to cure several cases of inoperable cancer with a diet (nuts, fruits, and biscuits) free of uric acid and its metabolic precursors. None of the patients recovered, but Haig refused to let his theory

[8] Haig, *Uric Acid as a Factor* (n. 2), pp. 154–156. Haig proposed a baffling biochemical rationale to explain how sexual activity acidified the blood. He also offered a uric acid interpretation of female sexual development: "The Causation of Anemia and the Blood Changes Produced by Uric Acid," *Brit. Med. J.*, 1893 (ii), 672–676.

[9] Haig, *Uric Acid as a Factor* (n. 2), pp. 111–112.

take the blame. His patients had either been too far advanced, or else lacked the intelligence and determination to stay on the unfamiliar diet. "Hospital patients," he concluded with some distaste, "are too ignorant or prejudiced to give this diet a fair trial in hospital, and they are too ignorant to provide what is required at home." A successful demonstration of his cancer therapy, he added, would have to be made "among the richer and better educated classes."[10]

Haig nevertheless hoped to make all classes better educated, to create a general public awareness of the toxicity of all foods containing uric acid or its purine precursors such as xanthine and hypoxanthine. Conversion of the human race to the "uric-acid-free diet" was his goal, though he recognized that even that sweeping a purification would not immediately rid the world of the poison. Uric acid is also produced by the body, through endogenous purine synthesis and catabolism, but precisely because it is endogenous, and thus a natural component of body chemistry, this amount of uric acid seemed unlikely to be harmful. Haig could still anticipate, though, that endogenous uric acid production would eventually disappear, as "the race evolves to a higher stage." In the meantime, unnatural uric acid, that resulting from erroneously selected food, had to be dealt with. The first step, of course, was identification of offensive foods, a process that conveniently incriminated the flesh foods Haig had already rejected on the basis of personal experiment. By the mid-1890s he also realized that chemical data branded as dangerous a number of vegetable foods he had been continuing to eat: beans, peas, asparagus, mushrooms, and wholegrain cereals also had to be eliminated because of their purine content. Haig was left, then, with milk, cheese, some vegetables, fruits, nuts, and—a unique position for a food re-

---

[10] Alexander Haig, "Uric-acid-free Diet in Inoperable Cancer," *Brit. Med. J.,* 1912, (ii), 81–3, p. 82. Also see Haig, "The Origin of Cancer," *Brit. Med. J.,* 1909 (ii), 1441; Haig, "Medical Treatment of Inoperable Cancer," *Brit. Med. J.,* 1911 (i), 111–112, 845; Thomas Horder, "Medical Treatment of Inoperable Cancer," *Brit. Med. J.,* 1911 (i), 785.

former—white bread. Additional blandness was imposed by the prohibition of coffee, tea, and cocoa on the grounds that they contained methyl xanthines (it was later found that caffeine and similar compounds are not metabolized into uric acid). And any rejoicing that at least alcoholic beverages were free of uric-acid-producing substances was quickly squelched by Haig's promise that his diet removed any need for stimulation and thus destroyed the taste for strong drink.[11]

Haig seems to have realized few people would be driven to such austere fare by gustatory impulses, for while he assured readers they could learn to enjoy the "uric-acid-free diet," he gave far more attention to the pleasures of uric-acid-free life away from the table. A disease-free, physically ebullient existence, a doubled life-expectancy, a painless death—all these were the common rewards of the diet. But, Englishman that he was (and having been a rower at college), Haig demonstrated most excitement over the sporting benefits of his regimen. *Diet and Food* was his contribution to the debate over athletics and nutrition. The book went through six editions in the years from 1898 to 1906, and predictably revealed that even athletic success was a function of uric acid intake. *Diet and Food*'s full theory of strength and endurance, however, must have surprised even the most jaded Haig-watchers. The premise on which the entire book was built was the idea that the energy for muscular motion was derived from the oxidation of protein to urea. That notion, first offered by Liebig half a century earlier, had long since been discredited and was no longer taken seriously—except by Haig. Yet he seems to have been unaware of his loneliness on this position, presenting the theory as if it were generally accepted, and even using his inimitable analytical skills to find a direct correlation between quantity of exer-

---

[11] Haig, *Uric Acid as a Factor* (n. 2), pp. 14, 132, 235, 838; Haig, *Diet and Food, Considered in Relation to Strength and Power of Endurance, Training and Athletics*, London, 1902, p. 47.

cise and excreted urea. He thus found himself at odds with Chittenden and other advocates of a low protein diet, but as usual he was more concerned about uric acid than protein. If the energy for exertion came from protein, Haig hypothesized, maximum strength and endurance required a free flow of protein-rich blood to the muscles. But vessels clogged with colloidal uric acid would not be able to supply a full complement of protein molecules to the tissues, nor to remove the waste of protein oxidation. The more uric acid food an individual consumed, therefore, the more physiological "friction" he would have, and the lower would be his performance in contests of endurance. That was undoubtedly why meat eaters usually succumbed to vegetarian rivals, but vegetarians, he continued, had no reason to celebrate. Their vessels too were contaminated, for beans, asparagus, and mushrooms yielded uric acid. Ordinary vegetarianism granted a relative advantage, but uric-acid-free vegetarianism was required for absolute superiority. Support for this point was provided by the record of the preeminent pedestrian of the day, Karl Mann. Mann was the vegetarian walker studied by Caspari at the Dresden to Berlin contest. He had been converted to vegetable diet in 1894, then switched to Haig's refined version in 1898. Within the year, Mann won an important seventy-mile race, but it was the 1902 Dresden-Berlin triumph that catapulted him into the international spotlight. Haig rushed to Berlin immediately, personally examined Mann just a few days after the race, and was pleased (but not surprised) to find him free of the cardiac hypertrophy that was supposedly epidemic among carnivorous competitors. "Athlete's heart," he concluded, was still another uric-acid-induced ailment (Mann, incidentally, travelled to Yale several years later, and nearly doubled Fletcher's record on the calf-raising machine).[12]

---

[12] Haig, *Diet and Food* (n. 11), pp. 2–3, 6, 23, 34, 95; Haig, *Uric Acid as a Factor* (n. 2), pp. 42–43, 99–103, 830–835; Haig, "Heart Failure as the Result of Deficient Food," *Med. Rec.*, *69*, 817–819 (1906); Wilhelm Caspari, "Physiologische Studien über Vegetarismus," *Pflüger's Archiv.*

Though Haig never used the term, he believed in a condition of "uric-acid-free heart," too. By this he would have intended heart in the full meaning of the word: the possession of strength, courage, hope, and mental energy. Haig's vision of total health, the end of his diet, was of a condition in which "exercise of mind and body is a pleasure, the struggle for existence a glory, nothing is too good to happen, the impossible is within reach, and misfortunes slide like water off a duck's back." In the end, Haig, like other health reformers, found moral force in his system, and came to regard it as a method for the perfecting of individuals and, consequently, the nation. His writings, in fact, convey a feeling of urgency for its application to contemporary social challenges such as physical and moral degeneracy, the declining birthrate in the upper classes, and the erosion of Britain's imperial standing. Ultimately, he hints, uric acid might be responsible for nothing less than the decay of English civilization.[13]

Two biochemical mechanisms for broad cultural disintegration were suggested by Haig. First, collaemia, by depressing circulation to the brain, might be expected to prevent clarity of thought, sap mental energy and endurance, and enfeeble will power. The social consequences of the subjection of an entire citizenry to cerebral starvation were frightening. No less unsettling were the effects of uric acid's second mode of action, its creation of an appetite for stimulants (though a theoretical mechanism for this effect was extracted from biochemistry only after the most ruthless torture). So arcane as to defy presentation except in its naked essentials, his argument took its start from the metabolic depression caused by uric acid. Physiological stimulation, it continued, necessitates a clearing of the compound from the

---

Physiol., 109, 473–595 (1905), p. 569; Jacques Buttner, *A Fleshless Diet,* New York, 1910, pp. 163–164, 173. There was limited testimony from others that uric-acid-free diet increased athletic performance; see W. A. Potts, "The Advantages of a Purin-free Diet," *Lancet,* 1905 (i), 1636–1638.

[13] Haig, *Uric Acid as a Factor* (n. 2), p. 321.

bloodstream. Experiment indicates that meat, tea, coffee, alcohol, and opium are all uric acid precipitants, hence are stimulants. The stimulation they effect, however, is only temporary, as the precipitated acid soon redissolves, and in greater quantity than before, thus making the sufferer more depressed than ever and with a renewed, stronger craving for stimulation. The more meat, tea, and coffee one takes, the more he wants, until finally meat alone can no longer satisfy the need. "And when meat begins to fail," Haig dolefully concluded, "alcohol is added; when alcohol begins to fail morphine or cocaine are called in and so on down the road to ruin."[14]

A uric-acid-free diet would cure the craving for alcohol, tobacco, and other stimulants, but making this plan of character rescue attractive to people already enslaved to stimulation, already debauched by uric acid, was a formidable challenge to even Haig's ingenuity and optimism. He occasionally envisioned a future "which will be ... truer, nobler and better, as man slowly realizes how much of his sordid past has had its origin in unnatural food." His more common mood, though, was gloom. Sprinkled through his writings are calls for "the nations which hope to survive" to open their eyes and see that uric acid "bids fair ... to menace our very existence." But would they listen? "No! I fear not! for history shows that things of this kind have been discovered and forgotten, rediscovered and reforgotten, and no doubt the process will be repeated yet many times; still I do think that possibly the representatives of *homo sapiens* (not of this race, for it will be mostly wiped out), in the 30th or 40th century may be a little more unanimous than they are today in believing that their natural food is after all that which is also best for them."[15]

It was Haig's son, however, who gave full expression to anxiety about the future of the nation. Kenneth Haig, like his father, suffered with migraine from an early age, and

[14] *ibid.*, p. 874.
[15] *ibid.*, pp. viii, 136–137; Haig, *Uric Acid. An Epitome* (n. 2), p. 99; Haig, *Diet and Food* (n. 11), p. v.

then, while a sixteen year old at Rugby, began to experience fainting spells. Conversion to the uric-acid-free diet brought a steady decline of his problems, though, as well as a growth of endurance that astonished even Haig *pere*. "At Oxford he won several college rowing prizes," father boasted, "and would, I believe, have been in one of the college boats, but that it was feared that his diet would demoralize . . . the rest of the crew."[16]

Kenneth's filial debt was unusually large, and he found deep satisfaction in partially repaying it with a 1913 volume entitled *Health Through Diet*. The title page also acknowledged his father's advice and assistance, so one might presume that Kenneth's comments reflected the concerns and opinions of Alexander. If so, both were terribly agitated by the country's falling birthrate, and saw uric acid as the cause. The younger Haig postulated that one clinical manifestation of uric acid precipitation must be an irritation of the vaginal wall, a "catarrh of the vagina" that dampened sensitivity and caused sexual apathy. As the degree of indifference should be proportional to the quantity of meat and other uric acid foods consumed, fecundity could be expected to decrease with rising social position—exactly the disturbing pattern which was being observed. A uric-acid-free diet, however, should enhance fertility by restoring natural function, a theoretical position confirmed by the woman who had been pronounced barren by her physician, but then conceived and bore a healthy child two years after adopting the Haig diet. Other women on the diet reported decreased menstrual flow and easier periods, prompting Kenneth Haig to wonder if ovulation "need . . . be accompanied by hemorrhage, or is the latter only a pathological symptom?" After also considering that rejection of uric acid would relieve morning sickness, allow less painful labor and safer birth, and improve lactation, he could no longer resist calling attention to the "national importance" of the "influence of the Uric-Acid-Free Diet on gynaecology and midwifery." His

---

[16] Quoted in Kenneth Haig, *Health Through Diet*, London, 1913, p. 77.

preface went further, proclaiming "that the rise and fall of nations is determined by the circulation." Nations, like armies, march on their stomachs, and "in the last resort their commissariat is their success or ruin."[17]

The investing of uric acid with cosmic influence stretched plausibility too thin for all but the most credulous, but the simpler idea that it caused a number of purely physical ills was able to achieve respectability in some medical circles and hold it for some time, and it was at least as popular in the United States as in England. To be sure, the Brahmins of the profession were scornful from the start. By the early 1900s, in fact, articles criticizing Haig comprised a distinct genre of medical literature, with remarkably consistent content. The comments of the editor of the *Journal of the American Medical Association* are representative: "Using methods that are known to be unreliable, he secured data that cannot be corroborated, and with these as a basis followed out a marvelous train of logic to the ultimate conclusion that practically all disease is due to uric acid.... No advance in physiologic chemistry and pathology, no amount of refutation of his claims, seems to have interested him or swerved him in the least, ... he ignores everything but his own cherished beliefs, and calmly follows them as they lead."[18]

But as exasperating as Haig's inattention to these frequent scoldings could be, uric acid critics were more disturbed by the naivete of rank and file physicians, so many of

[17] *ibid.*, pp. ix, 117–123.

[18] "Uric Acid Theories," *JAMA*, *43*, 550–551 (1904), p. 550. Also see Alfred Crofton, "Uric Acid Theories. A Critical Review, and Some Original Investigations," *JAMA*, *33*, 59–63 (1899); Frank Billings, "Uric Acid Fallacies," *Am. Med.*, *2*, 565–568 (1901); Lewellys Barker, *Truth and Poetry Concerning Uric Acid*, Chicago, 1905; J. J. R. Macleod, "Truth, Without the Poetry, Concerning Uric Acid," *Cleveland Med. J.*, *4*, 465–473 (1905); Arthur Luff, "Toxicity of Uric Acid," *Lancet*, 1905 (ii), 1864; Lafayette Mendel, "The Formation of Uric Acid," *JAMA*, *46*, 843–846, 944–947 (1906); "Uric Acid as a Business Proposition," *JAMA*, *46*, 1113–1114 (1906).

whom, it was claimed, had allowed themselves to be conditioned to diagnose "uric acid diathesis" reflexly if any uric acid were detected in the patient's urine. That the compound had been able to obtain what one commentator described as a "fixed hold" on the medical profession should not, however, have occasioned much surprise. Even the best educated medical scientists of the day had still only a nebulous view of metabolism and blood chemistry, yet all the while exuded confidence that both areas would be found to have important relations to disease. Standard pathology texts included coverage of the gouty diathesis, a loosely defined collection of symptoms commonly found among patients who never suffered an acute attack of gout, but whose families had a history of the disease. Uric acid was thus enveloped by just enough murkiness to give Haig's ideas an appearance of substance to the typical medical practitioner with a feeble grasp of biochemistry. In addition, his papers were published in prestigious journals—*Lancet, Practitioner, British Medical Journal, Medical Record,* and *Journal of the American Medical Association.* His books were impressively heavy tomes, written in technical language and filled with detailed graphs relating uric acid excretion to the ingestion of various foods and drugs, to exercise, menstruation, time of year, and even to the effects of a Turkish bath. His major work was revised six times in order to incorporate the results of his continued researches. By providing a simple, unifying theory, Haig met the needs of harried physicians who encountered on a daily basis patients with indeterminate symptoms and no definite pathology. Giving the devil his due, an American medical editor marvelled that, "no promoter of a commercial enterprise has ever been more skillful in enunciating, and pushing to a conclusion, theories as to the existence of a precious find in a mine than has Dr. Haig."[19]

[19] James Goodhart, "The Treatment of Uric Acid," *Practitioner, 76,* 9 (1906); Thomas Futcher, "Gout," in *Modern Medicine. Its Theory and Practice,* ed. William Osler, Philadelphia, 1907, pp. 808–844; Billings,

There is thus no cause for wonder that despite authoritative refutations, Haig drew a sizeable following. As early as 1901, a leading American journal contemptuously identified uricacidemia as the disease of the new century:

Now that 'malaria' is coming to be known among the backward members of the profession as a specific disease caused by a parasite, . . . a need is felt for some new catchword with which to mystify ourselves and the public. Judging from the glibness with which the "uric acid diathesis" is now talked of by both doctors and patients, this is apparently the coming disease. It explains numberless strange symptoms, gratifying the sufferer and having withal a comforting, scientific sound, which promises well for its usefulness and permanence. We know of physicians who are constantly making the diagnosis with pride, and who have not even dreamed that the matter needs any verification in the chemical laboratory. For these men it may be well to say that not by any means as much is known of the role of uric acid in the animal economy as might be supposed from the extravagant writings of Dr. Haig.[20]

Woods Hutchinson refused to apologize for presenting yet another attack on the uric acid theory because, he warned, "if we do not take it, it will take us." The fact that other medical celebrities, including Lafayette Mendel, Lewellys Barker, and J.J.R. Macleod, took the time to repeat these sentiments indicates that belief in the theory was indeed common, though we have the testimony of the believers themselves to finalize the point. Journal articles affirming the dangers of uric acid made heavy use of adjectives like

---

"Uric Acid Fallacies" (n. 18), p. 565; Reynold Wilcox, *The Treatment of Disease*, Philadelphia, 1907, p. 252; Haig, *Uric Acid as a Factor* (n. 2), pp. xiii–xvi; "The Toxicity of Uric Acid," *Ther. Gaz., 30,* 181–182 (1906), p. 181.
    [20] "Uric Acid from a Practical Point of View," *Pediatrics, 11,* 261–262 (1901), p. 261.

"lethal," "insidious," and "hydra-headed." One doctor reported swallowing a few drops of acid and immediately feeling a torrent of uric acid gushing into his big toe. A Massachusetts physician proposed heroic therapeutic measures to save a two-month-old child from uric acid poisoning, while a New York doctor exclaimed that "uric acid was the Devil himself." A final writer commented on a cartoon "in which a prominent society woman is represented as saying emphatically to one of her lady friends: *I do believe that I am just lousy with uric acid!'* Probably she was. Many of us are."[21]

As the last example suggests, the publicity given the uric acid theory also sparked an epidemic of self-diagnosis by the public. "Indeed," a Chicago physician complained, "among the laity it is the almost universal belief that a joint pain, myalgia, neuritis, neuralgia, etc. are due to uric acid. . . . How often does a patient say: 'My doctor says I have uric acid.' " By 1902, advertisements for Quaker Oats were referring to Haig to assure consumers the cereal would give "Home-Made Health."[22]

Whether or not Haig actually endorsed Quaker Oats, he agreed that diet was the only means of combatting uric acid. He also appreciated most people would have trouble converting to a uric-acid-free diet, because of habit, because past indiscretions had established a need for continued stimulation, and because his regimen was popularly confused with ordinary vegetarianism. There was no end to Haig's irritation, in fact, over many people's inability to discriminate between the garden variety vegetarianism (which in its "ignorance" produced only "unfortunate results") and his selective "physiological and purin-free diet." But though he felt "vegetarianism has been a great thorn in my side," stan-

[21] Woods Hutchinson, "The Meaning of Uric Acid and the Urates," *Lancet,* 1903 (i), 288–294, p. 288; *Uric Acid M., 1,* 275 (1901); *ibid., 2,* 404 (1902); *ibid., 6,* 21 (1906); *ibid., 11,* 16 (1911); J. B. Berkart, "The Alleged Perils of Uric Acid," *Brit. Med. J.,* 1917 (ii), 208–209, p. 208.
[22] Billings, "Uric Acid Fallacies" (n. 18), p. 565; *Dietetic Hygienic Gaz., 18,* xix (1902).

dard vegetarians responded favorably to his work, interpreting it as chiefly a condemnation of meat eating. Kellogg, for instance, gave considerable space in his writings to the dangers of flesh purines (and was no doubt attracted in good part by the claim that uric-acid-free diet eliminated constipation).[23]

To ease the transition from regular to refined diet, Haig devised a plan of gradual withdrawal from uric acid. His son Kenneth suggested eliminating uric acid from breakfast only for three weeks, then from lunch as well for the next three weeks, and so on. This plan included as one stage the removal of all tea from "afternoon tea." Converts also published at least two uric-acid-free cookbooks, while Haig opened a Sanatorium (Apsley House) at Slough, about half an hour from London by train. A gift from a grateful patient, it was "a fine Christopher Wren house, standing in lovely old-world grounds," equipped with garden and greenhouse, and adjacent to scenic countryside and three golf courses. Apsley House provided ideally congenial surroundings for the return to natural diet, but it was accessible to relatively few, and fewer still took advantage of it, or of the diet it offered. By Haig's own estimate, only a few hundred had "dared" to follow him, and his detractors implied the number was even lower. His diet was, in the common view, "a very joyless one, as well as being socially a nuisance." That valuation was, if anything, confirmed by those who adhered to the regimen. A correspondent of the *British Medical Journal* who identified himself only as "A Quondam Gourmet," confessed that, "I am a convert [to Haig's diet] in spite of myself." "I still," he elaborated, "hanker after the fleshpots. Caneton Rouennaise, with a bottle of Chambertin, still appears more attractive than Apsley Duck with salutaris, and English roast beef more savoury than mock beef

---

[23] K. Haig, *Health Through Diet* (n. 16), pp. 6–7, 48; A. Haig, "Vegetarianism and Physique," *Lancet,* 1908 (ii), 1632; John Harvey Kellogg, *Shall We Slay to Eat,* Battle Creek, Mich., 1905, pp. 38, 44–46; Haig, *Natural Diet of Man,* Battle Creek, Mich., 1923, pp. 89–91.

rissoles. Though my memory dwells with pleasure on many a past gastronomic treat, yet the improvement in my health and the increase in my power of endurance are such that nothing would induce me to revert to my former dietetic habits; and I know that mine is far from being a solitary experience." Such resigned followers of Haig were variously presented as "cranks," "martyrs," "disciples," and "shrivelled, juiceless, prematurely aged" beings; but they were never described as numerous.[24]

So as frightened as many people were of Haig's disease, the majority clearly considered Haig's cure to be even more discomfiting. But there was literally a ready solution to the dilemma. The therapy of gout had long included the administration of drugs presumed to be capable of dissolving uric acid and washing it from the body. Lithium compounds enjoyed a particularly high reputation, having been recommended by Sir Alfred Garrod himself after he observed lithium carbonate to have a powerful solvent effect on uric acid *in vitro*. But even though it had been established by the beginning of the twentieth century that lithium's solvent action did not occur inside the body, doctors continued to prescribe the carbonate, and other lithium salts, to combat gout and the gouty diathesis. And as uricacidemia established itself as a prevailing syndrome, lithium was promoted to the position of panacea. Medicine manufacturers stampeded into the new market, offering every imaginable synthetic preparation, as well as a line of natural, lithium-containing mineral waters. The manufacturers of one product—Thia-

---

[24] Gertrude Haig, *Some Recipes for the Uric-Acid-Free Diet*, London, 1913; Mrs. John Webster and Mrs. F. W. Jessop, *The Apsley Cookery Book*, London, 1905; Haig, *Uric Acid. An Epitome* (n. 2), pp. 146–147; Haig, *Uric Acid as a Factor* (n. 2), pp. 136, 837; K. Haig, *Health Through Diet* (n. 16), p. 56; "The Limitations of a Purin-free Diet," *Brit. Med. J.*, 1908 (ii), 1781; F. C. Eve, "Uric Acid and Diet," *Practitioner*, 75, 823–828 (1905), p. 823; T. Clifford Allbut, "Introductory Essay," *Practitioner*, 71, 1–5 (1903); Goodhart, "The Treatment of Uric Acid" (n. 19), p. 11.

lion (Figure 7)—actually published their own journal, *The Uric Acid Monthly*, and distributed it free of charge to all physicians in the United States and England. They later added *El Acido Urico* for the benefit of Spanish and Latin American physicians. Other uric acid solvents were promoted with less flamboyance, but promoted nonetheless, causing some physicians to charge that drug industry literature, embellished by detail men, was more important than Haig's writings for generating professional and public fear of uric acid. The irony of that development was that lithium compounds had no effect on uric acid, and even if they had, few preparations contained enough lithium to matter. Thialion's formula included less than two percent lithium citrate, and the highly touted Buffalo Lithia Water, it was eventually revealed, held only one-fifth the concentration of lithium to be found in Potomac River water; a patient would have had to drink at least 150,000 gallons of the mineral water daily to get a therapeutic dose! The *Journal of the American Medical Association* provided a sarcastic summary of the situation with the observation that drug manufacturers were growing rich "selling a 'solvent' which does not dissolve a substance that does not accumulate in the 'system' and does not cause a host of ills."[25]

As such assaults continued, uric acid's standing with the profession as a whole was steadily lowered. By 1915, physicians could jest that, "There was as much to be said for uric acid as there is for intestinal toxemia: it cured for a time its thousands, but the theory built about it caught cold and died." Already the year before, an American journal had concluded its brusque review of Kenneth Haig's *Health Through Diet* with the prediction that "the uric acid fad has

[25] H. Hare, C. Caspari, and H. Rusby, *The National Standard Dispensatory*, Philadelphia, 1905, p. 925; "Uric Acid Solvents," *JAMA*, 46, 1381–1382 (1906); "The Therapeutic Value of Lithium," *Ther. Gaz.*, 27, 242–243 (1903); "Uric Acid as a Business Proposition" (n. 18), p. 1113; Berkart, "Alleged Perils" (n. 21), p. 208; American Medical Association, *The Propaganda for Reform in Proprietary Medicines*, 9th ed., Chicago, 1916, pp. 205, 468; "Uric Acid Theories" (n. 18), p. 550.

had its day, and ... the present volume will not resuscitate it."[26] The younger Haig's volume was indeed the theory's last gasp. Alexander Haig also gave up the battle after 1914, spending his final ten years in quiet retirement. It would be wrong, however, to suppose that he had been cashiered from the profession. Even in his most passionate anti-uric acid days he commanded personal respect, and even affection, from medical colleagues. On friendly terms with some of the brightest lights in British medicine, Haig was regarded as honorable, and as generally competent when not astride his uric acid hobby horse. He was seen as quixotic, rather than quackish, and even the hard condemnations of his work often showed a soft side, whether expressions of gratitude for raising questions and stimulating research, or praise for his integrity and persistence. His obituary notices sounded the same tone, one describing him as "a man genial in nature ... [who] always seemed to maintain an even mental equilibrium under adverse criticism." The best summary of his life, however, was contained in one of Haig's own incidental remarks. The rhetorical question, "Is life worth living?," he wrote, is not adequately answered by the French response that it depends on the liver; actually, he announced with unintended prescience, "that depends upon uric acid."[27]

That realization had been the turning point in the career of another major health reformer. Eustace Miles' life had barely been worth living the first twenty-seven years. He had, to be sure, achieved a certain level of success as a classical honors coach at Cambridge and a skilled tennis player, but was often restless and depressed, slept poorly, suffered

---

[26] Clendening, "Review" (n. 2), p, 1199; *Ther. Gaz.*, *38*, 451 (1914). Public fear of uric acid seems to have carried into the 1920s, however: J. D. Allen, "Endogenous Uric Acid in Conditions Other Than Gout and Nephritis," *Kentucky Med. J.*, *22*, 240–242 (1924).

[27] T. Lauder Brunton, "Elimination and its Uses in Preventing and Curing Disease," *Lancet*, 1891 (i), 1361–1366; *Brit. Med. J.*, 1896 (i), 1149; *Ther. Gaz.*, *27*, 570–571 (1903); "Obituary" (n. 2), p. 826; Haig, *Uric Acid as a Factor* (n. 2), p. 322.

headaches, colds, and constipation, and had "a great liking for any form of alcohol." About 1896, though, he chanced to take a house with his good friend Hubert Higgins, the Cambridge anatomist who would go on to preach Humaniculture. Higgins introduced Miles to Haig's writings, Miles took up the uric-acid-free diet, and before long found himself feeling and looking better. His muscular flexibility and endurance improved, and even his memory grew stronger. Not least important, his thirst for alcohol disappeared.[28]

Miles' alcohol-free, uric-acid-free regimen allowed him to become one of muscular vegetarianism's best advertisements. He captured the national tennis championship in 1897, as well as a number of other major titles. His reputation as an athlete no doubt contributed to the popularity of his works in the United States as well as his native England. He in fact exemplified the principles of Progressive hygienic ideology as well as any American reformer.[29]

Those principles were not, however, identical to Haig's. Miles learned through experience that pulses—anathema to Haig—did not injure, but actually aided his vitality, and he soon ignored the uric acid theory's restrictions on certain vegetables. He became, in effect, a vegetarian, but he refused to be known by that name because he thought it had been sullied by mistaken practice. One of his many books, in fact, was dedicated wholly to the *Failures of Vegetarianism*, though those failures were hardly so numerous and complex as to require a separate volume. Most could be reduced to a simple ignorance of the nutritional needs of the body which, Miles believed, left too many vegetarians content with "an idiotic Potato-Cabbage Diet" that was woefully lacking in protein. His own diet, emphasizing legumes, grains, milk products, and high protein meat substitutes, he preferred to call "Simpler Food."

[28] Eustace Miles, *Muscle, Brain and Diet*, London, 1900, pp. 40–48.
[29] Jules Lefèvre, *A Scientific Investigation into Vegetarianism*, London, 1923, p. 163.

Choose the cheaper, Simpler Food
cheese and Protene, milk (if good),
Gluten, Hovis [a health bread], macaroni;
oats and other grains, and honey;
orange, apple, other fruits;
vegetables, pulses, roots.[30]

The same open-minded empiricism that had led him away
from Haig's confining diet, though, also recommended a
mixed collection of other health aids. Miles identified many
Avenues to Health in another work: exercise, muscle relaxation, deep breathing, hydrotherapy, positive thinking, and
so on up to the *Lebenswecker* (the last item, the "life awak-
ener," was the mid-nineteenth-century discovery of a German layman, Carl Baunscheidt; it was an instrument used
to make numerous small puncture holes in the skin, thus
providing an exit through which the body could expel any
contaminating matter. Miles was probably the last defender
of the *Lebenswecker*).[31]

Health avenues were many, but Simpler Food was far the
broadest. Miles saw it as the essential one, one leading to
states of extraordinary improvement. This was the doctrine
pushed in his monthly *Healthward Ho!*, which was dedicated to helping readers attain "All-round Efficiency." It
was the teaching imparted to boarders at "The Old House,"
his health retreat in the English countryside with a "de-
lightfully home-like atmosphere." One suspects that the
same dogma was somehow served with the bread at his restaurant, which hosted more than a thousand diners daily
and marked menu items to identify uric-acid-containing
dishes (apparently the quality of all the dishes was well
above the vegetarian standard; American gastronome James
Beard has cited Miles' restaurant as the only good vegetarian restaurant in his experience, and Miles himself, perhaps

---

[30] Miles, *Muscle* (n. 28), pp. 165, 227–229, 252–253, 334.
[31] Miles, *Avenues to Health*, London, 1902, pp. 216–220.

with Ella Kellogg in mind, rejected most vegetarians' meals as "execrably cooked").[32]

The philosophy advanced through all Miles' outlets was that health is a duty, "to ourselves, to our own Nations, to all Nations, and to posterity. It is, in a word, our duty to God." Health is also a virtue, he stressed, a positive state of mental and moral well-being generating in its possessor an "active tendency towards whatever is good" and an ability to "develope into the likeness of God." Along the way, one might also be fortunate enough to pass through a likeness to Rockefeller: Simpler Food saved money, time, and energy, gave endurance and optimism, and thus ranked as "one of the nearest approaches to wealth which are possible today." Miles gave no guarantees to the Simpler Food convert, but he assured him that, "the chances are that he will get wealth." If established as the national diet, Simpler Food would increase national prosperity, as well as physical and moral strength: during World War I, Miles came to see his system as vital "for the success and progress—nay, for the very existence—of our Nation and Empire." And this was the same man who had identified one of the failures of ordinary vegetarians as a tendency to "overstate their case."[33]

By the time of the war, Miles was straying even further from Haig ("Uric Acid Fetish" was his term), and amending his Simpler Food doctrine to concentrate on excessive carbohydrates as the chief dietary evil. Once bogged in this esoteric endeavor to prove "hyperpyraemia" to be even deadlier than uricacidemia, he quickly sank from sight.[34]

One of the avenues of health explored by Miles early in his career had been the "No Breakfast Plan." He had soon dropped it in favor of a "No Lunch Plan" of his own crea-

---

[32] Miles and Collings, *Uric Acid Fetish* (n. 1), pp. 268–269; Haig, *Self-Health as a Habit*, London, 1919, pp. 11, 190; Read, *Fads and Feeding* (n. 1), p. 102.

[33] Miles, *Muscle* (n. 28), pp. 19, 61, 155, 163, 227, 308; Miles and Collings, *Self-Health* (n. 32), p. 25.

[34] Miles and Collings, *Uric Acid Fetish* (n. 1).

tion, but for the masses the former proved much more attractive. Its author, Edward Hooker Dewey, was a regularly trained physician (University of Michigan) who began practice as a military doctor during Sherman's Georgia campaign. His year and a half experience in that capacity taught him that except for relieving his pain, there was nothing the physician could do for his patient by the administration of drugs. The lesson was repeated over and over in the civilian practice he began in Meadville, Pennsylvania in 1866, yet he continued to dispense standard remedies, in response to patient demand for medication, rather than hand recovery over entirely to nature. Not until after more than a decade of half-hearted dosing did he find the courage to break with convention. A young woman suffering with digestive troubles was unable to retain either food or the medicines Dewey prescribed. She had to be maintained on water alone, and at first seemed to decline. But before long her condition improved and after thirty-five days of fasting she was restored to full health. At this demonstration of the power of the *vis medicatrix,* Dewey finally abandoned the use of drugs altogether, even when his own son contracted diphtheria and neighboring physicians advised quinine and whiskey therapy.[35]

His son, and apparently all his other patients, recovered on Dewey's (rather nature's) "fasting-cure," but perhaps the greatest of all its wonders was the cure's suggestion of a new, "revolutionary" system of hygiene. If nature conquered disease by slowly using up superfluous matter, Dewey reasoned, disease was probably the gradually developing result of the consumption of excess food. And at what common meal was unnecessary food taken, if not breakfast? *"There is no natural hunger in the morning,"* Dewey decreed, because the resting body did not draw on food reserves. His "revolutionary" analysis truly was that uncom-

[35] Edward Hooker Dewey, *The No-Breakfast Plan and the Fasting-Cure,* Meadville, Pa., 1900, pp. 15–31.

plicated, but he dressed his simplicities in a fustian style that allowed them to pass as elegant insights before the eyes of the uncritical. Dewey himself was taken in, writing three sincere and earnest volumes (*The No-Breakfast Plan, The True Science of Living,* and *A New Era for Woman*), all first published in the 1890s and totaling more than nine-hundred pages of repetitive explication of the relation of a breakfastless regimen to every conceivable aspect of health. Distilled, his philosophy was merely that food in excess of body demand placed a drain on vital energy that weakened all tissues, and especially the blood (there were also hints of autointoxication from residual food in the intestine). It was a throwback to early hygienic doctrine, emphasizing quantity and largely ignoring quality of food (coffee was even recommended as the only item to be taken in the morning). The benefits of the No Breakfast Plan, though, were typical of ideological hygiene, with nearly unlimited physical improvement transcended by mental and spiritual perfection. There was a *"moral science* of digestive energy," Dewey maintained, and there were two areas of moral progress to which he applied that science with special interest. An obviously devout man, Dewey worried that "the gloomy, the irritable, the dyspeptic Christian is a dispenser of death and not of the higher life, and his religious faith does not spread by the contagiousness of example." He was most gratified, therefore, to save a missionary who had returned from the Congo with ruined health, and watch him go back to his post with twenty-four additional missionaries, all "converts to the new gospel of health." Other religious leaders, including a Reverend George Pentecost, no less, testified to the immense value of the No Breakfast Plan for their work.[36]

Dewey's own work of salvation was even more energetic in the field of female liberation, though his *New Era for Woman* bore no resemblance to the era envisioned by suf-

---

[36] *ibid.,* pp. 48, 84, 97; Edward Hooker Dewey, *The True Science of Living,* Norwich, Conn., 1902, pp. 1–18.

fragettes. The female bondage he strove to break was to ill health and its cause, domestic cares. Like Alcott, Dewey was sensitive to the Herculean demands placed on mothers and homemakers, and the eventual physical effects of daily grinding toil. His remedy was much simpler, though—the elimination of breakfast would improve the wife's nutrition, and also, by sparing her an early rising and hours of preparation and clean-up, allow her body enough rest to make remaining chores easy and nondebilitating.[37]

Liberated woman would not only be a healthier, more efficient homemaker, but also (and more importantly) she would be a healthier mother. At a time of grave concern about racial decline and the reproductive health of women, the No Breakfast Plan promised an end to the plagues of fallen wombs, menstrual irregularities, and difficult pregnancies. Dewey's analysis of that first problem will serve to illustrate his gynecological theory: "The womb by virtue of its dense vascular structure is peculiarly liable to trouble arising from weak nutrition [overnutrition]. The veins become enlarged, hence it is weighted with an abnormal amount of blood, so the heavy womb exerts an abnormal tension on the correspondingly weakened ligaments and we have falling . . . womb. How are we going to get it up again and make it stay?" Not with surgery or pessaries or other unnatural methods, Dewey protested, but by omitting the breakfast whose redundant food had overburdened the womb's vessels to begin with: "Physiological treatment you see."[38]

The *New Era* was subtitled "A Plain Pathway to the 'Kingdom of Health,' " and it was the leading of the rest of the race down this path that was the final responsibility of healthy woman. Dewey ended another book with an appeal to "the mothers of the land": "The No Breakfast Plan means

[37] Edward Hooker Dewey, *A New Era for Woman*, Norwich, Conn., 1898, pp. ix, 8, 22, 74–75.
[38] *ibid.*, pp. 175–190, 310–311.

for your children the best possibilities for the conservation of all the higher instincts and powers that will tend to save them from the saloon, the prison, the electric chair. If the Garden of Eden was abolished because you enticed man to eat the wrong food, it is for you to restore a new race of Adams in all the ways of health, of such health as will make the entire earth a 'Paradise regained.' "[39]

The number who explored Dewey's path to the kingdom cannot be determined. Already by 1895, Holbrook estimated that in a single New England town one hundred people were abiding by the No Breakfast Plan. That town seems to have been the exception, though, and a short-lived one at that. What Dewey disciples lacked in numbers, however, they made up in enthusiasm. A banker put his servant girl and dog on two meals a day, along with the rest of his family, and a publisher who was saved from lung disease gave Dewey credit as well for a more easily shaved beard. The "scientific reason" for that improvement, hypothesized along strict Dewey lines, was that "the pure blood which my digestive apparatus was making was strengthening and compacting all the atoms of the body, and in consequence of that, the skin was holding the beard in a firmer grasp, and this would make it cut more easily than it would when held loosely by the skin which had been fed by impure blood."[40]

Fletcher met Dewey in 1898, when he was at the beginning of his mastication experiments. Deeply impressed by him, he reduced his number of daily meals, and expressed his thanks by praising Dewey as an "Esculapian Luther" and sending him a copy of the "Chewing Song." Dewey in turn took Fletcher's advice to heart, making Fletcherism part of his therapeutic program and requiring patients to thoroughly masticate the food they were finally allowed after completion of their twenty- to thirty-day (and longer) curative fasts. Five years of testing the method convinced

[39] Dewey, *No-Breakfast* (n. 35), p. 207.

[40] *J. Hyg. Herald Health*, *45*, 46–47 (1895); Charles Haskell, *Perfect Health*, London, 1901, pp. 53–54.

Dewey that Fletcher had done "more for human weal than all the mere medical prescribers have given the world from Adam to the present moment."[41]

The mutual admiration society of dietary reformers also included Haig, who read Dewey, switched to two uric-acid-free meals a day, and soon felt still better in both body and mind. Other tribute that flowed to Dewey during his period of ascendance into the early 1900s included such exclamations as, "I really believe I have crossed Jordan, and am in ... a physical Canaan"; and the No Breakfast Plan is "the most important announcement made to the world, since the angels proclaimed the birth of Christ." A final glorifier placed Dewey's work somewhat closer to its true worth: although he began by calling it, "outside of the Bible, ... the *grandest book of the age,*" he ended with the declaration, "I would not do without its truth and light for $50.00."[42]

Rigorous fasting as a therapeutic measure was popularized by several other authors, but the ultimate in Progressive dietary fetishes, the most ingenuous confession of faith in the wisdom of nature, was the advocacy of uncooked foods. Also recommended under the headings of unfired food and the "Apyrotropher Diet," raw foods claimed the loyalties of several Progressive health reformers. Each of these Apyrotrophers had his own distinctive dogma, there seem to have been no firm organizational ties between them, but they nevertheless agreed on a range of doctrinal points. Primary among them was the assumption that nature is capable of carrying all foods to completion, and that human tampering with ripened fruits and vegetables will only undo that nutritional perfection. Otto Carqué expressed an idea popular among his peers when he attributed the perfection of naturally ripened fruits to the "free and uninterrupted exchange of the influences of light, heat and air, by which the electri-

---

[41] Dewey, *No-Breakfast* (n. 35), p. 105; Horace Fletcher, *The New Glutton,* New York, 1903, pp. 75, 77, 83.

[42] Haig, *Uric Acid as a Factor* (n. 2), pp. 761–763; Haskell, *Perfect Health* (n. 40), pp. 108, 115, 130.

cal forces of the sun are transmitted." Romantic excess and pseudoscientific speculation generally ruled apyrotrophic philosophy. When food was heated, explained George Drews (editor of *The Apyrotropher Magazine*), its natural chemical constitution was "perverted."

The sun energy (galama) is dissipated. The volatile essences are exploded. The tonic elements (organic salts) have been freed, mineralized and neutralized. The proteids are coagulated. The starches are rendered so soluble that they enter the circulation undigested. The atomic arrangement of sugar is rendered incongenial. And the oils are fused. Therefore cooked food readily ferments and decays in the alimentary canal [autointoxication!]; besides, its consistency does not give the proper exercise to the organs of comminution, digestion and absorption; and it has a tendency to puzzle, confuse and pervert the alimentary functions—thus laying the foundation for disease.

There were also more conventional forms of damage, such as uric acid irritation.[43]

Apyrotrophers were not necessarily vegetarians; some admitted raw oysters, and one offered his readers a passable recipe for steak tartare. But they did for the most part see themselves as refined vegetarians, and anticipated the same physical and spiritual blessings of correct diet. There was even some degree of "muscular apyrotrophy"—Gilman Low, a noted bodybuilder who lived on uncooked foods for awhile, performed some of his most spectacular feats of strength and endurance while on the diet.[44]

[43] Hereward Carrington, *Vitality, Fasting and Nutrition*, New York, 1908; A. Rabagliati, *Air, Food and Exercise*, London, 1904; Otto Carqué, *The Foundation of All Reform*, Evanston, 1904, p. 32; Gustav Schlickeysen, *Fruit and Bread. A Scientific Diet*, New York, 1877, p. 115; George Drews, *Unfired Food and Tropho-Therapy*, Chicago, 1912, pp. 11–12; W. D. McCurdy, *Eating to Live*, San Francisco, 1903, p. 35.
[44] Eugene and Mallis Christian, *Uncooked Foods and How to Use Them*, New York, 1904, p. 27.

Female emancipation was also an apyrotrophic project. As Eugene Christian, head of the Corrective Eating Society, pointed out, cooking was the most onerous of woman's domestic burdens. All those hours of inhaling the "poisonous odor" of cooking meat, and buried in "the grease and slime of pots and dishes" brought on "nervous exhaustion and premature old age"; it was "a worse bondage than the negro [had] suffered." The adoption of an uncooked diet freed her from all three meals, not just the breakfast Dewey offered, and gave her more time for "pure air and sunshine," for "new thoughts, new dreams, new hopes with which she may endow the race to be" and lightened "the leaden load that has been laid upon her by our civilization."[45]

Though small in numbers, raw food enthusiasts were not to be outdone, and they urged their millennial gospel with an evangelistic zeal that could only be envied by larger and better organized health reform programs. "Cheer up sisters and brothers and rejoice with me," a Gantryesque Drews appealed, "for I have found the key that unlocks the door to physical, mental, moral and spiritual salvation and I will tell you how to use that key if you will but listen."[46]

But listening was difficult in the Babel of Progressive hygienic ideology; there were so many keys to the doors to salvation—and not all of them were dietary.

[45] *ibid.*, pp. 50, 51, 75.
[46] Drews, *Unfired Food* (n. 43), p. 11.

CHAPTER NINE
PHILOSOPHY IN THE GYMNASIUM

☆☆☆☆☆☆☆☆☆☆☆☆☆☆☆☆☆☆☆☆☆☆☆☆☆☆☆☆☆☆☆☆

"EVERY VILLAGE THAT HAS TWO CHURCHES NOW," PRO-
posed a resident of Moses Coit Tyler's mythical village of
Brawnville, should "just put both congregations together, to
worship in one building and to practice gymnastics in the
other." Then

> there would be more godliness in this land, and more man-
> liness, too; the fashionable theology would be shamed out
> of its disgraceful Paganisms; and the diseased rubbish
> which was shot upon Christianity by forlorn old monks
> who had the stomach ache would be carted off by the scav-
> enger; and men and women would be more prayerful, and
> more charitable, and more virtuous, because they would
> have a more regular supply of the gastric fluids, and less
> torpidity in the liver, and fewer obstructions in the intes-
> tinal canal. Why, sir, it strikes me, as I go about the coun-
> try, that the particular kind of grace that we just now
> need to grow is the grace of a vigorous circulation and a
> sound digestion.[1]

Between 1860 and 1920, the grace of physical vigor won
through effort in the gymnasium and on the playing field
assumed unprecedented value in hygienic thought. One of
the original components of the traditional code of health, exercise had risen dramatically in status as nineteenth-century urbanization removed increasing numbers of people
from a life in which open-air exertion was a daily necessity.
Physician-authored handbooks of exercise and physical edu-

---

[1] Moses Coit Tyler, *The Brawnville Papers*, Boston, 1869, p. 20.

cation abounded during the second quarter of the century, with walking, riding, rowing, swimming, fencing, and skating being recommended to adults as well as children. Jacksonian health reformers stressed the need for regular exercise also, and some were even hardy enough to practice what they preached. Alcott often ran the mile between his home and the post office and was a capable pedestrian, once walking seventy-eight miles in a bit over two days.[2]

But exercise was subordinate to vegetable diet and sexual restraint among Jacksonian reformers; it was a necessary but still secondary principle of their doctrine. Only as the century moved into its second half did exercise take its stand as an independent and primary method of health building. Its coming of age as a distinct ideology was in large measure a manifestation of the emerging spirit of English "muscular Christianity," a form of social gospel that affirmed the compatibility of the robust physical life with a life of Christian morality and service and indeed contended that bodily strength built character and righteousness and usefulness for God's (and the nation's) work. Tom Brown, the archetype of the maturing muscular Christian, had been a popular fictional hero for half a century before Thomas Hughes immortalized him in the 1850s. But it was the novels of Hughes, and even more Charles Kingsley, which solidly established muscular Christianity as a cultural ideal in England—and in the United States.[3]

[2] *American Vegetarian, 1*, 141 (1851). For discussions of medical and general cultural attitudes toward exercise and health, see John Betts, "American Medical Thought on Exercise as the Road to Health," *Bull. Hist. Med., 45*, 138–152 (1971); Betts, "Mind and Body in Early American Thought," *J. Am. Hist., 54*, 787–805 (1967–68); Ralph Billett, "Evidence of Play and Exercise in Early Pestalozzian and Lancasterian Elementary Schools in the United States, 1809–1845," *Research Q., 23*, 127–135 (1952).

[3] Gerald Raymond, "The First, 'Tom Brown's Schooldays' (1804) and Others: Origins and Evolution of Muscular Christianity in Children's Literature 1762–1857," *North American Soc. Sport Hist., Proc.*, pp. 16–17 (1977); Bruce Haley, *The Healthy Body and Victorian Culture*, Cambridge, Mass., 1978, pp. 107–119.

Coined in 1857 by a critic reviewing Kingsley's *Two Years Ago*, the term "muscular Christianity" had quickly spread beyond the bounds Kingsley had had in mind. He had been preaching "the divineness of the whole manhood," the virtue of physical manliness and "healthy animalism." But an age enchanted by athletics and action could interpret muscular Christianity to mean a spiritual obligation to cultivate the body, and suppose that morality could be measured with a tape and weighed by athletic trophies. In fact, a "Christian Guild" organized in the north of England in the 1870s proposed making the winning of a town championship in running, wrestling, or rowing an entrance qualification. A decade earlier *Punch* had already warned that if trends at the universities continued. "Latin will be nowhere, Leaping everything; Geometry will yield to Gymnastics; Philosophy to Fencing; Paley to Pole-jumping; Homer to Hurdles; Cosines to Calisthenics; Trigonometry to Training."[4]

In the United States, the most one-sided of these mid-century competitions was the one involving gymnastics, a sport that outdid all rivals for the building of muscularity. To be precise, it was German gymnastics, the *Turnen* system developed by Jahn at the beginning of the century to promote national strength and unity, that led the advance of gymnastics in America. *Turners* practioners of the system, came to this country in two waves, each an aftershock of political repression in Germany. The first stirred a flurry of interest in the new exercises in the Boston area between 1825 and 1830, but the attention was not lasting; as a cynical physician analyzed it, the system was "better adapted to the Spartan youth than to the pallid sons of pampered cits, the dandies of the desk, and the squalid tenants of attics and factories."[5]

---

[4] Haley, *Healthy Body* (n. 3), pp. 107–109, 214, 221.

[5] Robert Barney, "German Turners in America: Their Role in Nineteenth Century Exercise Expression and Physical Education Legislation," in *A History of Physical Education and Sport in the United States and Canada*, ed. Earle Ziegler, Champaign, Ill., 1975, pp. 111–120; Bruce

Pallid dandies still proliferated in the 1850s, but the post-1848 influx of *Turners* was much larger and more persistent. Establishing gymnastic societies (*Turnvereine*) all about the country, more than seventy by the end of the 1850s, German immigrants generated interest in physical fitness throughout the larger population. And the strong and daring youth who were actually won to the practice of gymnastics translated that preoccupation with physical culture into an ideology of perfection. The exercises themselves were perfectly balanced, the parallel and horizontal bars, horse, weights, and climbing equipment combining to test all the muscles and force a complete range of motions. The gymnasium was relatively inexpensive, accessible in all seasons, and so diverse as to satisfy any taste for exertion with its "endless variety of manly competitions." Swinging about its apparatus, the adept soon discovered the full meaning of health: "Health is perpetual youth,—that is, a state of positive health. . . . Health is to feel the body a luxury as every vigorous child does."[6]

With health, one resisted and threw off the assaults of disease that levelled nongymnasts. There was additionally a mind-relaxing play that accompanied gymnastic muscle building and served to counteract "the one great fundamental disorder of all Americans . . . nervous exhaustion." Finally, this "only thorough panacea" which made "the whole voyage of life perpetually self-curative," saved its devotees from spiritual decay as well: "Physical exercises give to energy and daring a legitimate channel, supply the place of war, gambling, licentiousness, high-way robbery, and office-seeking. . . . It gives an innocent answer to that first demand

Bennett, "The Making of Round Hill School," *Quest*, monograph 4 (1965), pp. 53–63; James Johnson, *The Economy of Health*, New York, 1837, p. 104.

[6] Betty Spears and Richard Swanson, *History of Sport and Physical Activity in the United States*, Dubuque, Iowa, 1978, p. 121; Thomas Wentworth Higginson, "Gymnastics," *Atlantic M.*, *7*, 283–302 (1861), p. 301.

for evening excitement which perils the soul of the homeless boy in the seductive city."[7]

One young man saved by the gymnasium from a life of humiliation, if not dissipation, was George Windship (often rendered Winship), America's first popularizer of weightlifting for health. Windship might well have been a biographical model for the twentieth century's Charles Atlas: the next to smallest student in his Harvard class in the early 1850s, he was bullied by a classmate who threw his books down stairs and subjected him to other indignities. Resolving to rid himself of his tormentor, Windship turned to daily workouts in the gymnasium and within two years had so built himself up that the former nemesis backed down from his challenge rather than risk a thrashing. Since he had chosen gymnastics primarily to increase his strength, Windship found weight lifting the most fascinating exercise. Thus shortly after matriculating as a Harvard medical student in 1854, he began to apply himself seriously to weight training and to eventually become (as Dr. Windship) "the Roxbury Hercules." During that training period, incidentally, he experienced a period of slow progress that he thought might be due to the animal food in his diet. "I read anew the works of Graham and Alcott," he relates, "and conceiving that my strength had reached a stagnation point, I gave up meat." For once, muscular vegetarianism failed. Windship actually lost ground, until he returned to "beef-steaks, mutton-chops, and loins of veal." On the more stimulating diet, his strength advanced again, and by 1861 the five-foot seven-inch, 143-pound "Hercules" was able to lift more than two thousand pounds from the ground (Windship's lifts involved "merely" clearing the weight from the ground; they were not what modern weightmen call "dead lifts," which require the lifter to return to the fully erect position while holding the weight). He had also become so eloquent a lecturer on physical culture by then as to spark a "lifting

---

[7] Higginson, "Gymnastics" (n. 6), pp. 286, 287, 296.

mania" in America: "Like mushrooms after rain," a contemporary marvelled, "lifting machines sprang up in parlors and offices and schools everywhere." The lifters parroted Windship's motto—"Strength is Health"—and strained to accomplish the same escape from nervousness, headaches, and indigestion that the leader claimed he had achieved.[8]

But even the ancient Greeks had produced only one Hercules. Windship's success was difficult to duplicate, and even impossible for the half of society most in need of physical improvement. Something other than Windship's "hobby" was needed, one which would be "perfectly safe for a lady to drive." The answer, however, was not in the remaining exercises of German gymnastics, for ladies were deemed as incapable of vaulting the horse and handling the trapeze as hoisting the dumbbell. The only proper gymnasium equipment for females, apparently, consisted of "a few settees where sweethearts and wives may sit with their knitting as spectators."[9]

Dioclesian Lewis begged to differ. Like Alcott, Dio (his preferred name) Lewis practiced medicine for a period (in the 1840s), but soon gave up treatment for prevention. An animated and inspirational speaker—one could "inhale hygiene in his presence"—he became a commanding figure on the temperance platform from the 1850s into the 1880s. He also authored works on sexual hygiene (*Chastity; or Our Secret Sins*) and nutrition (*Our Digestion; or My Jolly Friend's Secret*). But his most cherished work was the system of "New Gymnastics" that swept the country in the early 1860s.[10]

The "old gymnastics" was inadequate, Lewis felt, not sim-

---

[8] George Windship, "Autobiographical Sketches of a Strength-Seeker," *Atlantic M.*, 9, 102–115 (1867); Dudley Sargent, *An Autobiography*, Philadelphia, 1927, p. 98.

[9] Higginson, "Gymnastics" (n. 6), pp. 288, 300.

[10] Mary Eastman, *The Biography of Dio Lewis*, New York, 1891; Fred Leonard, "The 'New Gymnastics' of Dio Lewis (1860–1868)," *Am. Phys. Ed. Rev.*, 11, 83–95, 187–198 (1906), p. 88.

ply because it shut out women. While an athletic young man himself, he had enrolled as a student of German gymnastics and quickly been impressed by the unsuitability of the exercises for children and old or fat men as well. Even young and fit men ran risks—a former student of Charles Follen, one of the introducers of *Turnen* in the 1820s, recalled his gymnastics days by stating he could remember "precisely who were injured." Lewis had also become convinced that the strength built by gymnastic work was not the true measure of muscular health. The gymnasts and the weight lifters were not gaining freedom from disease or insuring longer life with their bigger muscles, for their movements were too limited and strenuous, and not integrated to give balanced exertion. The body is "an exceedingly complicated machine, the symmetrical development of which requires discriminating, studied management"; "bodily symmetry," for all ages and constitutions, and both sexes, required "the New Gymnastics."[11]

Lewis began formulating his system about 1854, while in the process of curing his wife of tuberculosis with walking, wood-sawing, and other conventional exercises. His goal was to find exercises that would have the excitement of free play but could be combined to develop whole body flexibility, coordination, agility, and grace of movement. Exceptional muscular strength was not an object; mental and moral improvement were. Lewis' *idee fixe* was that physical education was the indispensable foundation of all other education, and that the American school system could never succeed at its task until it gave physical education as central a place as intellectual and character training. The first question that should be asked of a young lady when she enters a school, he suggested, was not "how have you progressed in latin but, 'Miss Mary, how is your spine?' "[12]

[11] Leonard, "New Gymnastics" (n. 10), p. 88; Dio Lewis, "The New Gymnastics," *Atlantic M.*, *10*, 129–148 (1862), pp. 131–132; Lewis, "New Gymnastics," *Am. J. Ed.*, *11*, 531–562 (1862), *ibid.*, *12*, 665–700 (1862).
[12] Lewis, "New Gymnastics" (n. 11), pp. 532–533.

The program Lewis formulated to save Miss Mary's spine was structured around several sets of light apparatus exercises. Among the more stimulating, apparently, were the bean bag games (he invented the bean bag to replace the large rubber balls which his early students were always allowing to bounce through windows). More than thirty distinct bean bag exercises were worked out by Lewis, though the distinctions between some were almost too minute to count: partners tossed bags back and forth through a suspended hoop, for example, in one exercise always catching with both hands, in a second with the right hand only, and in a third with the left every time. The bean bag was actually surpassed, though, by the rings, "the best [equipment] ever devised." Wooden circles six inches in diameter and one inch thick, the rings could be used in more than fifty exercises. Several were variations of partners holding rings between them and pulling firmly while twisting their arms in time to music (Figure 8). Others were more strenuous, and along with wooden dumbbell and wand exercises, dancing, and marching, rounded out the Lewis system. When performed to musical accompaniment, it was apparently more exhiliarating than a brief outline can convey: an English observer described a Lewis demonstration as "a sort of physical jubilee, a carnival of the emotional and vital powers."[13]

Comparable excitement typified the intital public review of this democratized gymnastics. In 1860, Lewis presented his system (exercises and goals) to the Boston convention of the American Institute of Instruction. The august body of educators responded with "frequent applause and hearty cheers," and a resolution that the Lewis gymnastics were "eminently worthy of general introduction into all our schools, and into general use." They also supported his plan for a Normal Institute for Physical Education, which was incorporated (in Boston) in the spring of 1861, and turned

---

[13] Eastman, *Biography* (n. 10), p. 84.

out within six months the first class of physical education teachers in America. The graduates were already in demand, for the gentle Lewis gymnastics had quickly made its way into schools around the country.[14]

Exactly half of that first graduating class of fourteen were women, and the percentage of female gymnasts increased in subsequent years. Lewis made a special effort to recruit women, even setting their fees 25 percent lower than the men's. The official justification for the reduction was "because of the unjust disparity of compensation which everywhere obtains between male and female labor." But Lewis' greater concern was for the disparity between male and female health: it was Miss Mary's spine that was in such need of attention, not Master John's. Lewis' gymnastic exercises were offered to all, but his fondest wish was that they could be made attractive to girls rendered anemic by corsets, heavy skirts, and socially prescribed inactivity.[15]

To that end he opened, in 1864, on the battle ground at Lexington, a school that he hoped would set off a new revolution, a winning of physical independence for women. Calisthenics and light gymnastics for women had been recommended by earlier reformers, most notably Catherine Beecher (and many of Beecher's exercises had been adopted and modified by Lewis). But the Family School for Young Ladies was a new departure. There Lewis intentionally accepted "delicate" girls of average age seventeen, girls who could not "go upstairs without symptoms," and put them on a schedule heavy with exercise and study, with no allowance made for their "periodicity." Each day began with thirty to ninety minutes of gymnastics, and the rest of the day was ordered to give fresh air and sun, plain (but not vegetarian) meals, nonrestrictive dress, pleasant social life, and regular hours. His young charges were also instructed to chew each

[14] Leonard, "New Gymnastics" (n. 10), p. 90; John Philbrick, "City School Systems in the United States," United States Bureau of Education, *Circulars of Information*, 1885, no. 1, pp. 99–103.

[15] Leonard, "New Gymnastics" (n. 10), p. 92.

bit of food thoroughly, as "the only direct contribution they could make to their digestion must be made in the mouth" (one must suspect that Lewis' *Five Minute Chats with Young Women* was one of the books scanned by Fletcher during his early search for health counsel). Saturdays were devoted to countryside tramps. Lewis even painted distance markers on trees and walls, at quarter mile intervals, so progress could be accurately measured. Girls who had labored up a flight of stairs at entry, graduated able to "walk from five to ten miles on Saturday without inconvenience." The school burned in 1867 and was not resurrected, but for that brief period it was a shining demonstration of the potential for female vitality. Nearly three hundred girls were trained there, and according to Lewis every one left with better health than she had brought.[16]

As proud as he was of his female pupils' flouting of convention, Lewis did not offer them strength so they could break their social bonds. Woman needed health in order to be a better mother and housekeeper (Catherine Beecher had been no more daring), and she was still something of a bauble to his eye (and to Beecher's, who grumbled that many of Lewis' exercises were too "ungraceful" to be suitable "for young ladies"). Lewis' argument for coeducational gymnastics rested on the premise that, "Girls are disinclined to exercise. We shall never reach satisfactory results in their physical development while we deny them the presence and participation of the more vigorous magnetic boys." Likewise, wooden rings should be made of expensive rosewood

[16] Catherine Beecher, *Physiology and Calisthenics for Schools and Families*, New York, 1856; Patricia Vertinsky, "Sexual Equality and the Legacy of Catherine Beecher," *J. Sport Hist.*, 6, no. 1, 38–49 (1979); Roberta Park, " 'Embodied Selves': The Rise and Development of Concern for Physical Education, Active Games and Recreation for American Women, 1776–1865," *J. Sport. Hist.*, 5, no. 2, 5–41 (1978); Lewis, *Five Minute Chats with Young Women*, New York, 1874, pp. 379–401; Lewis, "The Health of American Women," *North Am. Rev.*, 135, 503–510 (1882); Eastman, *Biography* (n. 10), pp. 89–111.

and carefully finished and polished—"The interest of young ladies is thereby greatly enhanced."[17]

And the health those young ladies acquired with the rings greatly augmented their attractiveness to young men. Gymnastics spokesman Thomas Wentworth Higginson reported that a friend in a neighboring settlement where the gymnastic revolution was well along, had told him that "in his town, if a girl could vault a five-barred gate, her prospects for a husband were considered to be improved ten per cent." But ultimately, the significance of giving more attention to female health attached to children, not husbands: "Unless they [women] are healthy," Higginson continued, "the whole country is not safe. Nowhere can their physical condition be so important as in a republic. . . . The fate of our institutions may hang on the precise temperament which our next President shall have inherited from his mother."[18]

Lewis' system was not only appraised as "the most important single step for the physical education of American women," but also as "the hobby of the day" for the other sex. That hobby's most energetic rider (next to its author himself) was the "professed Don Quixote of athleticism," Moses Coit Tyler. Tyler would eventually become a distinguished historian (the first professor of American history in the United States, in fact), but in his youth his highest honor was that of valedictorian of the 1863 class of the Normal Institute of Physical Education. From there he journeyed to England to popularize successfully the "musical gymnastics," then returned home to edify Americans with his *Brawnville Papers* ("Being Memorials of the Brawnville Athletic Club"). Originally presented in the pages of the *Herald of Health* (whose editor would name his only son Dio

---

[17] Beecher quoted by Edward Hartwell, "Physical Training in American Colleges and Universities," United States Bureau of Education, Circulars of Information, 1885, no. 5, p. 27; Lewis, *Five Minute Chats* (n. 16), p. 26; Lewis, "New Gymnastics" (n. 11), p. 700.

[18] Thomas Wentworth Higginson, "The Health of Our Girls," *Atlantic M.*, 9, 722–731 (1862), p. 731.

Lewis Holbrook), his fictitious community was populated with eager athletes who sang as they sweated, rending the air with the exuberant "Song of the Gymnasts":

> Now, gymnasts strong, lift we high a song
> For our art and its triumphs glorious,
> That leads the van for the health of man,
> And is over ills victorious!
> *Chorus*
> Then work away till a better day
> On our pill-cursed race is shining;
> For the "bell" and the "ring" shall defiance fling
> At the fiends of Disease and Pining.[19]

By the end of the third stanza it becomes clear that this was not the song, but the hymn of the gymnasts, who were themselves muscular Christians cast in the mold of their leader, Judge Fairplay: "Muscular Christianity," the judge pronounced,

> is Christianity applied to the treatment and use of our bodies. It is an enforcement of the laws of health by solemn sanctions of the New Testament. . . . It says that since every part of our nature is the sacred gift of God, he who neglects his body, . . . who allows it to grow up puny, frail, sickly, mis-shapen, homely, commits a sin against the Giver of the body. . . . Round shoulders and narrow chests are states of criminality. The dyspepsia is heresy. The headache is infidelity. It is as truly a man's moral duty to have a good digestion, and sweet breath, and strong arms, and stalwart legs, and an erect bearing, as it is to read his Bible, or say his prayers, or love his neighbor as himself.[20]

The identification of morality with muscularity was to grow as an article of hygienic faith through the final third of

---

[19] *ibid.*, p. 730; Higginson, "Gymnastics" (n. 6), p. 300; *National Cyclopedia of American Biography*, 1909 vol. 12, New York, 12:334: Tyler, *Brawnville Papers* (n. 1), pp. 97–98.

[20] Tyler, *Brawnville Papers* (n. 1), pp. 162–163.

the century and the Progessive years, though the arena
would become congested with competing programs of health
building. Lewis gymnastics eclipsed the *Turnen* variety for
a while, but the German system came back into favor in the
1870s as Lewis returned to temperance campaigning. By
that time military drill, encouraged by the Civil War, had
also become popular, as had the free exercises of Swedish
gymnastics. Adding to the variety were several systems of
weight training and the postwar growth of numerous sports
and games. The most effective propagators of muscular
morality, though, were members of the medical profession,
specifically those members who dedicated their careers to
birthing the modern physical education movement. Alcott had called his doctrine "physical education," but he
had had in mind a didactic exercise, a tutoring of the young
in the laws of health. He assumed that the teaching would
encourage play, but exercise was an implication, not the essence of the program. The definition of physical education in
the post-Lewis decades, though, began with movement and
effort; it was a philosophy practiced in the gymnasium first
and foremost, and only supplementarily taught in the classroom.

The philosophers of physical education were a lively set of
men, nearly all of them physicians with a preventive inclination. First in their ranks, in terms of seniority, was Edward Hitchcock, Jr., son of the "dyspepsy forestalling"
health reformer of the 1830s. Appointed Professor of Hygiene and Physical Education at Amherst in 1861, Hitchcock is generally credited with introducing physical education at the collegiate level. And by occupying that chair for
fifty years, "Old Doc" wielded an influential hand in the
subsequent development of the discipline. Students in the
early days of his tenure were put through a schedule of light
gymnastics similar to those of Lewis (they even used dumbbells manufactured by Lewis); toward the end of the century Hitchcock followed the national trend to spice the formal drills with more athletic competitions. Throughout, he

acted on his conviction that health was a duty to God, and a prerequisite for effective service to Him.[21]

The second professorship in physical education was assumed in 1879 by Dudley Allen Sargent, the acknowledged Newton of his field. Sargent began lifting weights at age fourteen, soon advanced to gymnastics, and served stints as a circus acrobat and private gymnasium operator before taking his position at Harvard. He had also found time to earn a medical degree from Yale in 1878 as a logical step in his pursuit of the "gleam which I must follow . . . preventive medicine." The Sargent System that he instituted at Harvard's soon to be famous Hemenway Gymnasium was structured around exercises on pulley-weight machines (many of Sargent's invention) that could be adjusted to the strength of the invididual and focussed on the cultivation of specific muscles. The system also involved "mimetic exercises," more than fifty activities designed to imitate the movement of various forms of labor and sport. By putting boys through graduated training in the system, Sargent asserted, "I developed manhood."[22]

Sargent and his system were the turning point for physical education as a profession. The discipline's stature in American colleges prior to the Harvard program is indicated by a story Sargent liked to tell on himself. Shortly after his appointment to the university, he met his first dignified Harvard alumnus: eagerly introducing himself as the new professor of physical education, he was chilled by the response, "Ah, they had a nigger when I was there." (Sargent had been preceded by a black boxing coach). But by 1885, his weight machines and mimetic exercises had been adopted by nearly fifty colleges and clubs. The demand for instructors of his gymnastics had compelled him to organize a teacher-training program at Harvard in 1884. And his

---

[21] J. Edmund Welch, *Edward Hitchcock, M.D., Founder of Physical Education in the College Curriculum*, Greenville, N.C., 1966.

[22] Sargent, *Autobiography* (n. 8), pp. 145, 149, 202.

ideas had been given general public circulation by the remarkably popular guide to muscle building, William Blaikie's *How to Get Strong and How to Stay So* (1879). In 1887, Sargent began his Harvard Summer School of Physical Education, which became a mecca for continuing education for teachers. Fifteen years later, he could report a total of 270 colleges giving physical education a place in their programs; 300 city school systems requiring physical exercises of their students; 500 YMCA gymnasia with 80,000 members; and more than 100 gymnasia connected with athletic clubs, hospitals, military bases, and miscellaneous institutions.[23]

Others instrumental in this flowering of physical education included Edward Hartwell, M.D., who was converted to the cause by Sargent and carried the Sargent System to Johns Hopkins; William Anderson, M.D., the director of the Yale Gymnasium who tested Fletcher and who led the move to establish a national physical education association; Luther Gulick, M.D., a graduate of Sargent's program who guided the growth of physical training within the YMCA and promoted both the playground and Campfire movements; and R. Tait McKenzie, M.D., also a Sargent student, who directed physical education at the University of Pennsylvania and was the most eloquent medical spokesman for athleticism. The work of these men and their colleagues was not merely the quantitative achievement of carrying physical education into so many institutions, but was also a qualitative transformation, an enlargement of the meaning of physical education. By their estimation, at any rate, physical training prior to the last quarter of the century had been adequately described by the designations "physical culture" and "gymnastics." It had aimed at the strengthening and refining of the body as an end in itself, with no thoroughgoing plan to use that physical improvement as the basis for mental and moral elevation. Admittedly, the muscular

[23] *ibid.*, p. 161; Hartwell, "Physical Training" (n. 17), pp. 56–58; Sargent, "Ideals in Physical Education," *Am. Phys. Ed. Rev., 6,* 110–121 (1901), p. 110.

Christianity doctrine of gymnasts and physical culturists assumed a necessary link between physique and character, but it was faith, an intuitive insight that had not been given a physiological rationale. Nor had muscular Christianity encompassed a definite system for cultivating the mental and moral with the physical. But the generation of physical educators headed by Sargent believed they had such a system in physical education and self-consciously distinguished it from its less ambitious and scientific predecessors—gymnastics, physical culture, and physical training. The latter terms continued in use, but they were understood to have acquired the enlarged and modern wholistic meaning.[24]

Thus Gulick could take a stage less than thirty years after Lewis and unveil "Our New Gymnastics." It was more accurately a new "new gymnastics," one that worked "for the salvation, development and training of the whole man complete as God made him." The triangle emblem of the YMCA was designed by Gulick too, and was meant to symbolize "spirit upheld by body and mind." The search for wholeness and harmony was also inspired by a pagan example. Physical educators of the turn of the century were virtually unable to discuss their work without describing it as nothing less than a crusade to establish within American society the Greek ideal of a sound mind in a sound body. A University of Pennsylvania instructor's summary of "the soul and body in physical training" expressed physical educators' Hellenic mission with typical optimism: "Beginning therefore with Greece, we will travel in a circle, and, exemplifying the saying that history but repeats itself, we will return at last to our point of departure and rest with our faces turned toward the land of nimble minds and exquisite bodies."[25]

[24] Fred Leonard, *A Guide to the History of Physical Education*, Philadelphia, 1917, pp. 268–380; Norma Schwendener, *A History of Physical Education in the United States*, New York, 1942, pp. 111–160.

[25] Gulick quoted by Leonard, *Guide* (n. 24), p. 322; Ethel Dorgan, *Luther Halsey Gulick, 1865–1918*, New York, 1934, p. 35; A. Holmes, "The Soul and Body in Physical Training," *Am. Phys. Ed. Rev.*, 14, 479–489 (1909) p. 479.

Physical educators' dreams were nevertheless held under tight rein by reality. They appreciated that the historical circle was far from being closed and that turn-of-the-century America bore little resemblance yet to Periclean Athens. Indeed, much of the impetus for the advance of physical education derived from the Progressive conviction that American society had degenerated to the point where it was facing a physical and moral emergency. The salvage plan of bodily renovation thus incorporated the same anxieties and hopes that left their marks on dietary ideologies, though the philosophy of physical education was less complex. As diverse as were the problems with which it grappled and the triumphs it promised, it could be reduced almost entirely to concern for a single difficulty—the menace of the city. Civilization and nature remained at odds, for the public at large as much as for hygienists. The American conscience was being tortured by the sociocultural turbulence and uncertainties of urbanization. Never had cities been so noticeably crowded and soulless and alien. The farmer's and villager's long-festering distrust of crowds and bustle and rapid change was being brought to a head by the ugliness of uncontrolled industrial expansion and the sight of waves of immigrants with foreign ways breaking over urban slums. The draining away by the city of much of the better stock among country youth provided additional cause to fear the nation had lost its stabilizing agrarian anchor and was drifting into degeneracy. When these pervasive social apprehensions were combined with the hard, ancient fact that city life is less invigorating and tranquil, a physical educators' revolt against the city became a certainty.

The revolt began at its traditional point, dismay at the physical condition of urban man. "Is it not shameful," McKenzie asked, "to think of a big, well-built man, brought up on the farm ... spending his days pushing a small pen or whispering into a dictaphone?" He inevitably became, in another's words, "that most modern product of all, the manikin of the city" (a "pale, wizened, undersized creature").[26]

But pity for the manikin extended beyond his inferior stature. The city not only demanded less of muscle, it required much more from the nervous system, and physical weaklings could not be expected to stand up to the unceasing process of "nervous katabolism" which was inherent in urban life. The prevention of neurasthenia was another object of physical education, expected to be achieved in the most direct way: stronger muscles, especially a stronger heart, improved circulation and increased the supply of food and oxygen to all cells, including nerve cells. Exercise built up nervous reserves, and it also interrupted the depletion of those reserves. In gymnastics and sport, the pressures and petty annoyances of life were temporarily forgotten, giving the body a respite from nervous taxation. According to Sargent, the purpose of muscular exercise was largely "to break up morbid mental tendencies, to dispel the gloomy shadows of despondency, and to insure serenity of spirit."[27]

Strengthening of the nervous system inevitably suggested improved mental functioning, another requirement for coping with city life. Physical educators were convinced by experience and intuition that muscle power generated brain power: the mind-clearing and -refreshing effects of exercise

[26] R. Tait McKenzie, "The Quest for Eldorado," *Am. Phys. Ed. Rev.*, *18*, 295–303 (1913), p. 300; Hans Ballin, "The Ethical, Physiological, and Psychological Aspects of Physical Training," *Nat. Ed. Assoc., Proc.*, 765–770 (1901), p. 769.

[27] A. B. Poland, "Scientific Value of Physical Culture," *Nat. Ed. Assoc. Proc.*, 230–239 (1892), p. 236; William Stecher, "Modern Viewpoints Regarding Physical Education," *Am. Phys. Ed. Rev.*, *23*, 225–231 (1918), p. 231; Sargent quoted in "Physical Training in College," *Outing*, *5*, 137–138 (1884–1885), p. 138. Also see Grace Kingsbury, "Physical Education in its Bearing on LIfe," *Education*, *26*, 224–230 (1905), p. 230; and William Herdman, "Recreation in its Effects Upon the Nervous System," *Bull. Amer. Acad. Med.*, *7*, 277–285 (1905–1906).

were an empirical truism corroborated by the premise of the body's organic unity basic to physical culture philosophy. Sentences such as "the whole body co-operates in developing energy for the support of mental as well as motor activity" were regularly prefaced by "of course," as though the proposition were unchallengeable common knowledge. Any who considered challenging it might be referred to the experiment performed at the Elmira, New York State Reformatory. Eleven inmates who were "coarse, stupid, insensitive, unambitious dullards" were placed upon a five-month program of calisthenics and dumbbell drills; all showed progress in build and posture, naturally, but also in "mental power and self-control."[28]

The common-sense mind-body connection was strengthened with a variety of more sophisticated arguments: a favorite exercise for physical education theorists was elaboration of the body's "myopsychic relations." Regular exercise and consequent improved circulation hastened the excretion of body toxins, ran a common rationalization, and prevented cerebral stagnation and "sluggish mentality." A Lockean hypothesis maintained that since all knowledge is derived from sensory impressions, the organs of action—of sensation collection—had to be highly trained; muscles had to be made fit "channels of intercourse between mind and body." Such reasoning could finally lead to the supposition that as "the chest, neck and shoulders enlarge . . . the convolutions of the brain grow deep and thicken.[29]

[28] M. V. O'Shea, "The Relation of Physical Training to Mental Activity," *Am. Phys. Ed. Rev.*, *9*, 28–35 (1904), p. 31; Edward Hartwell, *Report of the Commissioner of Education, 1897–1898*, Washington, 1899, p. 551.
[29] G. V. N. Dearborn, "The Relation of Muscular Activity to the Mental Process," *Am. Phys. Ed. Rev.*, *14*, 10–16 (1909), p. 13; Henry Ling Taylor, "Exercise and Vigor," *Am. Phys. Ed. Rev.*, *3*, 249–257 (1898), p. 251; Ballin, "The Ethical, etc." (n. 26), p. 765; *J. Hyg. Herald Health, 44*, 72 (1894). Also see Dudley Sargent, "Physical Training as a Compulsory Subject," *School Rev.*, *16*, 42–55 (1908); and William Krohn, "Physical Education and Brain-building," *Nat. Ed. Assoc., Proc.*, 818–823 (1903).

Psychosomatic intercourse was also conducted through muscular channels for the purpose of motor acts expressing the mind's "thought and feeling, judgment and volition." That process suggested an intimacy of mind and body, Hartwell expanded, which allowed the inference "that physical training is an essential element in the development of mental health and power." The notion of mental power, of course, led directly to will, an inexpressibly important virtue at a time when European as well as American social critics believed Western civilization to be degenerating because of a failure of will. Self-control and resolution were needed by the individual and the race to overcome decadence, and while gymnastics unquestionably cultivated the will by providing difficult-to-reach goals, it also worked in more subtle ways. G. Stanley Hall, the prominent educational philosopher, made a deep impression upon physical educators with his argument that since "the muscles are the only organs of the will," the means by which the will expresses itself in action, will power is practically only as great as muscle power. "Just in proportion as muscles grow weak and flabby," he explained, "the chasm between knowing and doing the right, in which so many men are lost, yawns wide and deep; and as they become tense and firm doing becomes . . . the best organ of knowing. Rational muscle culture, therefore, for its moral effects, often for the young the very best possible means of resisting evil and establishing righteousness, is the gospel, I preach to-day."[30]

It was a gospel many had preached before, for strengthened will was expected to direct the individual and his society toward Christian perfection. In as concise a statement of muscular Christianity as can be found, Hall spoke for Progressive physical educators as a group: "We are soldiers of Christ, strengthening our muscles not against a foreign foe, but against sin within and without us. We would bring

---

[30] Hartwell quoted by Stecher, "Modern Viewpoints" (n. 27), p. 229; G. Stanley Hall, "Christianity and Physical Culture," *Pedagog. Sem., 9,* 374–378 (1902), p. 375.

in a higher kingdom of man, regenerate in body; make it more stalwart, persistent, enduring, taller, with better hearts, stomachs, nerves, and more resistful to man's great enemy—disease. . . . Men are, happily, just now beginning to learn what a power can be brought to bear against the kingdom of evil in the world by right body keeping."[31]

The capital of the kingdom of evil was the city, where temptations to sin proliferated. The use of physical education to strengthen morality was therefore but another attempt to overcome the degenerative forces of urbanization. Calisthenics and sports were not merely substitutes for dissipation. While it was true that boys "would rather play football than get down in a cramped position to play craps," comfort and fun were secondary factors in wholesomeness. The effort of athletic endeavor, first of all, burned off the excess energy of youth, preventing its eruption in sensuality. Hence the common rejoinder to the 1890s attacks on football as too brutal: *"Football has ended a career of debauchery for more than one youth."* More important, though, was the vital energy generated by exercise, the energy spurring its possessor to accomplishment and making his life an exciting adventure that could not be side-tracked for even occasional self-indulgence. "Bodily vigor is a moral agent," Gulick contended, "it enables us to live on higher levels, to keep up to the top of our achievement. We can not afford to lose grip on ourselves." Exercise built moral fiber as surely as it did muscular fibers; the paradox of "the weaker the body the more it commands; the stronger the body, the more it obeys" achieved the status of a bromide among physical educators. It was the "sick, devitalized man" who needed the artificial stimulations of drink and narcotics and debauchery; but physical health cured him of such cravings. The aforementioned Elmira inmates were judged to have attained a better "moral attitude" through their program of exercise. Gymnastics restored physical vigor and "moral health" to the

---

[31] Hall, "Christianity" (n. 30), pp. 377–378.

patients at a Massachusetts Hospital for Dipsomaniacs and Inebriates. And at the University of Pennsylvania, undergraduate sexual morality became "incredibly higher," it was attested, after students became involved in athletics. But exercise had to be of the gymnastic sort, directed toward even, not excessive, muscular development. The prejudice against heavy weight lifting continued, and the ghost of Dio Lewis must have been overjoyed to learn that the mighty Sandow, despite his awesome musculature, was unable to hold down his appetites: he "eats and drinks and smokes regardless of consequences," a gymnastics gossip disclosed, "and is far from being an intellectual or moral giant."[32]

Gymnastics' value for character training rested only partly in its ability to strengthen one to resist temptation. That strength kept the man from becoming bad, but did not in itself make him good. When physical educators proclaimed that "the vocabulary of sport has become the terminology of ethics," they were thinking less of the passive ethics of self-restraint than of the aggressive ethics of action for the good of society and the race. They saw the gymnasium as a microcosm of life, a training ground in which a boy learned to set goals and work resolutely toward them, to endure through fatigue and pain, to accept responsibility for his actions, and to take a pride in his success that would translate into dignity. When the exercise was expanded into team sport, in the gymnasium or on the field, other socializing elements were brought into play. Hitchcock also rallied to the defense of football, proposing that the undeniable danger of the game was actually one (but only one) of its virtues: "To

[32] Percy Grant, "Physical Deterioration among the Poor in America and One-Way of Checking It," *North Am. Rev.*, *184*, 254–267 (1907), pp. 264, 265; B. W. Mitchell, "A Defense of Football," *J. Hyg. Herald Health*, *45*, 91–96 (1895), p. 93; Luther Gulick, *The Efficient Life*, New York, 1909, p. 107; Millicent Hosmer, "The Development of Morality Through Physical Education," *Mind and Body*, *21*, 156–163 (1914–1915), p. 157; Edward Cowles, "Gymnastics in the Treatment of Inebriety," *Am. Phys. Ed. Rev.*, *3*, 107–110 (1898); W. L. Schenck, "Exercise—its Physiologic Functions," *JAMA*, *22*, 417–421 (1894), p. 420.

play football a man must look out for and protect himself. He must also be the aggressor against the other side, and so must hold his temper and learn withal to be righteous with his opponent. He must expect defeat again and again, and must meet it like a man. And these, we claim, are necessities for a greater part of the public conditions of all our lives; and whatever disciplines us for this work early, helps us to be the better fitted for the stern work of life that assails us all at some time." The team play of sports, many others emphasized, was an especially valuable type of education in a democratic society, and the necessity of submitting to rules bred respect for the law. And it was a particularly urgent matter to extend it to the city youth, whose task-free life cut off from exposure to the elements denied him the opportunity to develop the manly qualities that were the birthright of the country boy.[33]

Gymnastic philosophy thus saw the *mens sana* as in large measure produced by the *corpore sano,* though the time-honored phrase from Juvenal was finally found to be inadequate to express physical educators' aims. Preferable, in McKenzie's view, was the goal of *"mens fervida in corpore lacertoso"*—"the ardent mind in the muscular body." The term best describing that fusion of powers was efficiency. Gulick entitled his lengthy manual on health building *The Efficient Life.* McKenzie interpreted his own work as a "quest for Eldorado," "the Eldorado of efficiency" inhabited by "the perfect man." Sargent (who had somewhat more respect for highly developed muscular strength than did the typical physical educator) combined exercises to determine the individual's speed and endurance as well as strength; the

[33] William Faunce, "Athletics for the Service of the Nation," *Am. Phys. Ed. Rev., 23,* 137–143 (1918), p. 138; Edward Hitchcock, "The Gymnastic Era and the Athletic Era of Our Country," *Outlook, 51,* 816–818 (1895), p. 817; James Hughes, "Physical Training as a Factor in Character Building," *Nat. Ed. Assoc. Proc.,* 911–919 (1896); H. W. Foster, "Physical Education vs. Degeneracy," *Independent, 52,* 1835–1837 (1900).

total score on this "Universal Test," the measure of the subject's all-round health, he termed the index of "physical efficiency."[34]

Efficiency was the Progressive synonym for our contemporary ideal of wellness, but efficiency went far beyond wellness in its glorification of work. While wellness is sought primarily for physical and spiritual self-fulfillment, the purpose of efficiency was achievement. "Our work will be productive of results that would otherwise have been quite beyond our reach," Gulick vowed. The results included personal success, of course, physical efficiency being absolutely indispensable for performing adequately in the busy and strenuous urban business world. Those "who have gone to the top," it was accepted, made it "because of their vitality, their ability to do things, to push, to stand strain." Even the gymnastic look could help one up the corporate ladder, according to the more calculating physical educators: "Muscular development and poise create an impression of manliness, strength and individuality which may stand one in good stead as a business value."[35]

The social value of work was held in far higher esteem, however. Sargent emphasized "the value of physical exercise as a means of attaining fitness for efficient service," and defined that service in classical moral terms: physically educated men would be better equipped "to fight the battles of the weak, to meet the game of the unprincipled strong, and wrestle with the great moral, social, political and financial problems that await them in the world." Not the least of these problems was the fate of the nation. Progressive physical educators too feared that American civilization was at bay, or at least soon would be unless physical deterioration

---

[34] R. Tait McKenzie, "Constructive Patriotism," *Am. Phys. Ed. Rev.* *17*, 245–254 (1912), p. 246; McKenzie, "Quest" (n. 26), p. 303; Sargent, *Universal Test for Strength, Speed and Endurance of the Human Body*, Cambridge, Mass., 1902.

[35] Gulick, *Efficient Life* (n. 32), pp. 12, 180; Kingsbury, "Physical Education" (n. 27), p. 225.

were halted. "A nation that is in physical decay is doomed," the head of Boston's Posse Gymnasium declared; "A nation that has no endurance can not clinch the nails it drives." Endurance and its parent efficiency were vital to the life of the country. Economic productivity and military strength required hardy bodies and agile minds, so physical education was a patriotic duty.[36]

Embodied within the concept of physical efficiency as a duty to the country was the notion of duty to the race. General human deterioration was deplored, but the decline of American stock was of most glaring concern. The common prescription was judicious marriage, selection of a physically fit mate, but the occasional ardent eugenicist among physical educators could carry his doctrine to rascist extremes. The 1910 convention of the American Physical Education Association, for example, was harangued by a speaker on racial hygiene to help society build better blood through physical training, and to preserve Teutonic blood from contamination by "less fortunate races." We need in America an aristocracy of blood," he concluded, "of rich, red blood, not the aristocracy of blue blood, ... but the aristocracy of strength, of health and of efficiency."[37]

The manufacture of an aristocracy of health was, however, threatened by urbanization. Even without the teeming, non-Teutonic masses that were its most visible obstacle to racial health, the city posed an evolutionary challenge. It was a new environment for human habitation, an industrialized jungle where men fought for survival with nerve power rather than muscular strength. Muscle was being lost both by these changing forces of natural (or rather civilized) selection, and through the abandoning of strength-building living habits. But nervous force adequate to the new demands had not yet been accumulated, since on an evolution-

[36] Sargent, "The Future of Physical Education," *Putnam's 7*, 14–20 (1909), pp. 18, 20; Rose Posse, "How Physical Training Affects the Welfare of the Nation," *Am. Phys. Ed. Rev., 15*, 493–499 (1910).

[37] W. W. Hastings, "Racial Hygiene and Vigor," *Am. Phys. Ed. Rev. 15*, 515–525 (1910), p. 525.

ary scale the change in selective forces had been very recent. The escape from this trap was for man to take control of his own evolution, and by the cultivation of physical vigor manufacture the nervous and mental vitality required by the modern environment. Bodily strength thus remained as essential for survival in the modern city as in the primeval forest.[38]

In undertaking the direction of complete individual, social, and racial development, physical educators attempted to be just what Gulick called them: "biological engineers." But despite their presumptuousness, a respectability attached to physical educators that saved them from being labelled faddists. The bulk of their attention was given to improvement of the body; the physical improvements anticipated were plausible, and they did not break in any major way with established scientific opinion (indeed, many European physicians held very similar hopes for the effects of exercise on their societies).[39] If they dreamed of creating a better world through physical culture, it was the dream of a man enthusiastic about the potentialities of his field of endeavor, not the wild imagining of a fanatic. The physical education excitement was sometimes satirized, but with the intent of keeping a basically sound movement within bounds, and not with the contempt that was shown for Grahamism or vegetarianism.

The popularity of physical culture, though, all but insured more radical interpretations of the hygiene of exercise by health-conscious zealots outside the physical education ranks. Hartwell called attention in 1899 to the variety of "systems and systemettes" of physical training being forwarded by "would-be reformers and minor prophets" as "schemes for hastening the millennium." He added that

[38] See, for example, Poland, "Scientific Value" (n. 27).
[39] Gulick, "The Problem of Physical Training in the Modern City," *Am. Phys. Ed. Rev.*, *8*, 29–34 (1903); on European physical education, see Robert Nye, "Degeneration, Hygiene and Sports in Fin-de-siècle France," paper read at the meeting of the Western Society for French History, Eugene, Oregon, Oct. 24–26, 1980.

"they can not be made to serve the ends of general physical education," but his dismissal notwithstanding, unorthodox physical culture did win a popular following and affected the public understanding of physical education.[40]

Some of the Progressive physical culturists were pure hucksters, "Get Strong Quick fakirs" as McKenzie called them. Some were genuine, if monomaniacal, campaigners for better health for all. At least one was both. Bernarr Macfadden, at any rate, combined an honest and boyish faith in the power of exercise with an entrepreneurial talent that carried him from rural poverty to the command of a vast publishing empire. His health was a rags to riches saga too. Born in 1868 to an alcoholic father and tuberculous mother, he was orphaned before his teen-age years. Weakness and illness also plagued his adolescence, but he fought back with dumbbells and distance walking and gradually built himself into a man capable of teaching gymnastics and winning professional wrestling matches. His self-image was naturally transformed as well, as demonstrated by the name change he adopted in the early 1890s. He had been christened Bernard (with stress on first syllable), a dandified name unacceptable for a man of muscle. By replacing the final "d" with an "r," and shifting the accent to the second syllable, he produced a name ending with a roaring sound. The effect was completed by changing his original "McFadden" to "Macfadden": the expanded first syllable evoked the power of the Mack truck (which was then being introduced), and the image was accentuated by decapitalization of the "f."[41]

Macfadden crowned his new name with a new title—"pro-

[40] Hartwell, *Report* (n. 28), p. 550.

[41] McKenzie's comment was made in the introduction to Sargent, *Autobiography* (n. 8), p. xvi. Biographical information on Macfadden is to be found in Mary Macfadden and Émile Gauvreau, *Dumbbells and Carrot Strips, The Story of Bernarr Macfadden,* New York, 1953; Robert Taylor, "Physical Culture," *New Yorker,* Oct. 14, 1950 (pp. 39–51), Oct. 21, 1950 (pp. 39–52), Oct. 28, 1950 (pp. 37–51); James Harvey Young, "Bernarr Macfadden," In *Dictionary of American Biography, Supplement Five, 1951–1955,* New York, 1929, pp. 452–454.

fessor of kinesitherapy"— but soon enlarged his pedagogic work to embrace the preventive health-promoting doctrine he called "Physical Culture." A magazine of that name was launched in 1899, the first project of a Physical Culture Publishing Company that would spread during the 1920s into the realms of romance and detective magazines and sensationalist tabloids, and make Macfadden a multimillionaire. His pen and presses were also responsible for a gamut of health handbooks stretching from *Hair Culture* through *Strengthening the Spine* to *Foot Troubles* and many, many others. His *Encyclopedia of Physical Culture* gave a five volume exposition of the system practiced at his several Physical Culture "Healthatoriums" (including one in Battle Creek across the street from the San) and his short-lived adventure in communal hygiene, Physical Culture City. Macfadden's system, also called "Physcultopathy," was largely a modernized version of Jacksonian health reform, its blend of unstimulating diet, exercise, sunshine and fresh air, cleanliness, and no medicine being rationalized by subjective interpretations of contemporary biological science. Its object was to secure "absolute purity" of the blood, a condition that would make disease "virtually impossible." "Even the dread disease germs of the bacteriologist" were impotent in healthy blood, Macfadden believed; though invading by the millions, they soon died without reproducing in an environment free from any peccant matter to sustain them.[42]

Pure blood was possible only with pure diet, but despite an abiding hatred for white bread, the "staff of death," Macfadden was not a latter-day Graham (nor was he a Kellogg, even though his Battle Creek days were given to promoting his new breakfast cereal, Strenthro). Though cynics laughed that he was trying "to light the path [to purity] by means of the blazing carrot," and Macfadden himself was wont to dec-

[42] Bernarr Macfadden, *Vitality Supreme*, New York, 1923, p. 179; Macfadden, *Macfadden's Encyclopedia of Physical Culture*, 5 vols., New York, 1914, 1:526–527.

orate his Christmas trees with carrots, Physical Culture did not require vegetarianism. Meat was more stimulating than vegetables, Macfadden held, and deposited more impurities in the body, but the proper practice of Physical Culture gave one the efficiency to control the stimulation and expel the impurities and live as healthfully as any vegetarian. Personal experience indicated meat gave strength and energy, and Macfadden apparently had a craving for flesh that had to be periodically subdued with lupine feasting. His justification was that appetite is an expression of natural (therefore healthful) instinct. Any overindulgence of appetite could be quickly corrected by fasting, a practice for which he admitted indebtedness to Dewey.[43]

Macfadden differed with Graham also with respect to priorities. As implied by the title of his third wife's marital (or should it be martial) memoirs—*Dumbbells and Carrot Strips*—exercise took precedence over diet. The motto of *Physical Culture* magazine was "Weakness is a Crime," and a favorite simile was exercise is "the tonic of life." Physical Culture, he elaborated, "means muscular strength.... Strength or power of some kind is what runs the human machine," so that "the man who is looking for health, but does not want muscles, will search in vain." For those who did want muscles, he provided endless pages of detailed instructions, drawings, and photographs of the calisthenics and weight-lifting exercises that had sculpted his own exquisite muscularity (Figure 9). "He was a superb male specimen," the third wife confided, who revelled in posing nude not only for her, but also (though in discreet profile) for the readers of his books. No muscle was left uncultured; indeed, no organ escaped his attention. Twisting and bending movements of the trunk stimulated the stomach and improved di-

[43] Bernarr Macfadden, *Strength From Eating*, New York, 1901, pp. 73, 133; Macfadden, *Virile Powers of Superb Manhood*, London, 1900, p. 144; Macfadden, *Macfadden's Encyclopedia* (n. 42), 3:1230; Taylor, "Physical Culture" (n. 41), Oct. 14, 1950, p. 46; Macfadden and Gauvreau, *Dumbbells* (n. 41), pp. 130, 226.

gestion. Other viscera were exercised by an "Inner Strength Course" of hand pressure on appropriate parts of the body. Gripping the middle section of a folded towel between the teeth and pulling the ends with forward, upward, and downward movements was recommended for dental health. Pulling the hair was his technique for scalp culture.[44]

A final exercise illustrates the most striking difference between Macfadden and Graham. One of the physical culturist's pieces of exercise equipment was a glass tube, "somewhat larger than the average male organ," which was placed around the organ and than attached to a vacuum pump. "As the air is removed," he promised expectant readers, "the blood is drawn down into the organ, gradually enlarging and drawing it out to its greatest possible size." Although he recommended extreme caution in the use of the instrument, the fact that he would attempt to give "new life and vigor" to the sexual organs, and even augment "unnaturally small" ones, sets Macfadden at the opposite pole from Jacksonian health reformers (he also invented, but apparently failed to patent, an electric "peniscope" that drew fresh, vitalizing air from outdoors and fed it to the needy organ through a long rubber tube).[45]

The late-Victorian loosening of attitudes toward sexuality found a sturdy champion in Macfadden. Virility was actually a criterion for complete health in his philosophy, a power closely interwoven with the exercise of other bodily parts. Muscular exercise, by quickening the circulation, "vastly" increased "the supply of new, rich blood" to the genital organs and gave them "renewed life." But whatever nourishment virility withdrew from muscular vitality was returned with interest: "The great importance of strong sexual powers cannot be too strongly emphasized. Their influ-

[44] Macfadden, *Macfadden's Encyclopedia* (n. 42), 1:512, 520, 2:585; Macfadden, *Vitality Supreme* (n. 42), pp. 111–114, 121, 162–163; Macfadden and Gauvreau, *Dumbbells* (n. 41), p. 6.

[45] Macfadden, *Virile Powers* (n. 43), p. 111; Macfadden and Gauvreau, *Dumbbells* (n. 41), p. 203.

ence on life is marvelous. If a fine, vigorous man acquires a complaint that weakens his sexual organs, his powers in every way will begin to decline—his muscles will grow weaker, his nerves will be affected, and unless a change is quickly made, he will soon become a physical wreck." In short, "a man to be of any importance must first *be a man.*"[46] One could unfortunately be too much of a man. Macfadden continued to warn of the dangers of marital excess, though if his wife's inuendos about his sexual appetite are to be accepted, his standard of excess was somewhat above the Graham-Alcott tolerance. For others he recommended "moderation," which apparently allowed several contacts a month (still a liberalization of traditional limits). But he was definitely concerned about the weakening effects of overindulgence. Both overactive partners could suffer, he supposed, but the female (as ever) demanded special consideration. Perhaps more than any health crusader yet discussed, Macfadden was preoccupied with breeding a vigorous new generation. His longest marriage seems to have been joined primarily for the purpose of breeding a "physical culture family," and the experiment proved so prolific that his wife came to refer to him as "the Great Begatsby." A nation of physical culture families was the long-term goal, but its realization required a nation of physical culture mothers: "Since woman bears the children, the very life and energy of the race depends upon her and her health." And that health was not to be misspent in inappropriate activities such as working and voting. Bearing and rearing robust babies was the sum of female existence in the physical culture world: "She is the mother of the race," Macfadden solemnized, "and in this function we shall find embodied her supreme power."[47]

His respect for physical culture motherhood was most

[46] Macfadden, *Virile Powers* (n. 43), pp. 13, 104, 125.

[47] Macfadden and Gauvreau, *Dumbbells* (n. 41), pp. 5, 75, 100, 125; Macfadden, *Macfadden's Encyclopedia* (n. 42), 2:994, 5:2461; Macfadden, *Womanhood and Marriage*, New York, 1918, lesson 1, p. 13.

shamelessly expressed in his worship of the female bosom. "Superb womanhood" (for Macfadden) was indicated by "a good bust." Well-formed breasts were evidence of muscular health, sexual attractiveness, and, most of all, reproductive fitness. These organs of nurture for the next generation were so vital a component of female and racial health that Macfadden boldly defied all propriety in presenting exercises for their improvement. In *Superb Womanhood*, he even published a series of photographs of bare-breasted women exercising in sometimes provocative stances![48]

Those photographs, and his discussion of superb womanhood and *The Virile Powers of Superb Manhood*, were part of Macfadden's attack on "the curse of prudishness" still stifling public discussion of sexual matters. Regarding sexual vitality as so elemental a facet of total health, he was forced to challenge convention, and even law, to get his physical culture message across. In 1907 he was arrested by postal officials for mailing an issue of *Physical Culture* that included an "obscene" article on the modes of transmission of venereal disease. The $2000 fine and threatened prison term following his conviction no doubt deepened his loathing for those who would keep man ignorant of his body (and thus his health), and perhaps suggested the penal imagery he used to denounce them. Prudes, in his judgment, were "murderers of womanhood and manhood, ... and I would take grim pleasure in seeing every last one of them struggling in the throes of death at the end of a hangman's noose." Macfadden failed to get his wish, but his candid encomiums to sex as a healthy, and health-giving, recreation helped open the American press to freer expression and make the public more comfortable with sexuality.[49]

His own fascination with sex did not divert Macfadden from the quest for material gain, though, and he made suc-

[48] Macfadden, *Womanhood* (n. 47), lesson 52, p. 12.

[49] Bernarr Macfadden, *The Power and Beauty of Superb Womanhood*, New York, 1901, p. 63.

cess in the marketplace as attractive a reward of physical culture as success in the bedroom. The formula was the usual—exercise and right diet bred endurance and energy and acuity, which amounted to efficiency. And "efficiency, first of all, means power," the power, he vowed to the aspiring businessman, that is "so essential to his rapid and permanent advancement."[50]

But the noblest end of the physical culture life was beyond sex and success. It was health, or better, "health plus." Volume one, chapter one of Macfadden's *Encyclopedia of Physical Culture* began with a paean to that ideal, "the most desirable possession of mankind," which puts into the shade all similar efforts before or since:

Health means vim, vigor, snap and energy. Health means clarity and strength of mind; purity and beauty of soul. The healthy person is unconscious of discomfort; he rises superior to it—is absolutely the monarch of all he surveys. He dominates life instead of allowing it to dominate him.... He is a unit—a being—a man, whole, complete, vigorous, perfect, happy—because healthy. To such a man work is a joy; obstacles but opportunities for endeavor; difficulties but a means for enlarged triumph.... Health is what gives manhood to man; womanhood to woman.... It is that which blesses the world with joyous, happy, vigorous, beautiful children, who, were there none other, would bring forth the millennium in a generation.[51]

Macfadden's varied overtures to the millenium, ranging from his siring of a physical culture family as a model for popular emulation to campaigning for the Republican presidential nomination in 1936, are too numerous to detail. What must be said of him in summary is that the kingdom of health which he sought was not merely an external society

---

[50] Macfadden, *Vitality Supreme* (n. 42), p. xi; Macfadden, "Health Made and Preserved by Daily Exercise," *Cosmopolitan, 34,* 708 (1903).
[51] Macfadden, *Macfadden's Encyclopedia* (n. 42), 1:1–3.

(a "New World" he called it), but a more glorious state of grace within the individual. Narcissus that he was, Macfadden saw health as primarily a duty to the self and a reward for one's self. Anticipating the direction hygienic religion would take in the second half of the twentieth century, he advocated a philosophy of human potential or self-actualization. "It lies with you," he challenged readers, "whether you shall be a strong, virile animal ... or a miserable little crawling worm." Blessed with the greatest potential of all creatures, humans must not "fail in your duty to yourselves," but strive to become "surfeited with power." For final inspiration Macfadden composed a stirring air—"Manhood Glorified"—to be sung "with majesty":

> The world resounds, demanding human glory
> The cry for health prevails throughout the land
> While grovling [sic] through life's mire
> Seeth not the strength, grace and poise
>   offered to all men.
> Thy head hold up and claim thy divine kingship,
> For thrones of mighty strength await thee
> Claim thine heritage, tingling with pow'r,
> And like a roaring lion fight,
> For manhood's great rewards.[52]

His misspelling of groveling is final dramatization of the inability of this lion of the gymnasium to pay heed to anything beneath full manhood.

[52] *ibid.*, 1:120, 2:1071–1072.

☆☆☆☆☆☆☆☆☆☆☆☆☆☆☆☆☆☆☆☆☆☆☆☆☆☆☆☆☆☆☆☆☆☆

CHAPTER TEN
THE HYGIENE OF THE WHEEL

☆☆☆☆☆☆☆☆☆☆☆☆☆☆☆☆☆☆☆☆☆☆☆☆☆☆☆☆☆☆☆☆☆☆

MACFADDEN WAS NOT ONE TO REST CONTENT WITH ONLY THE pleasures of the gymnasium. He played many outdoor sports as well, and enthusiastically recommended games to others interested in keeping their blood pure. But even without Macfadden's backing, sport was a more popular hygienic option than gymnastics by the end of the nineteenth century. Lewis seems to have honestly believed that his gymnastics were "not less fascinating than the most popular games," but for many participants the fascination soon turned to tedium. The rigidly prescribed drills lacked the spontaneity and unpredictability of free play, were more duty than fun, and had, moreover, a touch of the absurd about them. The various posturings required made a group performance of Lewis gymnastics take on successively the appearance of "a series of windmills,—a group of inflated balloons,—a flock of geese all asleep on one leg,— . . . a whole parish of Shaker worshippers,—a Japanese embassy performing *Ko-tow.* "[1]

An activity more entertaining to spectators than practitioners was doomed to passing popularity, and as the newness of the "New Gymnastics" faded, physical education advanced, as Hitchcock described it, from the "gymnastic era" to the "athletic era." Gymnastics maintained a standing of importance within physical education programs, but it yielded the position of top priority to "athleticism." As

---

[1] Dio Lewis, "New Gymnastics," *Am. J. Ed.*, *11*, 531–562 (1862), *12*, 665–700 (1862), p. 535; Thomas Wentworth Higginson, "Gymnastics," *Atlantic M.*, *7*, 283–302 (1861), p. 288.

Hitchcock (and others) experienced this transition, he came
to believe that although

> a man may get simple muscular development in a gymna-
> sium, and be strong in arms, legs, lungs, and back, ... he
> cannot get the real brawn, effective muscle, capacious
> lungs, a tough skin and the best of digestion, or a really
> reliable heart, unless he gets more of the natural process
> of health from mother earth and her surroundings of air,
> water, temperature, ozone, and the actual touch of soil and
> grass. ... Man needs outdoor discipline as well as that of
> the training master indoors, if he would secure the bodily
> condition and the physical power that make him the best
> man to conduct a business, to edit a newspaper, or to make
> the most effective use of high intellectual attainments in
> any calling.[2]

All the wonders of outdoors exercise notwithstanding, the
perennial problem remained—the new sports were confined
to an elite group. Fat men should not row, older men could
not play football, women could not play much of anything.
Just as the New Gymnastics had been needed to democratize
the gymnasium, some new enjoyable and invigorating, but
not too strenuous form of exercise was needed to democratize
the outdoors. A sport for everyman and everywoman, could
such be found, was certain to draw forth new philosophies of
self-perfection and social advance through muscular development. It was thus that the 1890s became the epoch of the
hygiene of the wheel.[3]

"I am the spirit of the age," one imaginative bicyclist
quoted his machine, "the *fin-de-cycle* sprite." All poetic tribute aside, it was prosaic progress in engineering that enabled the wheel (as its devotees endearingly called it) to
capture the fancy of an age. Several versions of "celeri-

[2] Edward Hitchcock, "The Gymnastic Era and the Athletic Era of Our
Country," *Outlook, 51,* 816–818 (1895), p. 817.

[3] The subject is discussed in more detail in James Whorton, "The Hygiene of the Wheel: An Episode in Victorian Sanitary Science," *Bull.
Hist. Med., 52,* 61–88 (1978).

pedes"—two wheels connected by a beam, on which a rider
sat while running over the ground—had been marketed in
France and England by 1830, but all were so expensive and
exhausting that only young men of means could manage
them. The machine was therefore initially a fashionable affection rather than an instrument of hygiene, and even the
introduction of crank-driven "velocipedes" in the 1860s, and
high-wheeled "ordinaries" the following decade, only partially popularized cycling. The fear of "taking a header"
("by no means a difficult exploit," beginners were advised;
"indeed the difficulty is to avoid performing it") confined
the unathletic and timid to inelegant tricycles until the final
stage of evolution of the bicycle, the "safety." The pattern of
this machine, utilizing wheels of the same moderate size and
placing rider and pedals between the wheels, was worked out
gradually through the 1880s. With the addition of pneumatic tires in 1889, and the reduction of price to as low as
$75, the bicycle was at last brought to the popular level. Now
nearly anyone of middle-class status could afford a wheel,
and could learn to ride it safely; and nearly everyone, it appears, took advantage of the opportunity. Physicians and
clergymen began making their rounds on bicycles, instead of
horses; policemen and journalists mounted the machines in
preference to walking their beats; the army experimented
with wheels as replacements for cavalry horses; athletes
turned to long-distance cycle-racing as a challenging form of
competition. Most of all, the public at large greeted the
"safety" as an exhiliaring recreation (or at least adopted it
in fashion-conscious imitation). By the mid-1890s, the "bicycle era" was in full flower: "We have become a race of Mer-
curys, . . . and the joy which is felt over the new power
amounts to a passion."[4]

[4] C. Turner, "The Wheelman's Faery Queen," *Outing, 30,* 207 (1897);
Robert Smith, *A Social History of the Bicycle,* New York, 1972; Freder-
ick Alderson, *Bicycling, A History,* Newton-Abbot, Eng., 1972, p. 55; F.
Prial, "Cycling in the United States," *Harper's W., 34,* 669–672 (1890);
Joseph Bishop, "Social and Economic Influence of the Bicycle," *Forum,
21,* 680–689 (1896), p. 680.

That passion was fueled largely by visions of improved health. Because cycling was fun, unlike the ritualized drudgery of calisthenics, it "is inducing multitudes of people to take regular exercise who have long been in need of such exercise, but who could never be induced to take it by any means hitherto devised." Cycling not only inspired otherwise inactive people to exercise, but provided more effective exercise than other sports. "The rider of a wheel takes exercise in the most even, steady way I know of"; "by [the cycle's] use the muscular system is exercised and developed with a uniformity that cannot be achieved by any other means"; "the exercise is well and equally distributed over almost the whole body, and . . . when all muscles are exercised, no muscle is likely to be over-exercised": these were widely shared opinions among physicians excited about the bicycle. When taken in the proper dosage, this exercise not only strengthened the voluntary muscles, but healthfully stimulated the heart, lungs, and digestive system, and encouraged the excretion of accumulated morbid matter. Even the nervous system would benefit both from the general invigoration of the exercise, and from the watchfulness the sport required. "The rider must constantly use the senses of hearing, seeing, and feeling in order to avoid collisions, direct his machine, and keep his equilibrium." Gradually the nerves acquired a new tone. "Every rider has felt it. He may not appreciate it now, because he is accustomed to it; but let him stop his riding, and the result is soon apparent in sluggish memory, or annoying organs, or easily tired limbs—in short, a loss of balance." With good reason, apparently, could sanitarians proclaim that the bicycle had advanced "the sanitation [personal hygiene] of this country . . . a hundred years," and expect "that the 'cyclo-antrhopos' of the twentieth century will suffer less from his nerves and will be more muscular than the man of the nineteenth."[5]

[5] H. Williams, "The Bicycle in Relation to Health," *Harper's W.*, 40, 370 (1896); T. N. Gray, quoted in Luther Porter, *Cycling for Health and Pleasure*, New York, 1895, p. 14; "Some Thoughts on the Hygiene of the Wheel," *Wheelman*, 1, 90–93 (1882–1883), p. 91; Seneca Egbert, "The

It went almost without saying that an exercise so effective at improving the health of the normal must restore the health of the debilitated. Merely a cursory gleaning of the medical literature of the 1890s yields an imposing list of ailments pronounced curable by the wheel. Dyspepsia, anemia, obesity, curvature of the spine, asthma, varicose veins, heart disease, and diabetes were the more frequently mentioned. Even the "over-riding of the right great toe by its minor neighboring toe" was corrected by regular pedaling. In the treatment of bilious diseases, another physician announced, "bicycle exercise . . . surpasses even calomel" (calomel, mercurous chloride, was one of the most frequently prescribed items in nineteenth-century therapeutics). When it was revealed in 1897 that the death rate from consumption among Massachusetts females had been steadily falling for five years, the announcement included the proposal that as women had been using cycles for about that length of time, the decline of consumption could be attributed to the invigorating respiratory exercise of wheeling. By the end of the decade it could truthfully be said that "it will soon be difficult to mention an ailment whose victims, provided they are not bedridden, may not, in somebody's opinion, derive benefit from the use of the bicycle." Indeed, the excitement with which some doctors and hygienists praised "the new remedy, 'Bicycle'" knew no bounds. It should be put into the "Materia Medica at the head of the 'Ferrum' preparations," urged one; it is "a preparation of steel and rubber . . . far more beneficent in its health and life giving properties than all the pills and potions ever invented," eulogized another; one could "throw physic to the dogs," all its proponents concluded, for "the bicycle has done more for the good of the

---

Bicycle in its Relation to the Physician," *Univ. Med. Mag.*, 5, 104–109 (1892–1893), p. 104; Henry Garrigues, "Woman and the Bicycle," *Forum*, 20, 578–587 (1896), p. 584; Benjamin Ward Richardson, *Vita Medica*, London, 1897, p. 247; Cesare Lombroso, quoted in "The Criminal Anthropology of the Bicycle," *Brit. Med. J.*, 1900 (i), 859.

human race than all the medicines compounded since the days of Hippocrates. . . . No, it seems hard, but we feel that the doctor's occupation is gone."[6]

But there was one affliction in particular for which the panacea seemed designed. As if by providence, the wheel had been introduced soon after the emergence of the disease of technologically advanced countries, neurasthenia. A cycling physician spoke for his profession as a whole when he lamented that Americans, especially, "are fast becoming, if we are not now, a race of nervous dyspeptics; in fact, many amount to little more than a rather unenviable . . . mass of organized nervousness." In recommending the bicycle as the proper remedy for this misery, the author flirted with paradox by stressing the wheel's congeniality with the hurried American way of life: "a large amount of exercise can be obtained in a short space of time, and . . . it gives the idea of doing something with a rush." Other writers were more apt to emphasize the escape from mental activity and worry afforded by cycling:

> I have the wheel of life;
> Soiled with my city's dust,
> From the struggle and the strife
> Of the narrow street I fly
> To the road's felicity,
> To clear me from the frown
> Of the moody toil of town.[7]

[6] J. James, "The Beneficial Effects of Cycling as an Orthopaedic Agent," *Brit. Med. J.,* 1896 (ii), 947–948, p. 947; E. B. Turner, "A Report on Cycling in Health and Disease," *Brit. Med. J.,* 1896 (ii), 38–39, p. 38; "The Bicycle and Phthisis," *Med. News, 71,* 535 (1897); "The Bicycle for Persons with Hernia," *N.Y. Med. J , 69,* 606 (1899); G. S. Hull, "Physicians and the Bicycle," *Outing, 3,* 57–58 (1883–1884), p. 58; W. T. Parker, "A New Remedy," *Outing, 3,* 59–60 (1883–1884), p. 59; "For and Against the Bicycle," *J. Hyg. Herald Health, 46,* 304–305 (1896), p. 305.

[7] "Some Thoughts" (n. 5), p. 92; "The Wheel," *Wheelman, 1,* 18 (1882–1883). Also see Graeme Hammond, "The Bicycle in the Treatment of Nervous Diseases," *J. Nervous Mental Dis., 10,* 36–46 (1892), and F. Fry, "The Bicycle and the Nerves," *Med. Mirror, 7,* 272–274 (1896).

With respect to the nervous system, the wheel could seemingly be either a tonic or a sedative, accommodating itself to the rider's needs.

In either event, cycling freed the individual from any craving for artificial stimulants or narcotics. The exercise itself was stimulus enough, and even were it not, all but the novice wheelman knew that "riding requires a steady head [and] *no drunken man can maintain his balance.*" So incompatible was smoking with steady cycling that America's consumption of cigars fell, according to 1896 industry estimates, by one million a day. Even morphine habitués soon "discovered that a long spin in the fresh air on a cycle induces sweet sleep better than their favorite drug." Cycling optimists were confident that opiate addiction was retreating before the wheel.[8]

It was unfortunate that weekend cycling cut deeply into church attendance, but it was futile for preachers to conjure visions of Sunday cyclists speeding uncontrollably downhill toward a "place where there is no mud on the streets because of its high temperature." Disciples of the wheel could not believe that brimstone awaited them for their worship of a machine that offered such opportunities for self-improvement. "In no other form of exercise," the typical apology began, "is there such a chance for good comradeship. From this comradeship grow a kindly expansiveness, a friendly enthusiasm, remarkable and pleasant to contemplate. There is no telling how much active moral force this expansive enthusiasm may in time generate." Expanded friendliness would be complemented by enlarged mentality. The intellectual challenges of bicycle touring—the reading of maps, the introduction to new places and people, the study of the history of areas visited—"makes each rider a Columbus," while developing his faculties of understanding and toleration. As the only physical exercise husband, wife, and children could

[8] C. A. Kinch, "The Bicycle and Tricycle for Physicians and Patients," *Wheelman, 2,* 361–363 (1883), p. 362; Bishop, "Social and Economic" (n. 4), p. 686; "Cycling versus Morphine," *Brit. Med. J.,* 1895 (ii), 1371.

conveniently take together, cycling strengthened "the whole family, [making it] one as it perhaps never was before." At the same time, it educated and moved people to civic and political responsibility, because of "something peculiarly democratic and independent about" it. So inexpensive as to be open to all responsible citizens, encouraging both cooperation and private initiative, and not requiring the employment of servants, the wheel made "democracy [take] a newer and more vigorous form; no longer the closet work of the student, or the idling of the voluptuary, or the intense but intermittent strain of the professional, but the healthy, regular, natural work of an American who understands that acting is living, and healthy action healthy life."[9]

Examples might be multiplied, but the visionary bent of cycling exponents is sufficiently clear. In their search for virtues in the wheel, no possibilities were left unclaimed. The bicycle ultimately appeared as the vehicle for the return to the Golden Age. The glory of Geeek civilization, a representative zealot preached, had been its union of mental and spiritual aspiration with physical striving. This organic wholeness had disappeared with the Greeks, and had become practically despised by Americans in recent years. But restoration was at hand: "All we [can] ask is done by the bicycle." It was not merely romantic sentiment that inclined cyclists to describe themselves so regularly as "knights of the wheel," but more substantially a genuine feeling that they were comrades-in-arms rescuing a civilization in distress.

> Good morning, fellow-wheelmen,—here's a warm,
>   fraternal hand,
> As, with a rush of victory, we sweep across the land! . . .
> For we are pure philanthropists,—
> Unqualified philanthropists;

[9] Bishop, "Social and Economic" (n. 4), pp. 683, 685; J. G. Speed, "The Bicycling Era," *Sci. Am.* 73, 124 (1895); "Bicycle Riding for Women," *Outlook,* 51, 1104 (1895); "Democratic Sport," *Outing, 4,* 222–223 (1884).

And would not have this happiness to any one denied;
We claim a great utility that daily must increase;
We claim from inactivity a sensible release;
A constant mental, physical, and moral help we feel,
That bids us turn enthusiasts, and cry,
"God bless the wheel!"[10]

Ironically, this instrument that drew such effulgent
praise from so many physicians was the source of unprecedented alarm to others. Doctors were still unsure of the medical implications of the physical training boom. The long-
term effects of repeated stress on the heart, lungs, and nervous system were anything but obvious. It was only natural,
considering the newness of mass athletics, to err on the side
of safety and find danger where a later, more experienced
and sophisticated generation would see only invigoration.
And it was also easy to rationalize pathology by the peculiar
positions and motions of cycling. Whenever an abnormality
was found in a patient who happened also to be a cyclist,
post hoc reasoning might lead to the placing of blame,
rightly or wrongly, on the patient's pastime. Many doctors
felt in addition a scorn for the extravagant claims of wheeling advocates. Under these conditions, an epidemic of presumed cycling diseases was nearly inevitable. From 1891 on
especially, the subject of the hygiene and pathology of the
wheel attracted a swarm of papers, letters, and editorials to
medical journals. France's Académie de Médecine devoted a
good portion of its time and energy in 1894 to opening up
the question of the bicycle and health. In 1896 the *British
Medical Journal* published a special, ten-part "Report on
Cycling in Health and Disease." At least a half-dozen authors explored the subject at book-length. These attempts to
involve the bicycle in the etiology of disease were a particularly strong medical backlash against hygienic extremism,

[10] H. H. M., "Greek vs. Modern Physical Culture," *Outing*, *3*, 211–216
(1883–1884), p. 216; Will Carleton, "Wheelman's Song," *Outing*, *4*, 5
(1884).

and illustrate conservative resistance to health evangelism.[11]

The uneasiness many physicians felt about the eventual effects of physical exertion put exercise hygiene in an exasperating situation: dull activities like gymnastics did not excite people to take sufficient exercise, but enjoyable ones like cycling seduced them into too much. The wheel was its own undoing, for the thrill of hurtling over the ground, the challenge of going even faster, and the assurance that all that effort was a helpful purge for body and mind, conspired to spur riders beyond reasonable limits of speed and distance. "Century runs" (nonstop rides of one hundred miles or more) became a test of manhood rivalled only by that of "scorching" ("we may define the term as an impulse overruling the cyclist's reason compelling him to overtake any and every moving object which may be in front of him"). Arrests for "furious riding" rose rapidly once the scorcher perfected his technique, magistrates accompanying fines with warnings that a speed in excess of six miles per hour "is not safe in the streets of a large town." The scorcher nevertheless continued "to slay miles and pedestrians," excite public outrage, and force increases in life and accident insurance premiums for all cyclists. But however abhorrent the scorcher, the medical profession could not ignore the injuries cyclists inflicted upon themselves. Initially, concern was directed almost exclusively at the damages from accidents. There was, of course, much inevitable bruising in learning to mount and steer the machine. The exquisitely battered legs of H. G. Wells' novice wheelman, Mr. Hoopdriver, was the fee that all paid to enter the world of cycling (even Macfadden took

[11] "The French Academy of Medicine on Cycling," *Lancet*, 1894 (ii), 643; E. B. Turner, "A Report on Cycling in Health and Disease," *Brit. Med. J.*, 1896 (i), 1158, 1211–1212, 1336–1337, 1399, 1510, 1564; 1896 (ii), 38–39, 98–99, 203, 469–470; Benjamin Ward Richardson, *The Tricycle in Relation to Health and Recreation*, London, 1885; Oscar Jennings, *Cycling and Health*, London, 1890; Porter, *Cycling* (n. 5); O. Laurent, *L'hygiene du Cycliste*, Brussels, 1897.

some bad falls trying to learn to ride a wheel, and it was surely the memory of those spills which made him give cycling only a tepid recommendation in his encyclopedia of physical activities). But even masters of the wheel were subject to losing control on crowded city streets, and collisions with other cycles, wagons, horses, and lampposts placed a new heading—"Death by the Wheel"—in obituary columns. And if most accidents were not fatal, they were at least frequent. New York and London averaged more than one recorded cycling accident per day in the 1890s, and it was estimated that only one-fifth of all accidents were reported.[12]

The fall and the collision, however, were hazards that could be anticipated by anyone before he adopted the sport, and the liberal opinion was that the informed individual should be permitted to risk limbs and life if he chose. As the novelty of the bicycle passed, the interest of physicians quickly shifted from the subject of acute injuries to that of chronic ailments, and considerations of posture, pressure, exertion, and excitement created a new medical category— "diseases of cycling." The obvious place for these diseases to begin was with the skeleton. The opinion was already strong that sports or exercises which concentrated muscular effort in a localized region of the body, and/or required positioning or movements not naturally practiced, were productive of musculo-skeletal deformities. Curvature of the spine was supposedly commonplace among gymnasts, fencers, and jockeys, and since the scorcher so studiously imitated the jockey, "doubling himself up like a capital C," he should be expected to suffer the same skeletal distortion. "Kyphosis bicyclistarum" was the technical name given this special

---

[12] "The Dangers of Cycling," *Lancet*, 1896 (ii), 133–134, p. 133; "A Tricycle Ride," *Brit. Med. J.*, 1882 (ii), 825; "Why Scorchers Scorch," *Med. Rec.*, 55, 662 (1899); "Bicycling and Insurance," *Brit. Med. J.*, 1896 (i), 1244; H. G. Wells, *The Wheels of Chance*, London, 1901, pp. 8–9; Robert Taylor, "Physical Culture," *New Yorker*, Oct. 21, 1950, 39–50, p. 39; "Cyclomania," *Living Age, 215*, 470–472 (1897), p. 470; "Editor's Table," *Sanitarian, 39*, 176 (1897); "Cycling and Vitality," *Lancet* 1892 (ii), 501–502, p. 502.

condition, but it was familiarly known as "cyclist's figure," "cyclist's spine," and "cyclist's stoop (Figure 10)." And not only did it afflict the wheelman of the present, distorting him into "Round-Shouldered Robbie, the Rough Rider of the Road"; its possible hereditary transmission threatened the future health of the race. With so many young married couples taking to the wheel, it seemed surely but "a figure of speech [to refer to] the rising generation."[13]

To forestall such a turn, two changes were required. First, adult cyclists had to be educated as to correct posture, and persuaded to adopt it in place of the injurious position of the scorcher. Manufacturers might hasten the conversion, it was hoped, by the invention of "a 'health bicycle' which could only be propelled by a person who sits erect."[14]

At the same time adults were being pulled back to the perpendicular, children would have to be lifted off their wheels altogether, or at least restricted in their activity. The craze for cycling had driven many parents to train their children in the sport at the earliest possible age, sometimes getting them started before the second birthday. The possible effects of the exercise on such young bodies, on soft bones and undeveloped ligaments, appalled even the proponents of wheeling. Ensuing discussion resulted in a broad range of recommendations for the proper age at which to begin cycling (from seven to twenty-one), but all agreed that a rider below the age of twenty-one should never attempt feats of unusual speed or distance lest his growing frame be stricken by kyphosis bicyclistarum or other deformities.[15]

On the question of injury to the mature skeleton, however, there was nothing like this consensus. Most physicians

[13] Fernand Lagrange, *Physiology of Bodily Exercise*, New York, 1898, pp. 314–326; "The Bicycler Should Sit Erect," *Med. News, 63*, 613 (1893); John Davison, "Is Bicycle Riding Conducive to Impotency?," *Trans. Colo. State Med. Soc.*, 225–229 (1895), p. 228; "Kyphosis Bicyclistarum," *Lancet*, 1893 (i), 1397–1398, p. 1398. Also see Benjamin Ward Richardson, "Cycling and Physique," *Asclepiad, 7*, 21–39 (1890).

[14] "Bicycling and Its Physical Results," *Med. Rec., 43*, 500 (1893).

[15] "Bicycling for Children," *Pediatrics, 7*, 357–359 (1899); Richardson, "Cycling" (n. 13), p. 22; Turner, "Report" (n. 11), p. 1337.

thought the scorching posture was unnatural, but some defended it as the best position for producing motion with a minimum of effort. An article in the prestigious *Lancet* announced as early as 1893 that kyphosis bicyclistarum "has already declared itself in many wheelmen," yet two years later the American physician Graeme Hammond examined fourteen professional cyclists, men who spent much of their lives in the scorcher's "bend," and could find no evidence of spinal deformity in any of them. "If any such condition has ever been observed," he concluded, "the number of cases of it must be very few indeed."[16]

Exactly the same reasoning which produced kyphosis was behind the connection of other ailments with the bicycle. By the mid-1890s, for example, many victims of appendicitis happened also to be bicyclists, and anatomical genius was hardly required to see that strenuous wheeling, particularly riding uphill, might twist the appendix over the edge of the contracted *psoas magnus,* contuse the appendix, and open it to infective agents. Similarly, the cyclist bent forward over his wheel had his abdominal contents pressed against the inguinal abdominal wall, and inguinal hernia might be expected as an easy product of pedaling strain. This injury was being charged to the bicycle by the early 1880s, though the specific entity "bicycle hernia" seems not to have been proposed until 1896. Throughout the period, cycling advocates disputed the charge, some arguing that men already suffering with rupture might safely ride (and without a truss!), others going so far as to advance cycling as a cure for hernia.[17]

---

[16] H. Campbell, "A Note on Cycling," *Lancet,* 1897 (ii), 1279; A. Gubb, "Precepts for Cyclists," *Lancet,* 1895 (ii), 942; "Kyphosis" (n. 13), p. 1397; Graeme Hammond, "The Influence of the Bicycle in Health and Disease," *Med. Rec., 47,* 129–133 (1895), p. 130.

[17] "Bicycling and Appendicitis," *Boston Med. Surg. J., 136,* 43–44 (1897); "The Bicycle and the Appendix," *Brit. Med. J.,* 1897 (i), 872; George Miel, "Bicycle Hernia," *Trans. Colo. State Med. Soc.,* 347–354 (1896); *Lancet,* 1879 (ii), 968; *ibid.,* 1882 (ii), 296, 337, 375.

Whether the wheel caused or cured hernia mattered little in practical terms. It apparently caused so many other ailments that the removal of rupture from the list might go unnoticed. From distortion of the foot, the wheel worked its malevolence upward through the anal veins and the kidneys to the rider's throat and face. "Cyclist's sorethroat" was the penalty for inhaling through the mouth while riding, the cold air, dust, and bacteria taken in by rapid breathing combining to irritate and inflame the respiratory passages. The throat discomfort, furthermore, must have contributed to the grotesqueness of a final condition—"bicycle face." In the words of its discoverer, this syndrome was characterized by "the peculiar strained, set look" produced by the "incessant tension" of maintaining balance on a two-wheeled machine. The sequelae of "bicycle face" were general nervousness, and "headache at the back of the head, where the balancing centre is situated."[18]

"Cyclo-phobia" surely reached its peak in the excitement over bicycle face and in the announcement by a New York physician of a new speciality, that of giving "advice regarding the medical and surgical diseases associated with the use of the bicycle." Not surprisingly, such positions were widely regarded as extremism. Every wheelman was now careful, the *Medical Record* jested, "to keep his brow smooth and his lip curled, so that no one can suggest the presence of the so-called bicycle face." *A propos* of the same topic, another medical editor predicted, "The medical man will soon have to worry about this question; hence he may deem it wise to read up on the subject. Then we may hear of the 'bicycle-face face.'"[19]

---

[18] "Cyclist's Sore Throat," *Lancet*, 1898 (ii), 95; *Med. Rec.*, *49*, 358 (1896); Jennie Chandler, "Sore Throat from Bicycling," *J. Hyg. Herald Health*, *48*, 243–244 (1898); A. Shadwell, "The Hidden Dangers of Cycling," *Living Age*, *212*, 827–834 (1897), p. 833; "A New Explanation of the Bicycle Face," *Med. Rec.*, *48*, 308 (1895).

[19] "A Medical Bicycle Specialist," *Med. Rec.*, *48*, 702 (1895); "A Physician on the Wheel," *Med. Rec.*, *50*, 557–558 (1896), p. 58; "Bicycle is King," *Med. Sentinel*, *3*, 402–403 (1895), p. 403.

It was not from such fringe areas as bicycle face that the great majority of medical opponents of the wheel made their assault, but from more solid central ground. Three points of attack were particularly favored—those of the cardio-vascular, nervous, and genito-urinary system. A rapid increase in the heartbeat being one of the obvious effects of cycling, concern for aged riders, or for those with undiagnosed heart disease was to be expected. But although reports of sudden death from heart failure while cycling were not unusual, acute attacks never provoked the fear that chronic injury did. Pulse rates were reported to soar as high as 200 to 250 during vigorous cycling, and while riders regularly survived such experiences, it was difficult to imagine their hearts could carry so heavy a burden for years without suffering damage. In the context of the 1890s, the condition of "bicycle heart" was a certainty, and men were actually rejected from military service on the basis of this diagnosis. Irving Fisher was told in 1896 that he had strained his heart "by hill-climbing on the bicycle." The diagnosis "frightened me. I feared sudden death, and I feared to hear my heart beat on my pillow." The anxiety caused him loss of sleep for two years, made him run down, and was therefore, he believed, a contributing cause of his tuberculosis.[20]

The analysis of the threat of cycling to nervous health covered considerably more territory than the "balancing centre" that was subjected to "incessant tension." It is, in fact, too complex to be explored here, except to take note of the condition of "cyclist's neurosis" that was supposed to result from the incessant pressure of the bicycle saddle on the nerves of the pelvic floor. Symptoms of the neurosis varied from tenderness of the perineum and testicles, constipation,

[20] "Cycling and Heart Disease," *Med. Rec.*, *47*, 186 (1895); "Bicycle Heart," *Brit. Med. J.*, 1898 (i), 908; A. C. Getchell, "Bicycling in its Relation to Heart Disease," *Med. News*, *75*, 33–37 (1899), p. 36; Fisher quoted by Christine Whittaker, "Chasing the Cure: Irving Fisher's Experience as a Tuberculosis Patient," *Bull. Hist. Med.*, *48*, 398–415 (1974), p. 400.

and "shrivelling and aching" of the penis to difficulty "in getting rid of the last few drops" of urine (with a resultant "uncomfortable trickle" down the leg). Direct mechanical injury from the pressing and jarring by the saddle was the mechanism assumed to be at the seat of a much longer list of genito-urinary problems. Strictured urethra, urethritis, prostatitis, and cystitis were all attributed to this "pommeling of the perineum." At least one loser in the battle of bicycle versus bladder was reduced to such unceasing agony that he shot himself, confiding to his wife before he died that "that bicycle brought me to this terrible end, yes it did."[21]

While the urethra, prostate, and bladder seemed to take the brunt of the saddle's punishment, other organs were also believed to be affected to some degree. Hemorrhoids, ischiorectal abscesses, and malignant testicular tumors, for example, were reported as wheel induced. There were also instances of priapism among cyclists, and although these were properly interpreted as the effect of impeded venous flow (rather than a sign of sexual arousal), erections in the saddle pointed to the unavoidable question of cycling as an aphrodisiac. The predictable answer was that the bicycle saddle, by rubbing and bouncing the perineum, must "call attention to the organs of generation, and so lead to a great increase in masturbation in the timid, to early sexual indulgence in the more venturous, and ultimately to early impotence in both." But surprisingly for this period when there persisted so

---

[21] W. H. Brown, "A Form of Neuralgia Occurring in Cyclists," *Brit. Med. J.*, 1898 (i), 553; Arthur Roper, "Perineal Pressure in Cycling," *Lancet*, 1896 (i), 1341–1343, p. 1341; John Robinson, "Bicycle Urethritis," *Med. News*, *73*, 428–429 (1898), p. 428; "Cycling and Traumatic Urethritis," *Med. Rec.*, *53*, 950 (1898); William Townsend, "Bicycle-riding Upon Improperly Fitting Saddles," *N.Y. Med. J.*, *63*, 243 (1896); G. H. Heard, "Bicycle vs. Bladder," *Med. World*, *16*, 495 (1898). According to a recent study by Robert Bond, "Distance Bicycling May Cause Ischemic Neuropathy of Penis," *Physician and Sports Med.*, *3*, 54–56 (Nov. 1975); but the wheel-induced numbness of the organ, fortunately, normally disappears overnight, and has no lasting effect on sexual function.

much uneasiness about sexual indulgence, both solitary and social, a majority of the medical profession seem to have regarded the wheel as an anaphrodisiac. "As it is well-known," a Denver physician explained, "that certain debased individuals resort to the stimulation of any of the parts mentioned to provoke and maintain the venereal cycle, resulting in due time in complete lack of response to any stimulus however intense, analogy of reasoning prompts us to believe that the bicycle stimuli produce in time an exactly similar condition of affairs."[22]

By whichever route—stimulation to venereal excess or depletion of nervous capacity—the wheelman's destination was the same: impotence. Since the same condition might also result from damage to the prostate or bladder, there is double meaning to the statement that sexual exhaustion completed the list of infirmities of the saddle. It was not merely the final addition to the list, but also the state to which other perineal injuries might lead. Whether or not they resulted in impotency, though, the number and range of these injuries were sufficient to back up the advice of Albert Gihon, retired medical director of the United States Navy. Because of the wheel, Gihon asserted, "I can give no more significant hint to the young man choosing his field than to make the perineum and its adjacencies the subject of his especial study."[23]

Unfortunately for any medical students who accepted Gihon's counsel, the budding specialty was already being nipped by the bicycle manufacturers. Responding to the medical demand for a saddle that would not pressure the

[22] "The Pathology of Bicycling," *Boston Med. Surg. J.*, *130*, 197–198 (1894); "Cycling and Ischio-rectal Abscess," *Brit. Med. J.*, 1896 (i), 1179; "Bicycle and Malignant Testicular Tumor," *Med. News*, *78*, 684 (1901); "The Effects of Bicycle Riding on the Perineum," *Med. Rec.*, *51*, 484 (1897); S. A. K. Strahan, "Bicycle Riding and Perineal Pressure, Their Effect on the Young," *Lancet*, 1884 (ii), 490–491, p. 490; Davison, "Bicycle Riding" (n. 13), pp. 226–227.

[23] Quoted in "Editor's Table," *Sanitarian*, *37*, 353–358 (1896).

perineum, manufacturers were selling wheels with a wide variety of "safety," "hygienic," and "anatomical" saddles by the mid-1890s. The design of these seems to have been carried out by mechanics, without medical consultation, and it is necessary to question the accuracy of descriptions like "anatomical" upon learning that at least one cycling mechanic desired a new style saddle because his old one kept "bruising my sternum bone." Nevertheless, the multiplicity of saddle designs was such that some were bound to meet with medical approval. The style that emerged with the highest praise was the one combining a widened back portion, to better accommodate the ischial tuberosities (which should properly bear the weight) with a slit through the peak or front section (Figure 11). When correctly slit, the front of the saddle assumed a concave form under the rider, exerted no pressure against the body, and freed him from "perineal servitude."[24]

But the new saddles did not immediately free the medical profession of their perineal anxiety. To be sure, concern for the wheel*man*'s genito-urinary system all but disappeared by 1900, and even by 1898 physicians could chuckle about the "time after the advent of the modern bicycle [when] the male perineum, as a medical and surgical subject of discussion, bade fair to rival its analogue of gynecologic and obstetric fame." Yet at the same time, that analogue, the female perineum, the object of such extraordinary medical solicitude throughout the Victorian era, was being recognized as the most vulnerable prey of all for the insatiable wheel. A new creature had been spawned by the cycling craze, the wheelwoman, and her presumed weaker constitution and more impressionable nervous system insured she would excite a level of apprehension never attainable by the male cyclist.[25]

It was not an easy ascent to such notoriety, for women

[24] "Injurious Bicycle Saddle," *Med. Rec., 56,* 395 (1899); "Cycling for Elderly Men," *Brit. Med. J.,* 1895 (ii), 561. Also see "An Improvement in Bicycle Seats," *Lancet,* 1893 (ii), 1193.

[25] Robinson, "Bicycle Urethritis" (n. 21), p. 428.

were actively discouraged from attempting the wheel. The epithet "unladylike" was, of course, the first obstacle to be overcome, but more formidable was the supposition of physical incapability. Ladies thus rode only the tricycle at first, but even that humble machine served to transport them to health. Many were the female invalids reported to have "found exercise with the tricycle better than medicines." That they were up to the still stronger remedy of the two-wheeler, however, was at first unthinkable. "Girls cannot ride the bicycle," a male cyclist pontificated; "That is undeniable." The only thing more difficult to deny, apparently, was the will of the "new woman" of the day to emulate masculine accomplishments. She had to parry moralistic charges that "the bicycle may be the first step ... towards a sportive life," that cycling gave her "horsey airs," or that she suffered from "actual dowdiness." She had, further, to endure the same anxious and pain-filled learning period as stronger male riders, but she persevered. By 1893, no up-to-date woman with self-respect would be caught pedaling more than two wheels.[26]

As women took to the roads, physicians took to their desks, turning out countless articles detailing either the value or the danger of cycling for female health. And on both sides the emphasis was placed where it had been put by other hygienists, on woman's reproductive capacity. Hence when optimists applauded the bicycle for forcing women finally to discard the corset for more comfortable cycling attire, and praised the wheel as "one of the greatest boons which [has] been conferred upon the sex in the present age," they could not avoid adding that the bicycle should "improve not only

[26] Minna Smith, "Women as Cyclers," *Outing, 6,* 317–321 (1885), p. 321 (also see Smith, "The Tricycle for American Women," *Outing, 5,* 423–426 (1884–1885); H. H. M., "Greek vs. Modern" (n. 10), p. 216; "Woman and the Bicycle," *Boston Med. Surg. J., 131,* 247 (1894); "A Plea for the New Woman and the Bicycle," *Am. J. Obstet., 33,* 575–576 (1896), p. 575; "Cycling for Women," *J. Hyg. Herald Health, 43,* 165 (1893).

the individual [woman], but the race generally." New York obstetrician Robert Latou Dickinson (later to be the medical counterpart to Margaret Sanger in the procontraception campaign) offered the most thorough exposition of the pelvic profits of cycling. From the observation that most of the work of wheeling is done by the legs, he advanced the argument that the adjacent area of the pelvis—its vessels, muscles, and organs—would share in the stimulus and increased blood flow during the exercise, and gradually develop a finer tone. With improved pelvic tone should come relief from the all too prevalent female complaints of chronic catarrhs, varicose vessels, hypertensive local nerves, and other chronic pelvic disorders. Lack of tone in the reproductive tract, he maintained, was the cause of women mistakenly thinking that "God intended [them] to suffer during menstruation and labor." As the best single exercise for strengthening the pelvis, bicycling, Dickinson concluded, was woman's best hope for restoration to reproductive normalcy. He even included the case histories of eight patients bothered by a variety of female disorders, all of whom had improved after following his prescription of the wheel.[27]

But for many other physicians that prescription seemed contraindicated by woman's biological role. She was not just subject to all the male cycling injuried, *de pied en cap*, from bicycle-foot to -face, and not merely more susceptible because of her natural delicacy and physically sheltered upbringing. The damages incurred by careless male cyclists might be regarded as largely their private affair, "but it is another matter when the welfare of that sex is concerned upon which depends the welfare of the race." And again it was the dreadful saddle that threatened the race's welfare. The modifications of saddles for the purpose of relieving perineal pressure have been related, but without notice that

---

[27] "The Sanitary Aspect of Cycling for Ladies," *Brit. Med. J.*, 1896 (i), 681; Robert Dickinson, "Bicycling for Women from the Standpoint of the Gynecologist," *Am. J. Obstet.*, *31*, 24–37 (1895), p. 25.

these alterations were designed for men. In fact, the manufacturers of the saddles of the early 1890s completely overlooked the broader pelves of the growing number of women riders and confidently offered to both sexes seats cut to the narrow contours of the male. As late as 1895, a Boston obstetrician surveyed the situation and found "that no serious attempt has as yet been made to produce a saddle that shall be adapted to a woman's anatomy." Some saddles were "absolutely unfitted" for female use, and virtually all the rest required many adjustments to be adapted to female riders. The chief inadequacy, he and other critics noted, was that the rear of the seat was not wide enough to support the average woman's ischial tuberosities, so that she sank and rested instead on her perineum.[28]

Consequently uterine displacements, distorted pelvic bones, hardened perinea that restricted parturition, and contracted birth canals were all expected to become increasingly common. The "Komphy," an elaborate perineal pad designed for ladies to wear beneath their cycle clothing, was invented precisely to prevent these conditions, but even it was ineffective against pedaling, which caused hypertrophy of the pelvic musculature and thus compressed the birth canal.[29]

The Hallers have analyzed American physicians' opposition to cycling as basically moralistic, stemming from fear for the modesty and delicacy of women abducted by the wheel from the protection and responsibilities of the home. It seems undeniable that uneasiness about the social implications of feminism fed doctors' suspicions of a physical pa-

[28] "Editor's Table" (n. 23), p. 355; James Chadwick, "Bicycle Saddles for Women," *Boston Med. Surg. J., 132,* 595–596 (1895), p. 595; Robert Dickinson, "Bicycling for Women," *Outlook, 53,* 550–553 (1896); James Prendergast, "The Bicycle for Women," *Am. J. Obstet., 34,* 245–263 (1896), pp. 249–250.

[29] T. R. Evans, "Harmful Effects of the Bicycle Upon the Girl's Pelvis," *Am. J. Obstet., 33,* 554–556 (1896); *Med. Rec., 47,* 573 (1895); J. McVitie, "Bicycling for Women: Its Effects on Parturition," *Lancet,* 1897 (ii), 51; "A Pneumatic Pressure-preventing Pad for Cyclists," *Lancet,* 1899 (i), 1164.

thology of female cycling. The very costume of the wheel-woman, a Bloomer-type outfit adopted for reasons of comfort and safety, seemed to brand her a suffragette. At the least, it was immodest. A Dr. I. Love, of St. Louis, thanked the wheel for prying women out of their unhygienic corsets, but regretted the ladies had stepped into a radical outfit "which lessened the respect of mankind for womanhood." In the midst of his worries over the low vitality of American women, the nation's declining birthrate, and the flooding of the country with immigrants of non-Anglo-Saxon stock, the physician must have been pressed not to regard the bicycle as an instrument of indulgence on which women shirked their social and racial responsibilities. The Seattle doctor who explained why female cyclists had not yet suffered the predicted obstetric difficulties surely struck a responsive chord with many of his colleagues:

> While bicycle riding may deform the pelvis, it will have little or no effect as regards the ease of childbirth. And why? For the simple reason that 'bike' riders do not have babies. Where or who is the physician that has attended a 'bike' rider in confinement? Will the female rider throw aside her wheel long enough to have a baby, let alone to rear a respectable sized family? The bicycle is a nuisance and a curse instead of a blessing. . . . The advent of this horrid means of locomotion is an instance in which the inventive genius of man has overtoppled itself.[30]

This distaste for women following mannish pursuits was publicly aired by more than one physician. Shadwell, discoverer of bicycle face, deplored the fair sex's fondness for "unsexing itself"; another observed that not only had the wheel "displaced the horse, [but] in women has, in a measure, replaced the uterus"; a third complained that women had become "wedded" to the bicycle, and as a result "they

[30] John and Robin Haller, *The Physician and Sexuality in Victorian America*, Urbana, Ill., 1974, pp. 174–187; I. Love, "The Bicycle from a Medical Standpoint," *Med. Rec.*, *48*, 464 (1895); A. Simonton, "Bicycling," *JAMA*, *31*, 1253–1254 (1898).

have little desire for matrimony which they come to regard as a ... kind of bondage. ... Consequently they prefer to remain spinsters, and a quasi third sex is formed. ... Womanhood in its physiological and motherly sense is sacrificed to narrow hips, atrophied breasts with retracted nipples, and a development of brachial, leg and abdominal muscles that would do credit to a lightweight."[31] Doctors were indeed faced with a dilemma. For her own, and the race's sake, woman had to be emancipated from weakness, neurasthenia, and pelvic disorders, and the wheel was an admirable means of lifting her to health—except that it threatened to also remove her from the home and its familial obligations and moral insulation. As fear of the latter possibility could easily be translated into condemnation of the bicycle on medical grounds, the wonder is not that so much pelvic damage was credited to the wheel as that so many physicians resisted the temptation. More often than not, the charges of pelvic injury were dismissed as imaginary, and sometimes with stinging commentary. At a time when hysterectomies were being performed with abandon, a New England physician wryly chided critics of the wheel: "The contents of a woman's pelvis should not be jarred [by cycling]; better a total extirpation than a jolt." The majority of the profession, whatever their feelings about the social and political liberation of women, welcomed the hygienic liberation offered by the bicycle. What they hoped was that the new female vitality would be channelled into traditional functions, and woman be made a more efficient homemaker rather than a rival of man. Their ideal was "Psyche," a woman "wheel missionary" who prized the health she had recovered through cycling because it improved her sweeping and bed-making.[32]

[31] Shadwell, "Hidden Dangers" (n. 18), p. 831; *Med. Rec.*, *53*, 949 (1898).

[32] "The Dangers of the Bicycle," *Boston Med. Surg. J.*, *131*, 352–354 (1894), p. 354; Porter, *Cycling* (n. 5), pp. 21–22. Haller, *Physician and Sexuality* (n. 30), pp. 86–87, also takes note of the medical profession's determination that the new woman be only an improved home economist.

There was a final aspect to the question of woman and the wheel that also touched on her reproductive fitness. Physicians of the 1890s were still edgy about the physical and moral consequences of masturbation, and some feared that that satanic saddle pressure might corrupt female cyclists. It looked, at least, like self-gratification might be readily and inconspicuously achieved by tilting the saddle pommel up and pudendum down. One woman, "who claimed a rather varied experience in sexual pleasures," actually admitted "that she could not ask for a more satisfactory development than could be obtained from the saddle of her bicycle." But for once on a question of masturbation, common sense prevailed. Doctors did not have to probe the matter very deeply to realize that while a chance existed that some girls might discover self-excitation if a bad saddle and poor posture led to "friction and heating of the parts," in most cases the rider would have to be consciously seeking gratification. And then, why complicate the act with a bicycle? Indeed, many concluded, the wheel was more likely to prevent the habit than generate it. Riding required concentration and diverted the mind from prurience; it induced fatigue, and it was positively uncomfortable when converted to clitoral stimulation. Gynecologist Dickinson went so far as to assert that the bicycle saddle compressed the pudic nerve in such a way as to quench desire—all but one of the wheelwomen patients who answered his inquiries testified "against sexual excitation, though one of them admits freely that she was formerly in the habit of relieving herself manually." The editor of a Canadian journal probably won some nods of approval for his claim that "the consensus of opinion is increasing overwhelmingly day by day that bicycle riding produces in the female a distinct orgasm." But the weight of medical opinion appears to have rested with the New York editor who responded that

> compared to Canada ... Sodom and Gomorrah were as pure as Salvation Army shelters. It appears that cycling ... is in Canada merely a means of gratifying unholy and

bestial desire. . . . Either the wheelwomen of Toronto are the vilest of their sex, or they are the victims of a contemptible slander. . . . The question of the healthfulness of cycling . . . is one that still admits of discussion; but the man who can assert or even suggest that the thousands, perhaps millions, of women throughout the world, who ride the wheel, are giving themselves over to self-abuse, puts himself beyond the reach of argument.

Nevertheless, the British birth control crusader and private sex counsellor Marie Stopes received a letter from an Irish clergyman as late as 1919 in which he complained about the relaxation of female mores in recent times: "I have been struck by watching girls in London outskirts riding cycles . . . —they elevated the peak of the cycle saddle and put it too high, in riding, it necessitated an overstretch of the leg at each downward stroke of the pedal, which rubbed the peak of the saddle where it should not be, those girls were always inclined to be fast."[33]

But when all was said and done, it was level-headedness that characterized the medical response to all the facets of cycling and health. There was extremism in both directions, born of the optimism of hygienists and the anxieties of a fledgling "sports medicine." Yet nearly all gravitated toward the central position that had been the essence of hygienic philosophy since Hippocratic times: temperance. Eventually the most common opinion about bicycling was that it was wholly beneficial to the person who was careful not to exceed his individual capacity, and harmful only to the one who indulged to excess. Replying to implications that the bicycle was "a machine more to be avoided than a roulette wheel," the editor of the *Boston Medical and Surgi-*

[33] Dickinson, "Bicycling for Women" (n. 27), pp. 33, 34; Prendergast, "The Bicycle" (n. 28), p. 250; "Bicycling for Women from the Standpoint of the Gynecologist," *Am. J. Obstet., 31,* 85–90 (1895), p. 86; "The Bicycle and Sexual Excitation," *N.Y. Med. J., 68,* 179 (1898); "Immorality in Canada," *Med. Rec., 50,* 681–682 (1896); Ruth Hall, ed., *Dear Dr. Stopes. Sex in the 1920s,* London, 1978, pp. 65–66.

cal Journal put the matter in proper perspective: "It is to be doubted whether such a beneficial exercise will perish because a few imprudent persons with cardiac lesions overdo themselves, or a French youth excoriates his perineum. There have been too many spindly children built up to healthy vigor, and too many chlorotic, languid girls made rosy and buxom by riding, for physicians to be easily alarmed and dissuaded from believing in 'wheeling.' "[34]

The true difficulty, as it developed, was not in winning the support of physicians, but in maintaining the participation of the public. The great attraction of the wheel, that it made exercising enjoyable and thus stirred to hygienic activity people who would otherwise have shunned exertion, was also its great weakness. For too many cyclists, improved health was a fringe benefit of the pastime. What actually drew and held them to the wheel was the speed and mobility, and feeling of adventure and fashionableness it provided. If another diversion should appear to offer the same qualities in greater abundance, many cyclists were ready to switch with little thought of the hygienic merits of the new pursuit. The bicycle, in fact, paved the way for its own obsolescence. It created a taste for rapid private transit at a time when the public appetite preferred mechanical to man power. The "motorcycle" was the inevitable supplanter of the wheel once it was made economical. By 1903, *Lancet* could detect a significant decrease in the number of cyclists, as well as in the quality of the sport for those who had remained in it. "The noise and dust and pace of the motor-car," it was lamented, "have taken the poetry completely out of a ride on the high-road." Articles on the hygiene and pathology of the wheel, once so numerous, had already become a rarity in the pages of medical, and public journals. The bicycle was being demoted to the status of a child's toy, while the automobile was coming in for its own share of hygienic praise ("With the motorcycle in use, the problem of street cleaning will be

[34] "Dangers" (n. 32), p. 354.

greatly simplified, and the health of our cities promoted"), and criticism ("A speed of fifteen or twenty miles an hour in a motor car causes [women] acute mental suffering, nervous excitement, and circulatory disturbances"). That the machine expected to free humankind from foul air and idleness should only foster another machine that would pollute the atmosphere and encourage sedentariness on a grand scale was the ironic conclusion of an originally auspicious chapter in hygienic ideology.[35]

[35] "Cycling and Motor-cars," *Lancet*, 1903 (i), 1460; S. Barton, "The Evolution of the Wheel—Velocipede to Motorcycle," *Sewanee Rev.*, 5, 48–62 (1897), p. 62; quoted by Frank Donovan, *Wheels for a Nation*, New York, 1965, pp. 8–9.

CHAPTER ELEVEN
A MODERN CONSPECTUS

SYLVESTER GRAHAM WAS RIGHT, OF COURSE. HIS FEAR that commercially baked, and adulterated, white bread portended a sweeping displacement of natural foods by artificial products has been realized to a disturbing degree in the twentieth century. Indeed, white bread—no longer cheapened with chalk, but denatured instead with benzoyl peroxide, tricalcium phosphate, and other additives—has become symbolic of a high technology food industry pressing ever more synthetic preparations upon a gastronomically illiterate public conditioned by advertising to welcome the artificial as necessarily an improvement over the natural. Things have come to such a pass that the manufacturers of Quaker Oats (so boastful of the naturalness of their cereal during Haig's day) have recently marketed an instant oatmeal enriched with "artificial Graham flavor!"

Artificial Graham flavor is delicious as an incongruity, but most unsettling as a reminder of the loss of integrity in modern diet. Undeniably, some of that loss is the unavoidable price of rapid population growth and urbanization. It is nevertheless justifiable to bemoan the necessity of breeding tomatoes that resist bruising during shipment but have the texture and flavor of cardboard, and to worry about the chronic health effects of the residues of pesticides, antibiotics, and hormones used to boost production. There are sound reasons to be dissatisfied with many modern foods.

There is also an unsound reason for dissatisfaction: the mere fact that a food item does not wholly conform to one's interpretation of "natural" is not, in and of itself, sufficient grounds for rejecting the food. But the religion of healthy-mindedness has always rested on that principle, that "Nature worketh all things to perfection." The premise accepted, any action altering natural process must thereby, inevitably, introduce imperfection. The giant strides in sophistication taken by the agriculture and food-processing industries through the first half of the twentieth century were thus certain to provoke a healthy-minded reaction, a broad-scale nostalgia for "natural foods." To give the various proponents of natural foods their due, they have voiced a number of legitimate concerns about the nutritiousness and safety of common food, and helped raise public awareness of serious dietetic issues. But because the natural foods agenda has been derived essentially from faith rather than science, insupportable positions have been just as readily taken. This promiscuous embracing of the spurious with the sound, and the natural theology that inspires it, is nowhere more evident than in the organic foods movement.[1]

Jerome Irving Rodale, the movement's seminal ideologist, was a man of impeccable hygienic pedigree. Born in 1899, he was a sickly child who finally conquered his nagging colds and headaches with the aid of Bernarr Macfadden's bodybuilding course. And though he went on to become an accountant, then a businessman, he never lost his interest in health promotion. Business profits allowed him to enter the field of health journalism in the late 1930s, but his early publications were as undistinguished as they were short-lived. Not until 1941 and his introduction to the work of an English agriculturalist who advocated the use of animal manure as fertilizer, did Rodale find his niche in popular hygiene. Within a year a new Rodale journal, *Organic Gardening and Farming,* was sent forth to proclaim that organic fertilizer was superior to synthetic preparations because it was natural. That simple message was of course

---

[1] See Sidney Margolius, *Health Foods. Facts and Fakes,* New York, 1973, for a survey of the modern health foods scene. Also useful are "The Problem of Food Faddism and Cultism," *J. Am. Dietetic Assoc., 61,* 126 (1972), and Peter New and Rhea Priest, "Food and Thought: A Sociologic Study of Food Cultists," *J. Am. Dietetic Assoc., 51,* 13–18 (1967).

adorned with quasiscientific evidence that compost was better for the chemical, physical, and bacterial composition of the soil, and produced higher yields of more nutritious crops. But when experts in agricultural chemistry scoffed at Rodale's claims (as they continue to do), he ultimately took refuge in mysticism. "In organically grown food you have things you don't even know exist," he told an interviewer in 1971, shortly before his unexpected death; in foods grown with manufactured fertilizers, "there is a little gleam of something that is missing." And what is that gleam? "Who knows? It may be a form of matter that we don't know yet. Maybe something that's excreted by enzymes, or bacteria. Maybe the bacteria who live off these things are healthier and can work like they used to work in the old days, and they've lost this ability through the artificialization of the soil and what-not."[2]

The certainty that nature is always superior, often in a way which surpasses understanding—that "Only God can make an enzyme"—has essentially guided the expansion of the Rodale philosophy from agriculture into all other areas of life. The Prevention System for Better Health, the completed expression of the organic philosophy, is unable to present any stronger indictment of plastic plates than of chemical fertilizers, yet the plates are condemned as unhealthful along with aluminum cookware, fluorescent lighting, gas furnaces, synthetic carpeting, fluoridated water, and other symbols of unnatural, technological society. (Rodale also disapproved of too heavy reliance on technological transportation in place of movement requiring exercise, and surely would have been pleased with son Robert's launching

[2] Rodale quoted by Wade Greene, "Guru of the Organic Food Cult," N.Y. Times Mag., June, 1971, pp. 30–31, 54–60, 65–70, p. 58. For the orthodox scientific position on the Rodale philosophy, see Frederick Stare, " 'Health' Foods: Definitions and Nutrient Values," J. Nutr. Educ., 4, 94–7 (1972); Hilda White, "The Organic Foods Movement," Food Tech., 26, 29–33 (April, 1972); and Ruth Leverton, "Nutritive Value of 'Organically Grown' Foods," J. Am. Dietetic Assoc., 62, 501 (1973).

in 1978 of a new Rodale magazine: *Bicycling*. The philosophy of cycling, the junior Rodale declared in a paean worthy
of the 1890s, "meshes perfectly" with organic ideology. "We
believe that most people have vast, untapped potential to do
more for themselves—and we recognize the bicycle as the
most efficient 'tool' for self-fulfillment.")[3]

The restoration of natural diet is the Prevention System's
primary objective, however, and that requires not only the
elimination of foods produced with synthetic fertilizer
("devil's dust"), chemical pesticides, and antibiotics and
hormones, but also all refined foods such as white bread and
sugar. Among unprocessed organic foods, furthermore, certain items are granted favored status, recognized as being
extraordinarily nutritious, and often therapeutic as well.
Vitalism blends with tradition in the identification of these
"Fabulous Foods": sprouts (especially alfalfa, "the wave of
the future in preventive medicine") most clearly embody
the life force, being themselves alive and in a crucial stage of
vital development; sunflower seeds suggest an association
with the source of all earthly life; yogurt ("milk that went to
college") not only confers the benefits earlier identified by
Metchnikoff, but effectively combats cold sores, cholesterol,
and cancer as well.[4]

The valid recommendations of the Prevention System obviously are mixed with much unsubstantiable, even dangerous advice. Exaggeration is most rife in the realm of nutritional supplements, where vitamins and minerals are
promoted as the most "Fabulous Foods" of all. Rodale took
seventy supplement tablets daily, and his son and successor

[3] J. I. Rodale, *The Healthy Hunzas*, Emmaus, Pa., 1949, p. 46; Rodale,
The Prevention System for Better Health, 3rd ed., Emmaus, Pa., 1973, p.
16; Robert Rodale quoted by James McCullogh, " 'Bicycling.' A New Rodale Magazine," *Prevention*, *30*, 70–72 (April, 1978), p. 72.

[4] Rodale, *Prevention System* (n. 3), pp. 13, 17, 34; Michael Clark, "Alfalfa, the Wave of the Future in Preventive Medicine," *Prevention*, *26*,
141–147 (Nov., 1974); Jane Kinderlehrer, "Yogurt—Milk That Went to
College," *Prevention*, *26*, 78–85 (Oct., 1974).

Robert indulges in a similar orgy that includes rose hips, bone meal, and kelp tablets. Predictably, vitamin C must be in the form of rose hips, and other supplements taken as natural products. Despite the assertions of biochemists that synthetic vitamin C is identical to the naturally occurring compound, organic ideology brands the synthetic as inferior. Rodale, Sr. supposed the natural substance to have other, unknown nutrients adjoined—the "gleam" again—and to have some important difference in the stereoisomerism of its molecules. Behind the jumbled interpretation of biochemical theory, though, lay the same intuitive trust in nature. A Rodale associate's rationalization of the superiority of natural vitamins began with an admission that she and her comrades had long accepted that "Natural is beautiful—and better" as an article of faith.[5]

The eternal appeal of that faith notwithstanding, the Rodale system was slow to win a following. Even after a second magazine, *Prevention,* was added in 1950, the organic movement stayed sluggish until the late 1960s. Then the circulation of *Organic Gardening and Farming* shot up to 700,000 by 1971, and *Prevention* sales rose even higher, to more than 1,000,000. Rodale's meteoric climb in popularity was a predictable natural phenomenon. The turbulent cultural climate of the late 1960s was unusually favorable to the growth of interest and belief in radical hygiene. Long-building uneasiness about the untoward effects of scientific and technological advance (particularly environmental pollution and food contamination) was joined by the social idealism and hatred of entrenched authority bred by civil rights and Viet Nam protests. The antiestablishment, neo-Romantic utopianism that possessed so many rebellious young made the aquarian generation highly vulnerable to heretical philoso-

---

[5] Greene, "Guru" (n. 2), p. 54; Robert Rodale, "My Personal Plan for Healthful Living," *Prevention, 26,* 21–28 (Jan., 1974), pp. 24–5; Jerome Rodale, "Natural Foods," *Prevention, 26,* 199–204 (July, 1974); Jane Kinderlehrer, "Natural is Beautiful—and Better," *Prevention, 26,* 96–100 (Jan., 1974), p. 96.

phies promising a better, cleaner, peaceful world by a return to natural living. "Organic" was a key concept in the counterculture philosophy of life before Rodale was discovered; the Prevention System gave organic life concrete meaning and clarified how day-to-day activity should fit into the cosmic framework. (It could even alter well-established behavior; at least some Rodale converts quit using the drug LSD because it is a synthetic compound, but continued smoking natural, organic marihuana).[6]

But anxiety about the synthetic environment, desire to live in accord with nature, and uncritical awareness of science are crosscultural. Hence while Rodale drew many of his new disciples from the disaffected young, conversions occurred in the larger, conventional society too. The progress of a system so clearly dedicated to prevention has also been boosted by the phenomenal burst of interest in holistic healing during the past decade. The impersonal, dehumanizing tendencies of an orthodox medicine committed to specialization and sophisticated technology has set off a reaction demanding wholistic care, care that treats the whole patient as a complex individual whose health is determined by the interaction of his mind and spirit, as well as work and home environment, with his body. Medicine has always been wholistic in philosophy, but practice has too often strayed from theory in the twentieth century. And though much of the agitation for a renewal of wholism has originated within the medical profession, alternative healers (from chiropractors and naturopaths through yogis) have challenged the adequacy of the orthodox response, and affected a smug "holisticer"-than-thou attitude toward allopathic medicine. The term holistic (without the original "w") has come to be associated in the popular mind with these multitudinous alternative approaches to healing and health building, and to connote an entire set of principles beyond the fundamental imperative to treat the whole patient. Holism emphasizes

[6] Greene, "Guru" (n. 2), pp. 52, 68.

the body's innate recuperative power, the *vis medicatrix naturae*, and assigns all therapeutic intervention the humble role of assisting the grand healer within. The rigorous modalities of establishment medicine, with their too frequent adverse reactions, are thus challenged by gentler, more "natural" methods ranging from herbal preparations to musculo-skeletal manipulations. Allopathic paternalism is also blasted, and patients (consumers) urged to exercise greater independence in selecting a healer, and to assume an egalitarian healer-patient relationship. Health itself is understood as a positive condition—wellness—and the individual told to take responsibility for preserving and enhancing his own wellness by eating properly, drinking moderately, smoking not at all, exercising regularly, and avoiding stress. Prevention is given precedence over therapy, and the ideal physician visualized as a counselor whose advice prevents illness in his patients and guides them to "high level wellness."[7]

The core philosophy of holism is clearly not new, but its resurgence is both a sign of enlarged public receptivity to hygienic ideology, and a vehicle by which individual ideologies can move forward. Health programs such as Rodale's existed and were holistic in spirit long before the term came into vogue, but by identifying with the newer, broader movement, Rodale and others have acquired a currency of great value in gaining public support.[8]

The Prevention System (and other recent hygienic plans) was also ecological before the general populace became so enchanted with that ideal. Hygienic ideology in a secular and shrinking world is far less likely than in previous eras

[7] Examples of holistic philosophy are Donald Ardell, *High Level Wellness*, Emmaus, Pa., 1977; and Mark Tager and Charles Jennings, *Whole Person Health Care*, Portland, Ore., 1978.

[8] Numerous articles linking the Prevention System with holism are sprinkled through the pages of *Prevention* magazine. For example, see Mark Bricklin, "The Dogs Bark, But the Prevention System Moves on," *Prevention*, 27, 35–48 (Nov., 1975).

to identify the perfect society as Christian or American. Natural society is instead commonly a society in which one does not just live in obedience to natural law, but lives fully as a participant in nature, as a member of a species with its own definite place in the network of biological existence. The world of life has no religious denomination or nationality. Health in that world is achieved by one's adherence to the biological laws promoting personal physical and spiritual well-being and contributing to the well-being of all fellow humans and other creatures. Ethically it often equates with Christianity, but the ideology is directed not upward, toward heaven, but outward, to the natural, planetary environment of which the individual is an integral part, and inward, to the person who is a unique creation of that environment and whose existential potential must be realized.

It is not merely contemporary diet that Rodale sought to reform, then, but contemporary society, a polluted, noisy, crowded, competitive, unecological environment. One of his more than thirty plays (none of more than dubious literary merit) portrayed the modern city as *Streets of Confusion,* where "even the trees don't know how to grow. These are the streets where life has no purpose, where it was predicted that a fountain shall come forth . . . but it is a sterile, barren fountain. . . . My fellowman drinketh and is enfeebled from it. These are the Streets of Confusion." The remedy to this biological confusion, Rodale promised, was his Prevention System, that "takes an ecological approach toward human life." In testimony to Congress as early as 1950, Rodale implied the Roman Empire had collapsed because of its inattention to organic agriculture, and prophesied the adoption of his organic method would build "a civilization such as has never before been seen."

> The genuine organiculturist is not merely an organic gardener or farmer; he lives his whole life in the organic manner. The organic principles must be felt deep in one's heart, and in everything one does. . . . The organic way is

the golden rule way. It means that we must be kind to the soil, to ourselves and to our fellow man. Organic means goodness. A heart that is full of benevolence will create in the body a spirit of physical and mental well-being that will enable it to better absorb all the nutritional elements from organically grown food.[9]

Organic living has indeed become a "way", a quest for natural existence transcending the boundaries of Rodale's system. In fact, the best known and most influential popularizer of organic diet has been a crusader from outside the Rodale camp: Adelle Davis. Educated in home economics and then biochemistry, but only through the master's level, Davis offers a classic illustration of the dangers of a little learning. Her four treatises on popular nutrition (*Let's Cook It Right*, 1947; *Let's Have Healthy Children*, 1951; *Let's Eat Right to Keep Fit*, 1954; and *Let's Get Well*, 1965) are riddled with misinterpretations of nutritional science and bad advice. But her lively style (and even livelier personal manner, as frequently exhibited on television talk shows), coupled with a pontifical confidence in the correctness of her views, won her the status of "high priestess of popular nutrition" during the late 1960s health revival. A 1973 federally sponsored survey of the majority culture's nutrition beliefs discovered Davis' teachings had made the general public much more respectful of organic foods and vitamin supplements (another government agency identified her as the most harmful single source of nutrition misinformation).[10]

[9] J. I. Rodale, *Three Plays*, Emmaus, Pa., 1966, p. 65; Rodale, *The Complete Book of Food and Nutrition*, Emmaus, Pa., 1961, pp. 618–619; Rodale, *Prevention System* (n. 3), p. 12; Rodale, *Our Poisoned Earth and Sky*, Emmaus, Pa., 1964, p. 306.

[10] John Poppy, "Adelle Davis and the New Nutrition Religion," *Look*, *34*, 62–65 (Dec. 15, 1970), p. 62; Howard Schneider and J. Timothy Hesla, "The Way It Is," *Nutr. Rev.*, *31*, 233–237 (1973); James Harvey Young, "Adelle Davis," in *Notable American Women. The Modern Period*, ed. Barbara Sicherman and Carol Green, Cambridge, Mass., 1980,

Davis' writings were actually a mixture of much valid nutritional information with a bizarre assortment of claims for the therapeutic and health-enhancing value of organic foods, vitamins, and minerals. The B vitamins, for example, were offered as cures for baldness, and flat-chested women were assured they could become buxom with vitamin E supplements. Davis also fueled the fear of hypoglycemia, or low blood sugar, that became a form of national hypochondria in the 1970s. It was her version of autointoxication—take the irritability and depression produced by hypoglycemia, she warned, and "add a few guns, gas jets, or razor blades, and you have the stuff murders and suicides are made of." Fortunately, a sure method of preventing hypoglycemia was available in the form of liberal protein consumption. The modern National Research Council protein recommendations, so painfully won after Chittenden's experiments, were attacked by Davis as much too low. In fact, she decreed, it is "probably impossible" to eat too much protein. Her protein recommendation was necessary as well for a feeling of energy and drive, resistance to disease, and preservation of beauty and youthfulness. And even though her protein habits contradicted Fletcher's practice, the result was the same: odorless stools.[11]

Davis' works concentrated on the myriad of specific dietary components and their physical benefits and injuries, but through the mass of detail ran a transcendent ideological strain. In a society optimally nourished, she contended, political leaders and business executives will be less prone to foggy thinking and consequent costly mistakes. School chil-

---

pp. 179–180. Also see Jane Howard, "Earth Mother to the Foodists," *Life, 71,* 67–70 (Oct. 22, 1971); Edward Rynearson, "Americans Love Hogwash," *Nutr. Rev., 32,* supp. 1, 1–14 (1974); Rynearson, "Adelle Davis' Books on Nutrition," *Med. Insight, 5,* 32–34 (July–Aug., 1973); and Ruth Baker, "Encounter with Adelle Davis," *J. Nutr. Educ., 4,* 92–94 (1972).

[11] Adelle Davis, *Let's Eat Right to Keep Fit,* New York, 1954, pp. 15, 19, 71, 166; Davis, *Let's Get Well,* New York, 1965, p. 176.

dren will learn more efficiently. Children will even be born in better health, for the perfect nutrition of parents before the child's conception will insure healthy chromosomes that will combine to create a being of exceptional potential (would-be fathers were advised to give especial attention to their vitamin E intake if they hoped for intellectually vital children). The mental, as well as emotional and spiritual health promoted by right eating allowed Davis to have her own dream of an organic future: "That dream has to do with agriculture, but it is not of agriculture. It is a dream of world peace. This dream starts with a family which perhaps creates its Shangri-La on an acre of land, a family in which a high degree of health has laid the foundation for character, courage, integrity, serenity, graciousness, and love in the home. Enough such families can make up a community, a state, a nation, a world at peace."[12]

Yet there are numerous organic foods enthusiasts who would deny that Davis' world would be at peace. Her nutritional scheme, after all, included meat, a food she considered necessary to satisfy body demands for protein and vitamin B_{12} (vegetarian children are often brain-damaged by these dietary insufficiencies, she charged). But a world where animals are butchered for food clashes with the vegetarian concept of peace. The utopia of many vegetarians is the most expansive organic-ecological world view of any contemporary hygienic ideology.[13]

Such generalization is risky, for vegetarianism has continued as a highly complex movement. There is much diversity of diet between lacto-ovo vegetarians, lacto-vegetarians, ovo-vegetarians, vegans, and fruitarians. Numerous organized groups, as well as unaffiliated individuals, carry the vegetarian banner. Some are vegetarian through religious persuasion, others for ethical, economic, and/or hygienic

[12] Davis, *Let's Eat Right* (n. 11), pp. 17, 213; Davis, *Let's Have Healthy Children*, 3rd ed., New York, 1972, pp. 9, 44.
[13] Davis, *Let's Have Healthy Children* (n. 12), p. 141.

reasons. Many of the new vegetarians who have swollen the ranks since the late 1960s are motivated by their absorption in Oriental philosophy and religion. "I don't believe in vitamins," one such vegetarian has said; "yin yang and the Order of the Universe are the overriding principles."[14]

There is nevertheless a general acceptance among vegetarians of all types, vitamin skeptics included, that fleshless diet is the natural human diet, and is required for the highest physical health. Furthermore, the accumulation of much medical data to suggest an association between meat eating and heart disease, gastrointestinal cancer, and other serious health problems has allowed vegetarians to construct a rather compelling physiological case for their diet. Unfortunately, their plausible denunciations of cholesterol and sodium nitrate are too often joined with attacks on compounds of less probable injuriousness. Ptomaines (from autointoxication) and uric acid are still prominent features of anti-flesh discourses. To illustrate, vegetarians make better lovers, apparently, because uric acid (as Haig long ago instructed) lowers endurance; vegetable diet thus "gives a person more 'staying power.' " "helps your body to do its thing better," and transforms one's love-making from "a fifty yard dash [to] a five mile Olympic run."[15]

As deserving of ridicule as this sexual (and other vegetarian) physiology may be, the larger philosophy behind it has

---

[14] Johanna Dwyer, *et al.*, "The New Vegetarians," *J. Am. Dietetic Assoc.*, *62*, 503–509 (1973), p. 508. Also see Darla Erhard, "Nutrition Education for the 'Now' Generation," *J. Nutr. Educ.*, *2*, 135–139 (1971).

[15] Nathaniel Altman, "Can a Non-meat Diet Enhance Your Love Life?," *Vegetarian Life*, July–Aug. 1979, 1–3. Also see Friends of All Life, "Some Thoughts on Diet," *Vegetarian World*, *1*, no. 3 (1974), p. 2; Jacques deLangre, "The Physical Cost of Flesh Foods," *Vegetarian World*, *1*, no. 4 (1974), p. 8; Frey Ellis and V. Montegriffo, "The Health of Vegans," *Plant Foods for Human Nutrition*, *2*, 93–103 (1971); Kyu Lee *et al.*, "Geographic Studies of Arteriosclerosis," *Arch. Env. Health*, *4*, 4–10 (1962); O. Gregor, *et al.*, "Gastrointestinal Cancer and Nutrition," *Gut*, *10*, 1031–1034 (1969); Frey Ellis, "Incidence of Osteoporosis in Vegetarians and Omnivores," *Am. J. Clin. Nutr.*, *25*, 555–558 (1972).

an estimable nobility. Vegetarianism is an international humanitarianism. A flesh centered diet is renounced not just to spare innocent animals, but to free land for much greater productivity and thus save starving humans. Vegetarians call on the prosperous nations to sacrifice meat so the poorer nations can have bread, and hope that in the process respect for the dignity of all life will be learned. All will thus be better nourished spiritually as well as physically, and be restored to a peaceful, healthful natural order, assume a cooperative rather than exploitative place in the global ecology. The fervor with which this vision of bloodless coexistence is held is underscored by the seemingly quixotic efforts of many vegetarians to wean their cats, dogs, and other domesticated carnivores from meat. Numerous successes have been recorded, and have sparked the hope once dear to Kellogg: the vegetarian keeper of a vegetarian cat is "interested in peacefully and gradually raising the carnivores of this world to a higher level of existence that I believe they used to enjoy." Her own pet "has become a much more sensitive, communicative, loving cat," "a lover instead of a fighter." This feline reformation is a fatuous exercise, certainly, but it still betokens the admirable natural humaneness impelling the vegetarian mission. H. Jay Dinshah's keynote address to the 1975 International Vegetarian Congress capsulized this ethos in its title: "Vegetarianism is Good for Life," for individual, racial, and universal life.[16]

But progress through that chain of being begins with the individual, whose bodily improvement on fleshless diet augments his mental and moral powers. The coming of the vege-

[16] A thorough presentation of the humane-economic argument for vegetarianism is Frances Lappé, *Diet for a Small Planet*, 2nd ed., New York, 1975. The reclaimed cat is described in Penny Harper, letter to *Vegetarian World*, *1*, no. 4 (1974), pp. 12–13; a similar note in a nineteenth-century health journal reveals that dogs reared on a meatless diet not only "become kind and gentle," but also "improve in sagacity and perception." *J. Hygeio-Therapy*, *4*, 45 (1890). Dinshah's address is reported in "Vegetarianism is Good for Life," *Vegetarian Voice*, *3*, no. 1 (1976), pp. 1–3.

tarian millennium still awaits mass acceptance that the diet
is physically healthful. And as before, living examples speak
louder than theories. Vegetarian literature still abounds
with specimens of athletic success, from basketball star Bill
Walton ("The Vegetarian Vacuum Cleaner"), through
Alan Jones (whose 27,003 nonstop sit-ups won him a place
in the *Guinness Book of World Records*), to Chandgi Rham,
who captured the Indian national wrestling title with his
"kilos of vegetarian muscles."[17]

Yet another impressive entry in the list of contemporary
muscular vegetarians is Ambrose Burfoot, 1968 Boston Marathon champion and current distance running journalist.
His sport is not a new facet of hygienic ideology—health
promoters of the 1890s often recommended it as an alternative to cycling. Holbrook was a regular jogger who acclaimed
the recreation's effects on muscles, heart, blood, and care-
filled mind. He kept his enthusiasm within bounds, though,
as did most others who recommended the exercise. But there
was, even then, the occasional runner who saw his sport as
the best, the only complete, exertion. A correspondent of
Holbrook's journal, to cite one example, prescribed running
to prevent tuberculosis, heart disease, constipation, and
menstrual difficulties, and to improve overall physical and
spiritual vitality as well: "Start running and the breath
quickens, the pulse leaps, the brain brightens, as the freshly
oxygenized, purified blood begins to bound through it, the
eye sparkles and the charm of your boyhood has returned
once more."[18]

It is a sad thought that the gentleman's purified blood was
still insufficiently oxygenized to sustain his life until the

[17] Gregg McNeill, "Walton Joints Portland Trailblazers," *Vegetarian World*, 1, no. 2 (1974), p. 18; McNeill, "Jones May Soon Break 'All' Records," *Vegetarian World*, 1, no. 3 (1974), p. 19; "A Vegetarian Wrestler," *Indian Veg. Cong. Q.*, April–June, 1968, p. 45; "Kilos of Vegetarian Muscles," *Indian Veg. Cong. Q.*, pp. 33–35 (Jan.–June, 1969).

[18] *J. Hyg. Herald Health*, 44, 69–71 (1894); J. W. Lloyd, "Running as an Exercise," *J. Hyg. Herald Health*, 45, 126–130 (1895), p. 126.

1970s and the transfiguration of his recreation into a religion, "the religion of the runner" (the phrase is that of Bob Anderson, the editor of *Runner's World* magazine). As any distance-running worshipper (myself included) will insist, serious discussion of the subject must begin with a distinction between the true religion and the uninspired derivative sect of jogging. The unenlightened continue to confuse the two, and many joggers blasphemously call themselves runners (but never vice-versa!). The technical difference between the two is simple, a matter of pace—nine minutes per mile or slower is jogging, faster is running. But the runner does not just move faster; he goes farther, and with a far more serious intent. Jogging is merely a fad, one which has improved physical health as an end, but strives for no higher goals. Nine minutes per mile, after all, is little more than a brisk walk; it is hardly the pace of a person who is driving for some form of excellence. The jogger may, to be sure, be motivated by other considerations than cardiovascular improvement and weight reduction. There is a smart young professional set in which jogging is a cultural imperative, as essential to respectability as a Cuisinart or a hot tub. It is also a modish alternative to the singles bar, as witness the coquettish T-shirt inquiring, "Your pace or mine?"[19]

The runner alters his pace for no one. His conquest is not of others, but of himself. Aerobic conditioning, steady improvement of cardiopulmonary efficiency (rather than Windship's strength or Lewis' agility) is his immediate project of good works. Completion of the marathon, preferably in less than three hours, is the rite through which he must pass to demonstrate his worthiness. Along the way, nearly endless additional benefits accrue. The voluminous running literature of the past decade is a veritable cornucopia of promises of a more abundant life. Running reduces weight and blood pressure, combats asthma and atheroscle-

[19] Anderson quoted by Kenny Moore, "Taking Part: You Ain't Seen Nothin' Yet," *Sports Ill.*, *49*, 38–40 (Dec. 25, 1978–Jan. 1, 1979), p. 39.

rosis, can even make one immune to heart disease. It retards the aging process, strengthens sexual performance, and eases pregnancy and labor. The "positive addiction" of running cures the negative addictions of alcohol and nicotine, and relieves stress, depression, even schizophrenia.[20]

Running does have its dark side. Injuries are common, and the country is inundated with cases of runner's foot, runner's Achilles, runner's knee, runner's back, etc., to equal the worst that the bicycle was able to do. But even injuries are a blessing—they teach the runner patience and a more profound respect for the wholeness he will have when he recovers. And injuries are another experience with pain, the most elemental of sensations that every runner must confront again and again in order to appreciate his humanity. Pain is not only character training, although "learning to deal with pain is learning to deal with life." Much more significantly, pain is the bridge from the body to the spirit, a barrier against which the runner can test himself and learn the depth of his will and passion and courage. To conquer the pain of the marathon is to discover "the glory which only comes from being a fully aware human being." A "respectable" marathon, another has written, must be "suitably painful."[21]

But relaxed pain-free running has its glories too, including, it is claimed, the stimulation of imagination and creativity. In totality, it is another exercise in James' healthy-mindedness, and in fact we are informed that, "If you would be a marathon runner, study William James." He is the philosopher of joyful effort, of striving to fully unleash and experience "the energies of men." Even James, however, might

---

[20] The best source for articles presenting the countless virtues of running is *Runner's World* magazine.

[21] Donald Monkerud, "Putting Your Finger on the Source of Pain," *Runner's World, 14* 59–61 (Aug., 1979), p. 60; Garrett Tomczak, "Is the Pain Necessary?," in Editors of Runner's World, *The Complete Runner*, Mountain View, Cal., 1974, 12–17, p. 16; George Sheehan, *Running and Being. The Total Experience*, New York, 1978, p. 206.

have been put off by the grandiosity of running philosophy. The sport is relaxing, conducive to meditation, productive of joy. There is satisfaction in struggling against lactic acid, merited self-esteem in overcoming the formidable three-hour marathon challenge, and bliss in exhaustion. But while one learns much about his body and will during the closing miles of the marathon, those miles are not along the road to Damascus. It is jejune to write of *Holistic Running,* or worse, of *Running and Being.* Nevertheless, cardiologist George Sheehan, the sport's philosophical pace setter, has interpreted running to his following as the ultimate mode of self-discovery. In certain exalted moments on the roads, he writes, "there is a light and joy and understanding. For a time, however brief, there is no confusion. I seem to see the way things really are. I am in the Kingdom."[22]

More accurately, the kingdom is within him. The counterpoise to vegetarianism's planetary altruism is running's self-centeredness. Throughout radical hygiene of the past half-century there has been a steady drift of reform emphasis from society to the individual. Health reformers in the existential age have increasingly concentrated on the value of hygiene for self-actualization, and given relatively less attention to the lasting social changes that might be expected to follow. And if vegetarianism has most strongly resisted that rule, distance running is its extreme exemplification. Notoriously lonely, the distance running philosopher is content to let the rest of the world go as it may. He is a happy warrior against his own imperfections, a seeker of the maximum heroic self, a muscular existentialist. "I am fighting God," Sheehan thinks as he labors up a hill; "Fighting the limitations he gave me. Fighting the pain. Fighting the unfairness. Fighting all the evil in me and the world. And I will not give in. I will conquer this hill, and I will conquer it alone."[23]

[22] Sheehan, *Running and Being* (n. 39), pp. 204, 253.
[23] *ibid.,* p. 41.

Like all hygienic ideologies, the religion of running wins converts by appealing to our primitive intuition that the body and soul are intimately wed, and that self-denial purifies both to bring self-fulfillment. It reinspires the universal hope that the present body is far below the attainable body, that there was, and can be again, a world where the muscles and organs and the mind and spirit they encase will harmonize in unimpaired splendor. For the runner, that world is his self, but Sheehan was also speaking for the socially oriented ideologues of the Jacksonian and Progressive eras when he recently wrote that,

> Each of us is an experiment in human performance. Each of us reflects, for ill or good, the potential with which we were born. Each of us has the choice of doing the most or the least with what we have. . . . The idea of health and the concept of wellness are, in fact, much too bland. What we need . . . is something to arouse our emotions, inspire the imagination, address our more solid virtues. Human performance is just such an idea, concept and goal. . . . Once I discovered running, it became the key that unlocked all my energies. . . . [It opened] the world beyond health, fitness and wellness—the world of maximum human performance.[24]

The hygienic philosophers of the past century and a half have differed greatly in their interpretations of human potential, the means by which it can be realized, and the ends to which it should be directed. Yet whether running, gymnastics, or vegetable diet has been the key, the kingdom of health has in the final analysis been the world of maximum human performance. Whitman, himself a part-time devotee of radical hygiene, captured its spirit with a vividness that surpassed even James:

> One's-Self I sing, a simple separate person,
> Yet utter the word Democratic, the word En-Masse.

[24]Sheehan, "From Sheehan," *Runner's World*, 15 (Oct., 1980), p. 25.

Of physiology from top to toe I sing,
Not physiognomy alone nor brain alone is worthy
    for the Muse. I say the Form Complete
    is worthier far,
The Female equally with the Male I sing.
Of Life immense in passion, pulse, and power,
Cheerful, for freest action form'd under the laws divine,
The Modern Man I sing.[25]

[25] Walt Whitman, *Leaves of Grass,* New York, 1965, p. 1.

Index

Library of Congress Cataloging in Publication Data

Whorton, James, 1942–
    Crusaders for fitness.

    Includes index.
    1. Health reformers—United States—History.   2. Health
attitudes—United States—History.   I. Title.
RA418.3.U6W5   1982   613'.0973   82-47621
ISBN 0-691-04694-8   AACR2